BOTULINUM TOXIN

ILLUSTRATIVE MANUAL OF INJECTION TECHNIQUES

85 Illustrations
154 Photographs
27 Videos

BOTULINUM TOXIN
Illustrative manual of injection techniques

ISBN 978-88-97438-69-4

Publishing coordination: Giuseppe Roccucci
Editing: Rachele Villa
English translation: Annette Fowles
Design and layout: Massimo D'Onofrio - www.grafic-house.com
Illustrations: Davide Gamberini

Printing: Starprint srl
First edition: February 2022

PUBLISHER
Griffin srl unipersonale
Via Ginevrina da Fossano 67/A - 22063 Cantù (Como) - Italy
Tel. + 39 031.789085
customerservice@griffineditore.it
www.griffineditore.it

QR Code VIDEO System

To watch the videos scan the QR codes using the camera on your device or download a QR reader app

PREFACE

The use of botulinum toxin for the aesthetic treatment of patients is now firmly established as the first choice for facial improvements. Started in the 1990s, the use spread quickly from the United States to many other countries where clinicians witnessed, first-hand, the huge benefits for patients. Easy, fast, usually painless and with excellent results, the non-invasive treatment is far easier than using dermal fillers and has, for most patients, long lasting benefits over many months. The first product was licensed in 2002 in the United States as Botox® Cosmetic, but many more have now received regulatory approvals for facial treatments around the world.

In the past 20 years, clinicians have carefully refined how toxin is used aesthetically. The dosages, injection sites, the times between injections and related aspects have all received much attention. Detailed studies of facial anatomy have been of great benefit and, indeed, are essential in order to provide patients with optimal results. Training today, for new injectors, always involves anatomical details: accompanying cadaver studies have significantly increased injector confidence and understanding.

This new book, from the leading and most experienced clinicians in Italy using toxin for aesthetic improvements, provides the latest and best information available to the reader. After an introduction to toxin, including the much-discussed psychological impacts of use, all aspects of the treatment process and procedure are presented for consideration. Often, these are not dealt with in publications, but detailed information is provided here. The many uses in the face, not just those which are licensed but all so-called "off-label" applications, are then described in detail. Excellent anatomical drawings accompany before/after photographs of patients treated in the respective areas.

Of importance, the new treatment paradigm of micro-injection is then considered, the use of small doses in multiple locations for improvement of skin quality. In addition, the uses of toxin for dermatological therapy of acne, rosacea and wound healing have been included, aspects of toxin use that are currently developing quickly. The use for hyperhidrosis, known for 25 years, is included.

Today, use of toxin is often accompanied by dermal fillers, laser treatments or other therapies in a combination regimen for patients. Here, these aspects are discussed to give a global approach perspective. Though rare, the occurrence of complications is also discussed.

The authors have completed their work by presentation of the most frequent uses of toxin in therapeutic applications, such as cervical dystonia, facial spasms, drooling, migraine and bruxism. Particular applications for anal fissure, vaginismus and depression, a heavily-studied use, are presented. These provide the reader with a full, balanced perspective of uses in doses higher than used for aesthetic treatments.

I commend this book, bringing together important data and information to readers both experienced in the use of toxin, but also those interested to start working in the field of aesthetics.

Dr Andy Pickett
Director and Founder
Toxin Science Limited

INTRODUCTION

Writing a book about botulinum toxin probably isn't all that difficult. Over twenty thousand publications on the subject, years of experience in administering it, and a meticulous examination of literature definitely help when it comes to accomplishing something that is challenging to say the least.
Involving the leading Italian experts in the field in a multidisciplinary approach and studying everything that we really need to know about botulinum toxin step by step is much harder. However, after months of arduous but careful preparation, we have succeeded, and the approval received from Andy Pickett in his excellent preface bears witness to this.
Thousands of articles examined, personal experiences shared without jealousy but rather in the spirit of close collaboration, spaces reserved for the use of the toxin in other disciplines and, above all, the rich iconography, from explanatory drawings to photos of clinical cases and complications, along with technical videos, make this text a milestone in the complex process of learning about botulinum toxin.
Defining beauty and establishing unambiguous standards of evaluation is far from easy, but we are in no doubt that the toxin has contributed over the years to creating a facial harmony that is extremely hard to give up.
This is one of the reasons why specialists in this science, constantly in balance with the arts, have to expand and constantly update their knowledge, something which all the authors involved in this publication, through me, have installed into it.
But before turning the pages, let's take a moment to reflect upon the words of Oscar Wilde: «Beauty cannot be questioned. It has divine right of sovereignty».

Professor Giuseppe Sito
Aesthetic Surgeon and Physician

EDITOR

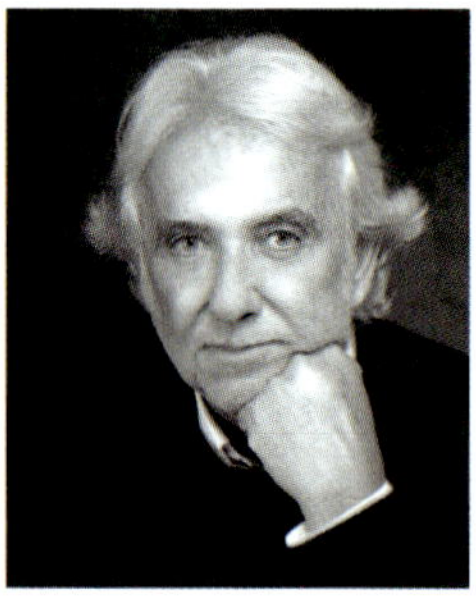

Giuseppe Sito

Born in Naples, he graduated with honours from the University of Naples. He then obtained diplomas as a specialist in General and Endocrine Surgery at the same university, and in Urology at Rome's Università Cattolica del Sacro Cuore. He attended courses in Aesthetic Surgery at the Société de Chirurgie Esthétique in Paris, obtaining the relevant diploma.
He is scientific director of Università Pegaso for the 1st and 2nd level master's degrees in Aesthetic Medicine and the Advanced Training Course in Aesthetic Medicine.
He is a member of the Società Italiana di Chirurgia Plastica Estetica.
He teaches at Agorà Postgraduate School of Medicine specialising in Aesthetic Medicine in Milan.
He has taught at the Scuola di Perfezionamento Universitario in Chirurgia Plastica ed Estetica of the University of Pavia.
He was one of the founders of the Associazione Italiana Terapia Estetica Botulino and held office at its Deputy President for several years.
He is reviewer for journals of Plastic Surgery and Aesthetic Medicine with a high impact factor in the United States. He is Editor in Chief of the *Journal of Plastic and Aesthetic Surgery*.
He is the author of over 100 publications and consultant to numerous publications in the field of Aesthetic Medicine.
He is legal medical consultant, specialised in Aesthetic Medicine, for the Court of Naples.

AUTHORS

Giovanni Brunelli
Surgeon specialised in Plastic and Reconstructive Surgery. He holds a European Diploma in Hand Surgery. He completed his training in Plastic Surgery and Hand Surgery in France, the United Kingdom and the United States.
Having practiced freelance since 1998, he directed the Hand Surgery service at the Istituto Clinico Città Studi in Milan until the end of 2018. He is author/co-author of 82 scientific publications.
He is a member of Aicpe (Associazione Italiana di Chirurgia Plastica Estetica), Sicpre (Società Italiana di Chirurgia Plastica Ricostruttiva ed Estetica), Isaps (International Society of Aesthetic Plastic Surgery), Sies (Società Italiana di Medicina e Chirurgia Estetica), Sime (Società Italiana di Medicina Estetica), Fime (Federazione Italiana Medici Estetici) and Aiteb (Associazione Italiana Terapia Estetica Botulino).

Lucia Calvisi
Surgeon specialised in Dermatology at the University of Cagliari. She has perfected her professional training working mainly in the field of aesthetic medicine, participating actively in the most prestigious national and international congresses and maintaining an active collaboration with the University of Brooklyn, New York. She currently teaches at the Università telematica Pegaso and is the author of numerous national and international publications.

Alberto Diaspro
Surgeon specialised in maxillo-facial surgery at the University of Turin.
He obtained a master's degree in Facial Plastic Surgery at Rome's "Tor Vergata" University, a master's degree in Aesthetic Medicine and Therapy at the University of Camerino and a Diploma as Expert and Consultant in Aesthetic Medicine at the Agorà Postgraduate School of Milan.
He is a member of Aicpe (Associazione Italiana Chirurgia Plastica ed Estetica), Eafps (European Academy of Facial Plastic Surgery), Aicef (Associazione Italiana

Chirurgia Estetica e Funzionale della Faccia) and Sicmf (Società Italiana di Chirurgia Maxillo-facciale).
He is currently Medical Director at Rigeneralab - Centro di Medicina Rigenerativa in Turin.

Maria Vittoria Giatti
Surgeon specialised in Plastic and Reconstructive Surgery.
She is a member of the Società Italiana di Chirurgia Plastica Ricostruttiva ed Estetica (Sicpre), the Aesthetic Multispecialty Society (Ams) and the American Society of Plastic Surgeons (Asps), and was formerly a member of the International Society of Plastic & Regenerative Surgeons (Ispres).
She has worked with internationally renowned plastic surgeons and lecturers in various theoretical and practical courses for doctors and specialists in the field. She has taken part in numerous national and international master's degree courses and scientific congresses and has produced several communications and scientific publications. Beauty coach and scientific consultant for innovative pharmaceutical and medical companies.
She has worked in prestigious clinics in Paris, Florence, Bologna, Verona, Rovigo and Ferrara. She currently works in her own practice in Bologna, where she also runs the Medical Academy for the training of medical specialists in advanced plastic surgery and aesthetic medicine techniques.

Claudia Ledda
Surgeon, in specialist training in Neurology at the University of Turin since 2019. She works mainly with movement disorders and treatment of dystonias with botulinum toxin, topics on which she is author of several publications.
She is a member of the Movement Disorder Society (Mds), the European Academy of Neurology (Ean), the Società italiana di Neurologia (Sin) and the Accademia italiana per lo studio della malattia di Parkinson e dei disordini del movimento (Limpe-Dismov).

Gabriele F. Muti
Surgeon specialised in Plastic and Reconstructive Surgery since 1996 and in Microsurgery and Experimental Surgery since 1999.

He has been an assistant at the Niguarda Milano burns centre, a fellow at the department of Reconstructive Oncology of the Istituto Nazionale dei Tumori in Milan and Medical Director at Multimedica in Sesto San Giovanni. Since 2001, he has been consultant in Plastic Surgery at the Istituto Dermatologico Europeo (Ide) in Milan and, since 2006, he has been practising Aesthetic Surgery and Medicine on a freelance basis.
He cooperates with international companies in the field of botulinum toxin, hyaluric acid and suspension threads. He is the author of numerous scientific articles on botulinum toxin and speaker at international congresses. He is a member of Isaps (International Society of Aesthetic Plastic Surgery) and Asps (American Society of Plastic Surgeons).

CONTENTS

For Lorenzo, Alessandra and Sissi
For my students
For those I love, and who love me in return

G. Sito

1

INTRODUCTION TO BOTULINUM TOXIN

Gabriele Muti, Giuseppe Sito,
Maria Vittoria Giatti

HISTORY OF BOTULINUM

Gabriele Muti

Botulinum toxin has definitely had an interesting and rather particular past, leading it to become the most widely used beauty treatment in the world today. Since time immemorial, man's history has been closely interwoven with botulinum toxin, resulting in the poisoning of people over time, and all that this has involved.

As civilisation progressed, the first attempts were made at preserving food safely, probably to the benefit of the body, but while the possibility to store food made people's lives so much easier, it also favoured the spread of botulinum toxin.

Over the centuries, a correlation between sausages and botulinum toxin was discovered, and a 10th century edict by Byzantine Emperor Leo VI actually forbade the production of blood sausages, pre-empting science in terms of prevention.

The history of India shows that the Maharajahs used the poison extracted from sausages to kill their enemies.

The first historical description of botulinum poisoning dates back to 1735. In Germany, in 1793, several people died after eating raw sausages. Initially there were suspicions that they had been poisoned with Atropa belladonna, due to a lack of knowledge of the pathogenic process which caused some confusion, but this theory was soon rejected. It was subsequently concluded that the consumption of "Blunzen", a popular local food made of pork stomach stuffed with blood and spices, was the cause of this food poisoning.

In 1802, the local government of Southwest Germany issued a public notice regarding the harmful consumption of blood sausages. Professor Johann Heinrich Ferdinand von Autenrieth (1772-1835), of Tuebingen University, was the first to analyse the symptoms of these cases of poisoning. Later, a German doctor named Justinus Christian Kerner (1786-1862) became the first to study botulism and called the new toxin "sausage poison", without, however, succeeding in completely defining the "biological poison". In 1895, Émile van Ermengem (1851-1932), professor of bacteriology at Gand University, finally isolated the *Clostridium botulinum* bacterium from some samples of a piece of ham which had poisoned a number of people at a dinner in the Belgian village of Ellezelles. He isolated the same organism in the ham and in the corpses of the victims, and called the toxin *Bacillus Botulinus*, from the word "botulus", which is Latin for sausage. Professor van Ermengem was the first to describe the situation in full: he proved that it was a poison and not an infectious disease, and that salt and heat were able to prevent it from being lethal.

When the food and food preservation industry were undergoing full development at the beginning of the 20th century, scientist Karl Friedrich Meyer (1884-1974) invented techniques to prevent the growth of the organism by deactivating the toxin with heat.

It would seem that, in 1941, it was used in operation Anthropoid to try to kill Nazi general Reinhard Heydrich.
Between 1932 and 1945, the Japanese Unit 731 carried out experiments on human guineapigs, administering botulinum to prisoners during the occupation of Manchuria.
In 1944, biochemist Edward Schantz 1944 cultivated *Clostridium botulinum* and isolated the toxin. Only after his discovery were different serotypes of the toxin discovered.
Some years later, in 1949, Burgen's group discovered that botulinum toxin was able to block neuromuscular transmission. Botulinum toxin is so poisonous that, in human beings, the LD50 (lethal dose 50, referring to the single dose of a substance capable of killing 50% of a sample population of guineapigs) is estimated to be just 1.3-2 ng/kg injected into the muscle/intravenously, and 10-13 ng/kg if inhaled. At that time, botulinum toxin was known as the most poisonous substance to exist and, as a result, numerous attempts at exploiting it as a biological weapon were made during the Second World War. The research of Carl Lamanna and James Duff led to the technical discovery of techniques to concentrate and crystallise the toxin.
Apparently, in operation Mongoose in 1961, the CIA soaked some of Fidel Castro's favourite brand of cigar in botulinum toxin. The cigars were never used but, when they were tested years later, they were still just as poisonous as they had been when they were originally soaked in the toxin.
It wasn't until 1980 that it was used in human beings, so many years after its discovery, by the ophthalmologist Alan Brown Scott to treat strabismus. In December 1989, the US Food and Drug Administration (Fda) approved onabotulinumtoxinA (Botox) for the treatment of strabismus, blepharospasm and hemifacial spasm in children under the age of 12. In 2000, the Fda approved its use for cervical dystonia.
It wasn't until 2002 that the Fda approved its use for cosmetic purposes, specifically to improve the appearance of glabella wrinkles. Two years later, in July 2004, its use in the treatment of underarm hyperhidrosis was approved. In 2010, approval was issued for its use to treat adult sufferers of chronic migraine and then, in 2011, to treat urinary incontinence associated with neurological conditions.
In 2013, the Fda accepted it for the treatment of crow's feet, making it the only Fda-approved remedy for this area. Botox is also an off-label remedy for eyebrow lifting, gummy smile, forehead lines, bunny lines, the platysma, chin muscles and even temporomandibular joint disorders and bruxism. It is used for a wide range of purposes today and is increasingly recommended in numerous medical specialisations.
Botulinum toxin B (MyoBloc) was approved for the treatment of cervical dystonia in 2000. Dysport and Xeomin, which came onto the scene only towards the end of the first decade of the 2000s, were approved in 2015 for the treatment of upper limb spasticity, but their use in aesthetic medicine has long been approved.

BOTULINUM TOXIN AND HOW IT WORKS

Gabriele Muti

As we have seen, botulinum toxin has always existed and been an active part of man's life. But what does the botulinum toxin molecule consist of? Botulinum toxin is made up of a neurotoxin, which represents the core of the molecule, and auxiliary complexing proteins. The core of the toxin is a 150 kDa (kilodalton) complex in which we have a 50 kDa light chain and a 100 kDa heavy chain, while the auxiliary proteins are both haemagglutinins and other non-toxic non-haemagglutinin proteins. A variety of botulinum toxins with different compositions are available on the market, as we will see in the following chapters, where the differences are explained.

The molecular weight of these different botulinum toxins varies according to the presence or absence of auxiliary complexing proteins. This is why we find proteins with molecular weights from 150 kDa up to approximately 1,400 kDa on the market.

The action of botulinum toxin is carried out without the use of auxiliary complexing protein chains. Based on various studies, freshly injected botulinum toxin comes into contact with tissue and a physiological pH, completely separating from the auxiliary complexing toxins within approximately 60 seconds to ensure complete effectiveness. When the botulinum toxin is injected into the tissue, it binds to the gangliosides and the SV2 protein receptor on the presynaptic nerve endings. This is achieved by means of the heavy chain that it is made of. The botulinum toxin is then transported into the nerve ending of the axon by the endosomes, which then allow the botulinum toxin to be internalised and made available for action.

Once the botulinum toxin has been translocated into the cellular space of the neuron (cytosol) and the heavy chain has completed its action, the light chain intervenes. The light chain is a metalloprotease.

The SNAP25 protein is attacked by the light chain of botulinum toxin. But what is the importance of the SNAP25 protein? It is a protein that binds to the neuronal membrane and is responsible for the exocytosis of the vesicles, acting on several subunits of the Ca channels. This protein is cleaved by the light chain of the botulinum toxin, so it is no longer able to release acetylcholine vesicles into the synaptic space.

By blocking the release of the neurotransmitter acetylcholine, the muscle is no longer stimulated, so it relaxes. In this way, not only can the muscle no longer contract, but it also loses its silent contracting tone, allowing the simultaneous relaxation of the skin and the reduction, smoothing or disappearance of wrinkles.

DILUTION AND DIFFUSION

Gabriele Muti

The diffusion of botulinum toxin (botulinum neurotoxin, BoNT) has been studied thoroughly in humans and animals using a variety of techniques, including compound muscle action potential (CMAP) and the potential triggered by neuron motion, histological determination of glycogen-depleted muscles, acetylcholine esterase staining, muscle fibre diameter variability and the quantitative electromyography (EMG) measurement of muscle activity.

Evidence of prevalence comes from studies carried out in both animal and humans.

In a study that uses muscle biopsy to identify diffusion, Borodic reported a BoNT/A diffusion gradient over a distance of 30-45 mm from the site of injection into the latissimus dorsi muscle of rabbits.

A study that investigated whether the volume of solution used to inject equivalent units of botulinum toxin A affects the diffusion of the toxin in the treatment of dynamic forehead wrinkles found that injecting botulinum exotoxin A at a lower concentration and higher volume resulted in greater diffusion covering a larger area. The toxin diffusion model was altered by muscle contraction in the sites injected.

Pickett suggested that confusion regarding the extent and clinical significance of diffusion between different botulinum toxins may be attributed to the incorrect extrapolation of information from studies carried out on animals in particular clinical settings. The testing of products with different dose ratios and the erroneous suggestion that products with larger complex molecular sizes migrate less may be due to poor study design.

It has been suggested that BoNT diffusion is influenced by a number of factors such as dose, concentration, volume, injection speed, needle size, distance of the tip of the needle from the neuromuscular junction, number of injections, selection of the target muscle, presence of muscle fascia, presence of tissue damage in the injection site, muscle contraction after injection and the protein composition and molecular size of the toxin formulation. However, dose, concentration and volume are probably the biggest contributors, in the sense that the higher the dose, concentration or volume, the greater the risk of migration.

Based on the principle that larger proteins diffuse more slowly through an identical aqueous medium than smaller proteins, Foster predicted that a botulinum toxin of greater molecular size or weight would be less likely to migrate outside the injection site than one of lesser size or weight.

On this matter, Carli claimed that there is no difference in the diffusion characteristics of different products. Furthermore, in a long-term clinical trial, the diffusion profile of onabotulin and incobotulin (which lacks complexing proteins, the largest and smallest molecules respectively) did not differ. This suggests that complexing proteins are neither necessary for the therapeutic effect of the toxin nor relevant to diffusion into the tissue. This is consistent with previous findings according to which 150-kDa neurotoxin is released from the 900-kDa complex in less than one minute when exposed to physiological pH values.

The migration of botulinum toxin can be dose-dependent and specific complications can be related to the choice of injection site. In one work on idiopathic spastic torticollis, dysphagia occurred when 150 units of onabotulin were injected into the sternocleidomastoid. This dysphagia disappeared if the dose was reduced to 100 units.

The volume of injection has also been implicated as a factor in migration. In one study, a five-fold increase in volume led to a 50% increase in the area affected.

Therefore, a possible consequence of the higher volume injected seems to be greater migration into the surrounding tissue with a consequent reduction in the duration and extent of the effect.

Other injection-related factors that can affect diffusion, but to a lesser extent, include needle calibre and injection speed. A needle that is too big or an injection that is too fast can cause trauma in the target tissue, with the result that the absorption of the toxin by the target area decreases, leaving more toxin to migrate to neighbouring areas.

Diffusion can also be influenced by the distance between the tip of the needle and the neuromuscular junction (NMJ), with increased uptake and reduced diffusion when the needle tip is close to a group of NMJs. Other authors have suggested that muscle conformation and distribution of muscle fibres may also influence the diffusion of botulinum toxin.

Perhaps the most useful technique for limiting migration is perfect placement on the target muscle. Several techniques using EMG and endoscopic guidance or imaging guidance are believed to increase the accuracy of targeting and consequently the reduction of migration. EMG, electric stimulation (ES), or ultrasound guidance, is used in children for muscle groups that are hard to locate. EMG is also commonly used to confirm the appropriate localisation of the needle in specific muscles immediately before injection. Ultrasound is a relatively convenient, painless and less time-consuming procedure. Sconfienza et al. reported that the use of ultrasound to guide needle placement before injecting botulinum toxin into the iliopsoas muscle in 10 patients with spinal lesions allowed easy and accurate needle placement. The use of ultrasound has also been shown to produce results that are superior to manually guided injections in the treatment of sialorrhoea in patients with Parkinson's disease.

It is generally accepted that reducing the migration of botulinum toxin is a desirable goal after injection. Numerous studies have been accumulated over time, suggesting that botulinum toxins have different diffusion characteristics. Meticulous placement of the toxin with the correct dosage, precisely targeting the right muscle to produce a precise treatment, offers the best chance of a good result.

Although botulinum toxin serotypes are structurally and functionally similar, specific differences in neuronal receptor binding sites, intracellular enzymatic sites and species sensitivity suggest that each serotype has its own unique pharmacological entity, sometimes due to distinct purification and production procedures. Doctors have to have a knowledge of the different serotypes, the different doses used for each formulation of each serotype and the side effects profile of each product in order to prevent adverse effects related to migration.

As far as dilutions are concerned, we are well aware that they are recommended by manufacturers, but the variety of treatments and often the personal preferences and experiences of doctors have altered dilutions in an attempt to achieve the best possible results. As we mentioned earlier, increasing the volume of the injection facilitates greater migration of botulinum toxin. The question is, is this always true? and, if so, to what extent?. If we stick to aesthetic medicine, there are two different ways to treat a flat muscle (frontalis or orbicularis muscle) and a muscle with a precise muscular belly (corrugator muscle). A muscular belly like the corrugator needs the right amount of toxin and we can reduce the dose to reduce the unpleasant sensation experienced by the patient. In a flat muscle such as the orbicularis, we have seen how certain studies have shown that the normal concentration or dilution of the correct amount of toxin does not change the result, whereas if we reduce the units and increase the dilution we can achieve the same effect. Probably in the first case, the amount of neurotoxin is sufficient to completely cover a sufficient number of neuromuscular plaques to achieve the desired effect. By contrast, if we reduce the units and increase the dilution, the toxin migrates more and probably has a more widespread action on the muscle, so the same result can be achieved.

IMMUNOGENICITY OF BOTULINUM TOXIN

Gabriele Muti

As stated in the product leaflets for the botulinum toxins available on the market (incobotulinum, onabotulinum and abobotulinum), repeated use of these toxins may reduce the desired effect or even fail to produce the desired effect due to an anti-botulinum toxin antibody reaction.

Another possible cause of immunogenicity is the presence of complexing proteins, which increases the causes of a possible immune response with the formation of neutralising antibodies.

We know that the immune system must be activated for antibodies to be produced.

Dendritic cells, which are the sentinel cells of the immune system, need a signal to stimulate T lymphocytes. Substances that can stimulate dendritic cells in botulinum products include both haemagglutinins and inactive botulinum neurotoxin, as well as the protein clostridial.

What happens to our immune system?

Activated T lymphocytes recognise antigens and stimulate the B lymphocyte response. In turn, activated plasma cells produce and secrete antigen-specific neutralising antibodies.

In practically every failed treatment, where either the doctor or the patient is unhappy with the result, the doubtable nature of the immune response has to be taken into consideration.

Approaches with a considerable amount of botulinum toxin such as the "whole face treatment" can trigger this kind of a reaction, so much so that scientific literature reports an increasing number of cases of failed aesthetic treatments.

After initial positive responses, patients may cease to experience clinical effects when botulinum toxin is administered, with unsuccessful secondary responses. It has been estimated that, in patients treated with high doses of the toxin, failure due to the production of neutralising antibodies may reach 6.6 % of the subjects treated.

Failure of the treatment to be effective can be subjective as well as objective, i.e.: the patient can report the lack of effectiveness and the doctor may or may not agree with this. While, on one hand, expectations may be too high, on the other, the response may only be moderate.

Lack of response is classified as partial or complete. It is defined as partial when no definite therapeutic effect can be obtained or when the therapeutic effect is reduced in intensity or duration. This partial response usually occurs within two to three years of beginning treatment. A complete lack of response occurs when a series of repeated injections fails to produce a discernible therapeutic effect. It was found that, in 81% of cases, this type of failure is preceded by a partial failure.

Reasons for a poor response to treatment

Our immune system recognises botulinum toxin as a dangerous foreign body. As mentioned earlier, this leads to the formation of antibodies that bind to the toxin and could therefore neutralise it. Neutralisation by the antibodies takes place by binding the botulinum toxin and preventing it from binding to the nerve ending.

Obviously by avoiding this link and the internalisation of the toxin, it is impossible to prevent the arrival of the cholinergic messages to the muscle, which will not relax. The toxin does not take effect and the muscle continues to contract.

Various studies have shown that this effect is greater in toxins that contain a higher amount of accessory proteins, which stimulate the immune system to a greater extent.

The greater the amount of foreign protein injected, the greater the risk of an immune response. Moreover, the greater the number of treatments and the shorter the distance between injections, the greater the possibility of an immune response.

In practice, we have seen how immunogenicity can lead to the failure of neurotoxin therapy.

There are two types of failure: primary and secondary. Failure is considered primary when a patient achieves no improvement even at the first administration. In this case, the toxin may continue to be unsuccessful even at higher doses.

Similarly, failure also occurs at lower doses, and this could also be due to an error in the botulinum toxin injection site. Muscle contracture may reduce the effectiveness of the treatment due to the high presence of lactic acid in the muscle. There may also be a fault in the storage of the toxin. A last cause could be a particular genetic predisposition of the subject to resist the toxin and to trigger immunogenicity.

The other possibility is secondary failure. In this case, the patient obtains an effect with the first dose, but the effectiveness gradually lessens over time. This tends to happen after a couple of injections. It could always be caused by a low dosage or an error in the injection point, but sometimes there is also a different perception of the effect between the operator and the patient.

Only a small proportion of these patients have antibodies that neutralise the toxin (NAbs). In this case too, ineffectiveness may be partial or complete. Assessments of NAbs antibodies are carried out using the ELISA test or immunoprecipitation assay; there are also various clinical tests which can be used for assessment.

In a meta-analysis including four studies which examined onabotulinumtoxinA in spasticity, only one of 317 patients (0.3%) developed new NAbs (measured by the MPA), despite higher mean doses in all indications.

In another study of 279 patients subject to long-term treatment of upper limb spasticity with onabotulinumtoxinA, only one of 224 patients examined (<0.5%) developed new NAbs via MPA (Membrane Proteon Array) associated with clinically reduced reactivity.

In an open study on the treatment of upper limb spasticity with three cycles of abobotulinumtoxinA, no antibodies were found via MPA in 41 patients. In

TABLE 1 - NAbs ANTIBODIES TESTING

UBI	Injection into the medial portion of the eyelid	May cause asymmetric corrugation
FTAT	Injection into the forehead	May cause asymmetry on the forehead
EDB	Injection into the short extensor of the fingers (with EMG)	>50% reduction in the CMAP of the muscle
SCM	Injection into the sternocleidomastoid (with EMG)	With %>2 SD reduction at maximum contraction
NST	Injection into the hypothenar eminence (with ninhydrin solution)	Reduction of the anhidrotic area

UBI = units brow injection, FTAT = frontalis antibody test, EDB = extensor digitorum brevis, SCM = sternocleidomastoid, NST = ninhydrin sweat test

the TOWER study, which examined increasing doses of incobotulinumtoxinA (400, 600, and 600-800 U over three cycles) in 155 patients with spasticity, none of the patients developed NAbs.
Looking at toxin-related antibodies, in 2010, a meta-analysis examined the rate of formation of NAbs with the use of onabotulinumtoxinA for various indications in 16 studies. For all the indications, 11 out of 2,240 subjects (0.5%) were found to have NAbs during treatment. Of these 11, only 4 patients (0.2%) lost clinical reactivity.
A recent meta-analysis on abobotulinumtoxinA found a prevalence of NAbs of 1.4% in 3,326 patients across 14 studies.
In the previous meta-analysis of 61 studies examining the immunogenicity of BoNT, incobotulinumtoxinA was found to have the lowest rate of NAbs formation.
Overall, immunogenicity rates of BoNT-A formulations (excluding the original batch of onabotulinumtoxinA) were low, with meta-analyses estimating prevalence from 0.5% for incobotulinumtoxin, 1.5% for onabotulinumtoxinA, and 1.7% for abobotulinumtoxinA.
Many studies have shown the formation of antibodies 10-11 months after the first treatment with the neurotoxin in up to 14% of patients treated.

What to do if the results of treatment are non-existent

It has been shown that antibodies (NAbs) can vanish over time, although subsequent repeated injections can reactivate them. Other studies have shown that using four times the dosage can reactivate the effect. The use of different formulations and/or a lower presence of complexing proteins could also be considered.

COMPARISON OF THE BOTULINUM TOXINS ON THE MARKET

Gabriele Muti

There are three botulinum toxins on the Italian market. The first to appear, in 1989, was the famous Botox (onabotulinum type A), which in 2006, following instructions from the Italian Drug Agency (Aifa), was renamed Vistabex so that it could be used not only in hospitals but also in private medical practices.

Meanwhile, in 1990, another botulinum toxin, Dysport (abobotulin type A), was being prepared. In 2009, it was named Azzalure. In 2005, Xeomine (incobotulin type A) came onto the market, and was subsequently renamed Bocouture in 2010, to allow its unrestricted sale.

Botulinum toxin molecules are extracted directly from Clostridium botulinum by defragmentation. Then, after being isolated via a purification process, they are transformed into commercially marketable formulations. Although they all originate from the same strain of Clostridium botulinum (the Hall strain), the purification process varies depending on the final botulinum toxin product: while incobotulinum is purified via chromatography, a crystallisation process is used to purify onabotulinum and abobotulinum. This forms the different molecules that make up the finished product which, as we know, are 900 kDa for onabotulinum, between 500 and 900 kDa for abobotulinum and just 150 kDa for incobotulinum. While the molecular weight of the pure toxin is 150 kDa, the presence of accessory chains which are not essential to the operation of the toxin changes the weight value.

There are excipients in the formulation that characterise the product. In addition to albumin, which is found in all three products, there is sodium chloride in onabotulinum, lactose in abobotulinum and sucrose in incobotulinum.

Another major difference is how the stabilisation of the final product is achieved: while onabotulinum is vacuum dried, freeze drying is used for both incobotulinum and abobotulinum.

Analysis of the product leaflets

The non-interchangeability of botulinum toxin units is supported by all companies due to the different valuation of the units, expressed as Allergan units, Merz units and Speywood units. These units certainly differ, but they have been compared in scientific literature, as we will see below.

They are all white powders for injectable solution, but with different therapeutic indications.

Incobotulinum is indicated for wrinkles in the upper third of the face in patients under the age of 65, where the severity of the wrinkles has an impact on the patient's psychological well-being. Abobotulinum is also indicated for patients under the age of 65, but only in the glabella region and for crow's feet. Onabotulinum is considered only for the wrinkles of the upper third of the face, with no age limit.

Use in paediatric patients is described

in the individual leaflets of incobotulinum, abobotulinum and onabotulinum. Aesthetic treatment is discouraged in patients under the age of 18 for all three.
It is hard to assess the potency of botulinum toxins which, for biological drugs, is measured using LD50 (Lethal dose 50), i.e.: the amount of neurotoxin that kills 50% of a group of mice, but is now assessed on highly sensitive cells. The test is carried out with the active pharmaceutical ingredient and the finished product (with the addition of excipients). This prevents a true evaluation of the potency comparisons and does not consider the type of mouse strains decided upon, the diluent and the dilution intervals.
If we look at the on-label treatments of toxins, we find some differences.
In the case of the glabella, four units are recommended for the five injection sites for incobotulinum, with the possibility of increasing this to 30. It is generally agreed that the effect starts to become apparent after 2-3 days and lasts up to four months. For onabotulinum, only the four units for each of the five injection points are mentioned. Lastly, for abobotulinum, 10 Speywood units are recommended per injection site, up to 50 units, paying attention to the levator palpebrae muscle to avoid eyelid ptosis.
Moving on to the periorbital region, four units of incobotulinum are recommended for the three points of administration, for a maximum standard dose of 12 units per side with activation by day six reaching peak activity on day 30, with completion of activity at four months.
For onabotulinum too, four units are recommended for the three injection points, with a maximum of 24 units in total between the two sides and activation within one week, with a duration up to the fourth month.
For abobotulinum, 30 Speywood units are recommended per side, with ten units per injection point.
Action on the lateral portion of the orbicularis muscle about one cm from the orbital margin is suggested for all three toxins, avoiding treatment of the zygomaticus major and the zygomaticus minor to avoid an asymmetric smile or ptosis of the modiolus of the mouth.
On the forehead, a dose of 10-20 units is recommended for incobotulinum, to be distributed in a horizontal line a couple of centimetres above the eyebrow, in five injection points. In this case, improvement is visible within seven days, with maximum action at 30 days and a duration of at least four months.
Onabotulin recommends a dose of 20 units to be distributed between two horizontal lines. The lower of the two should be at a median height between the highest point of forehead function and the eyebrow, at least two cm above the eyebrow, and the higher of the two should be halfway between the highest point of forehead contraction and the lower line. There should be two injection points on the upper line and three on the lower line.
The forehead is considered off-label for abobotulinum, so the product leaflet does not currently contain any indications for treatment.

In the general indications, should incobotulinum fail to be effective, the appropriateness of the treatment must be assessed. An additional treatment can be administered three months after the initial dose, and it is not recommended for use in patients over the age of 65.
Onabotulinum also envisages possible failure and a reassessment of the causes, with repetition of treatment after three months at the earliest. However, treatment cycles lasting more than a year have not been assessed.
Abobotulin always envisages subsequent doses after three months at the earliest, but the safety of the treatment has been assessed for 24 months with a total of eight treatment cycles for the glabella and four cycles over a total of 12 months for periorbital wrinkles.
The contra-indications are the same for all botulinum toxins. Obviously, hypersensitivity to the active ingredient is mentioned, but this can also be extended to its excipients. Neuromuscular diseases such as myasthenia, Lambert-Eaton syndrome and amyotrophic lateral sclerosis are considered pathologies in which the use of botulinum toxin is strongly discouraged.
All three indicate knowledge of the local anatomy as essential, obviously to guarantee safety but also to allow the recognition of wrinkles caused by skin slackness and/or photo-ageing, which could prevent the botulinum toxin from being effective.
The possibility of excessive migration of the botulinum toxin, leading to the involvement of neighbouring muscles (see cases of eyelid ptosis), is also described.
For abobotulinum, care should be taken not to inject it into a vein or artery, while for onabotulinum it is advisable to have adrenaline and a nasogastric tube on hand in case of dysphagia.
In all cases, excessively frequent use of botulinum toxin could trigger an immunity to the toxin, rendering its injection useless due to the formation of antibodies.
Considering interactions with other drugs, aminoglycoside antibiotics or spectinomycin, which interfere with neuromuscular transmission, should not be used in conjunction with botulinum toxins, which could theoretically enhance their effect. For incobotulinum, muscle relaxants should also be used with caution, and intermediate-acting drugs such as vecuronium and atracurium (cure-like agents) are recommended.
4-aminoquinoline drugs may also reduce the effect of botulinum toxin.
Obviously, as there is no data on pregnancy and lactation, all three advise against using botulinum toxins, except under exceptional circumstances. However, no data on a reduction in fertility in either men or women following use of the toxin is available. In cases of asthenia, weakness, impaired vision, dizziness and drooping eyelids, driving a car or operating potentially dangerous machinery is not recommended.
With regard to adverse effects, all three botulinum toxin manufacturers report not only local adverse effects at the injection point, such as pain, swelling, redness and bruising, but also more generalised effects. They describe cases of eyelid ptosis and Mephisto sign, headache, flu-like symptoms,

insomnia, dysphagia, urticaria, muscle contractions and spasms, and even facial asymmetry and dyspnoea, as well as swollen eyelids and dry eyes, and musculoskeletal and connective system disorders. In the event of adverse reactions, the recommendation is to report them on the Aifa website.

Reactions such as dyspnoea (which is described in the case of an overdose) may require respiratory assistance and even hospitalisation.

There are significant differences in the way the products are stored: while abobotulinum and onabotulinum must be kept at a temperature between 2 and -8 °C, also after reconstitution with saline solution, incobotulinum is very stable at room temperatures up to 28 °C.

All three manufacturers recommend reconstitution with NaCl physiological saline solution by suctioning the saline solution from the vial vacuum, avoiding the formation of bubbles and gently rotating the vial.

If botulinum toxin is dispersed into the environment, it should be neutralised with sodium hypochlorite (Javel's water). If it gets into the eyes, rinse thoroughly with water or an ophthalmic solution to dilute the botulinum toxin solution. If it comes into contact with open wounds, take the correct steps according to the amount of product spilled.

MORPHODYNAMIC ANATOMY

Giuseppe Sito

When botulinum toxin began to be used for aesthetic purposes, it was first used on the upper third of the face, which is the area most affected by ageing, neglecting its use on the lower areas of the face. Later, and actually not all that long ago, it was also injected into the middle and lower thirds of the face (fig. 1).

Consequently, in this chapter we will look at the anatomy of the upper third of the face, the middle third and the lower third, topographically subdividing the areas usually subject to injection with botulinum toxin.

General details on muscles

The whole face is covered by the skin and, underneath, the subcutaneous tissue, areas that are not usually affected by botulinum toxin. However, it should be noted that facial skin differs significantly from one area to another. For example, the skin of the eyelids is the thinnest and most delicate on the whole body, while that of the top of the head and the temporo-occipital region is much, much thicker. Other areas could be defined as histologically similar to the rest of the body.

It is a well-known fact that the target of botulinum toxin is muscle tissue, so we are going to devote these pages mainly to the study of the muscles targeted by botulinum toxin infiltration.

Most muscles are attached to the skeleton by means of fibrous structures called "tendons". If the tendon is cylindrical, it is called a tendon, but if it is flat, it is called an aponeurosis. Tendons and aponeuroses are supporting structures or connecting structures.

There are other muscular forms that do not originate from the skeleton but are embedded in the subcutaneous tissue of the face and neck. These are called mimetic muscles and include the superficial aponeurotic muscle system (SMAS), which consists not only of muscles but also of fibrous laminae (septa), which divide the face into loggias.

Muscles vary in shape and the striated muscles, those responsible for movement, can be named according to their shape (e.g.: triangular, rhomboid), the number of their parts or bellies (e.g.: biceps, triceps or quadriceps) and, lastly, their morphological characteristics (e.g.: major, minor).

Muscles usually shorten during contraction and lengthen during extension. It is also important to remember that muscles can be divided into agonists and antagonists, and this must be taken into account especially when using botulinum toxin, so that their contraction and flexion capacities are used in order to prevent asymmetries. Other muscle functions (e.g.: rotation, abduction, etc.) are of no relevance for the use of botulinum toxin.

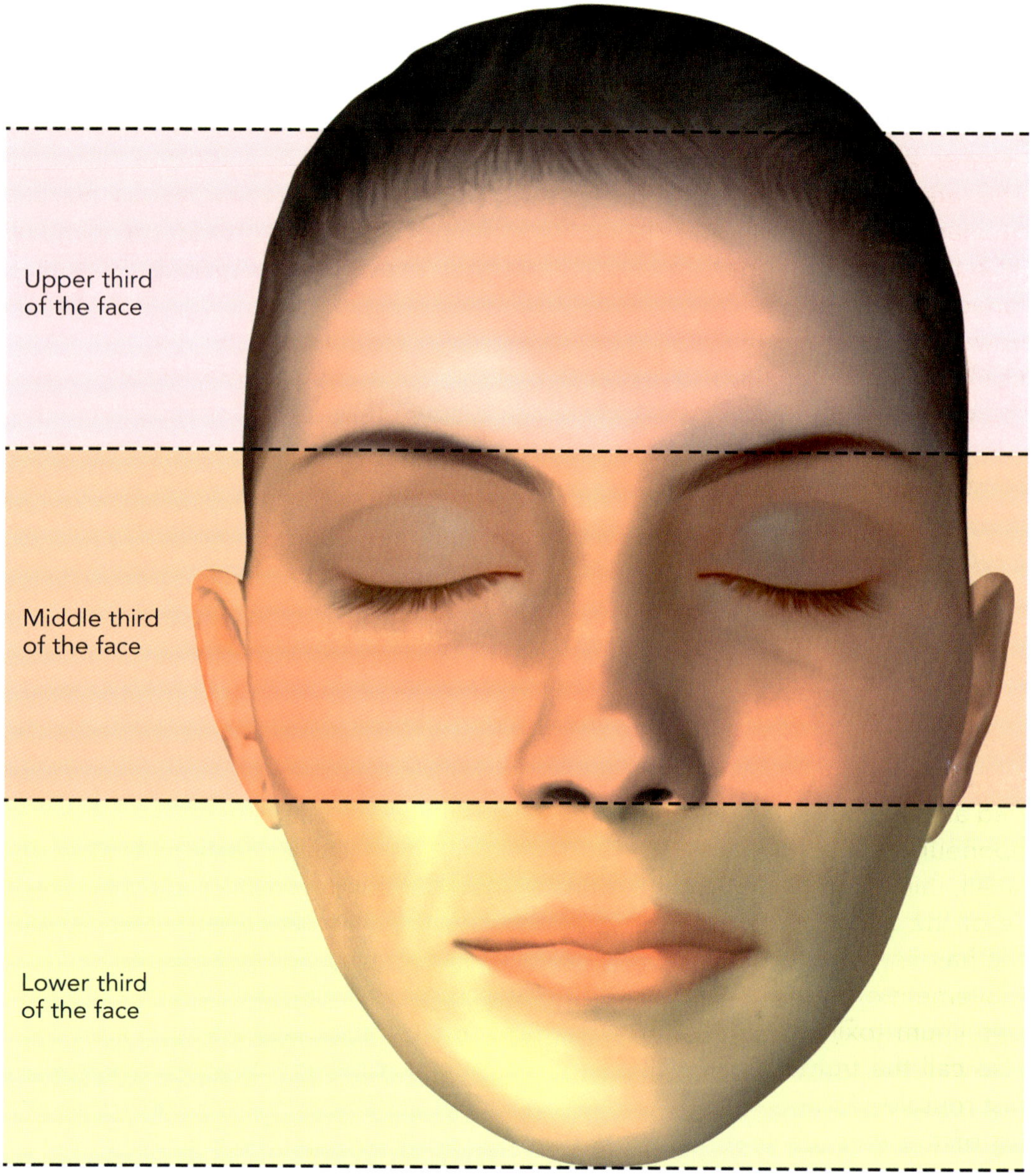

Figure 1 The three facial districts

UPPER THIRD OF THE FACE

The upper third of the face is usually considered to be the area between the capillitium (epicranial region) and a horizontal line that passes through the apex of the zygomatic protuberances (fig. 2).
This area mainly contains the mimetic muscles, also known as expression muscles. These are small fleshy subcutaneous bundles resulting from the upward division of an important superficial muscle originating in the neck, the **platysma** (fig. 3), and they are responsible for the movement of small areas of the face.
The muscles we are most interested in are the following.

Occipitofrontalis muscle

The **occipitofrontalis muscle** (fig. 4) consists of a large, thin frontal portion which occupies almost the whole frontal bone, with an often triangular-shaped area in the centre, occupied by an aponeurosis, sometimes crossed by small, thin muscle bundles. The purpose of the frontalis muscle is to retract the hair line and raise the eyebrows, a movement of considerable interest for botulinum toxin infiltration. We could also call the frontalis muscle the agonist muscle of the glabella area, made up of the muscles that we are going to specify.

The glabella muscle "group"

The **glabella** (fig. 5) is a small median depression in the frontal bone, above the frontonasal suture between the brow arches. It constitutes one of the main craniometric points: it corresponds to the upper craniometric point of the nose and is called the nasion (or the bridge of the nose). The muscles that cover it are the depressor supercilii muscle, the procerus muscle and the corrugator supercilii muscle.
The **depressor supercilii muscle** is a small fleshy bundle positioned deeply under the frontalis muscle, which forms the vertical glabellar lines when it contracts.
The **procerus** muscle, which forms the horizontal wrinkles at the top of the nose when it contracts, is a mimic muscle that mobilises the soft part of the nose.
The **corrugator supercilii muscle** (fig. 6) is usually 16 mm above the horizontal plane of the glabella and between 4 and 14 mm from the midline. It merges into the frontalis muscle and the dermis, about 30 mm above the plane of the glabella and about 16-34 mm from the midline. The maximum length in Caucasians is about 21 mm, while in Asians it is shorter. Morphologically, the corrugator muscle has two muscle bellies, the first being transverse and the second oblique. The oblique belly originates from the superior part, while the transverse belly originates from the superolateral part. The oblique belly joins the frontalis muscle in the superomedial part, not far from the glabella. Hypertrophy of the corrugator muscle determines the most severe wrinkles on our face. The glabella group contributes to the downward stretching of

the top of the eyebrows (fig. 7) and is the group with the most vigorous fibres in the upper third of the face. It is usually more hypertrophic in men than in women and this must be taken into account when administering the toxin.

Orbicularis oculi muscle

The **orbicularis oculi muscle**, the sole function of which is sphincteric, to open and close the eyelids, is located in a very delicate and slack subcutis, is richly vascularised and helps to draw the eyebrows medially and downwards (figs. 8-9). It is therefore considered as an antagonist of the frontalis muscle. There are slightly conflicting views on the anatomy of the orbicularis muscle. Most claim that it consists of two bundles, the palpebral and the orbicularis. Others, mainly of surgical extraction, such as the author, maintain that the orbicularis muscle also has a third bundle, the so-called suborbital, which extends to the limit of the Bichat fat pad and detaches a small bundle that forms the ciliary muscle of the Riolanus, the ciliary margin in contact with the eyeball, which must never be damaged, especially during blepharoplasty. Underneath the orbicularis muscle are the fat pads (fig. 10), two for the upper eyelid and three for the lower, which can be seen as we age due to the acquired slackening of the orbicularis muscle. The latter should never be weakened excessively with botulinum toxin, because there is a risk that it will no longer perform its primary function, forming an iatrogenic ectropion.

Levator palpebrae superioris muscle

The **levator palpebrae superioris muscle** (fig. 11) is a small muscular bundle, antagonistic to the orbicularis muscle, which originates in the optic canal, from a tendinous ring, running forward and upwards to the tarsus of the upper eyelid. This muscle does not have an aesthetic function, but it is the muscle affected by accidental infiltration that causes the most common and most feared side effect, eyelid ptosis.

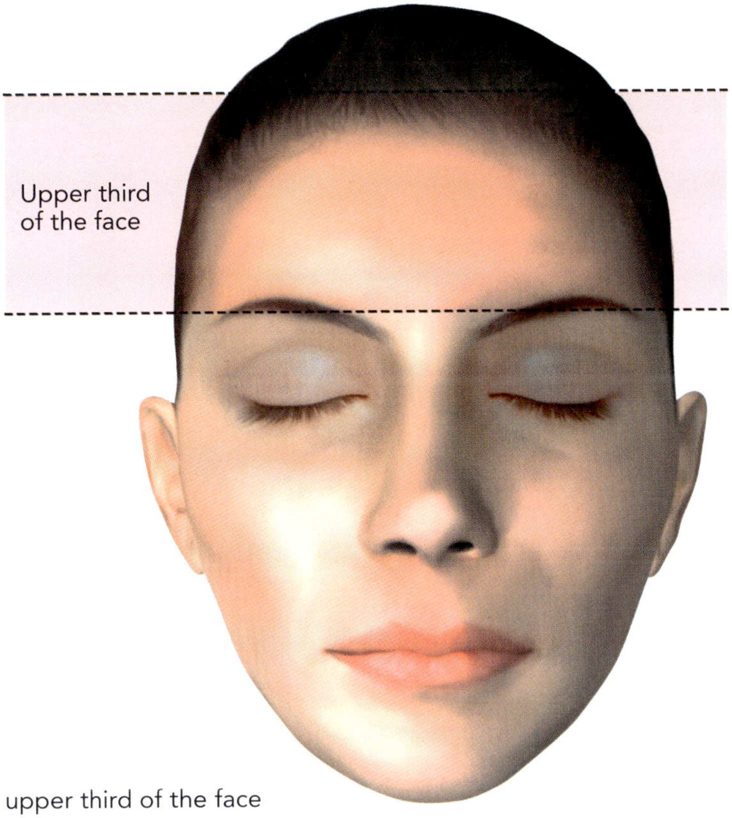

Figure 2 The upper third of the face

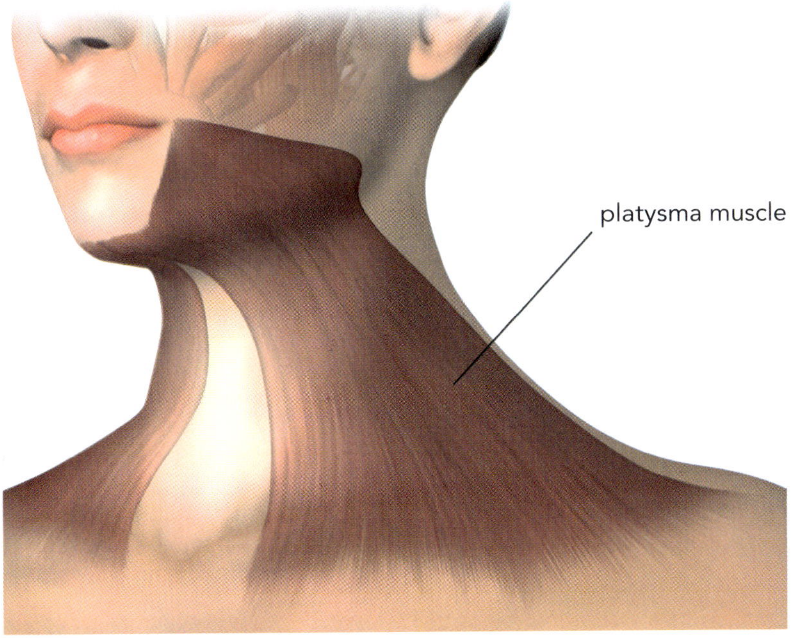

Figure 3 The platysma muscle

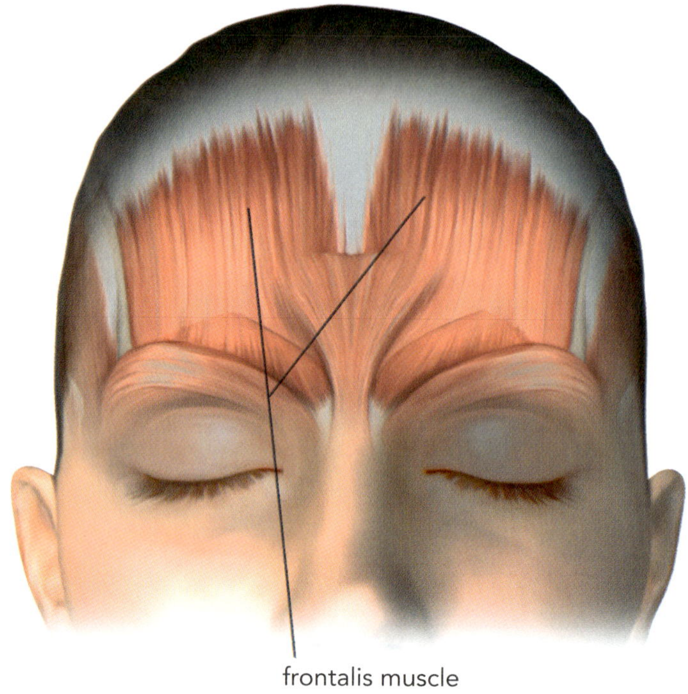

Figure 4 The frontalis muscle

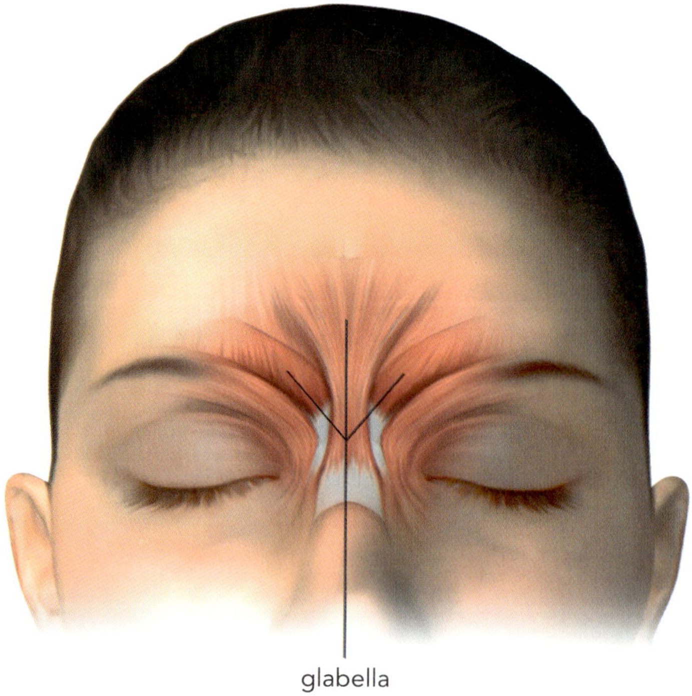

Figure 5 The glabella

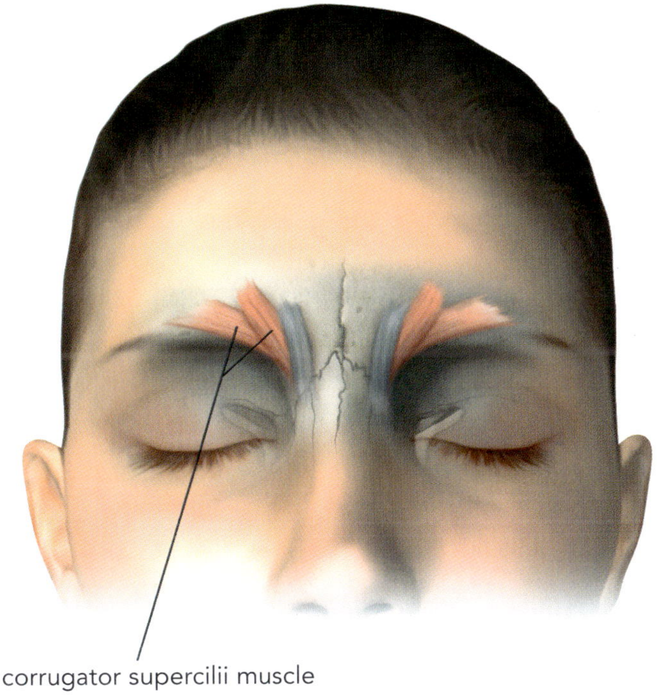

Figure 6 The corrugator supercilii muscle

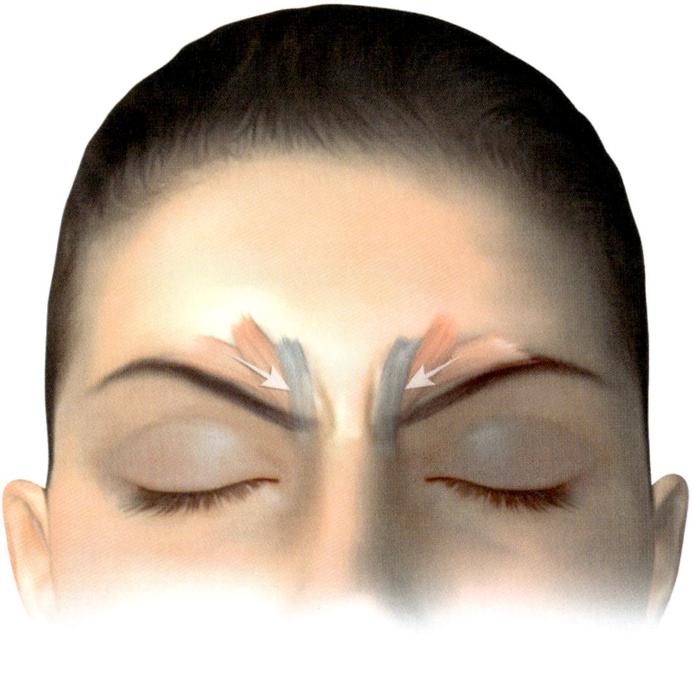

Figure 7 The action of the corrugator supercilii muscle

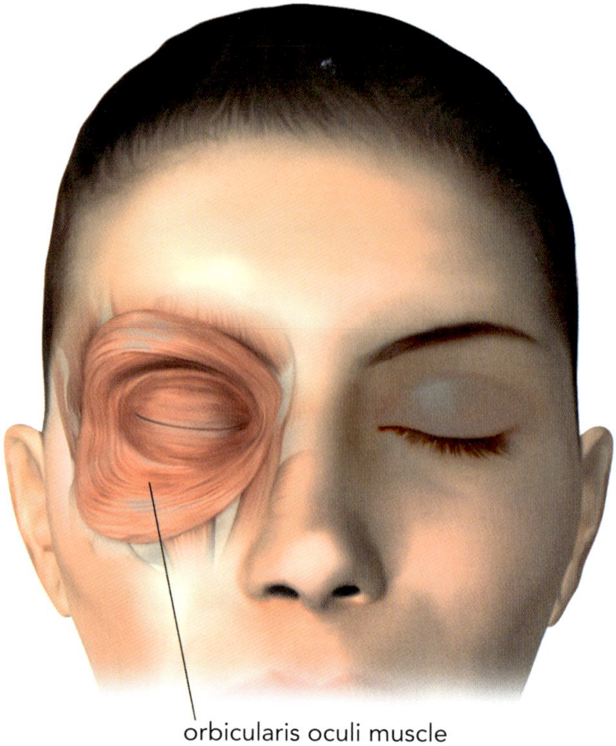

Figure 8 The bundles of the orbicularis oculi muscle

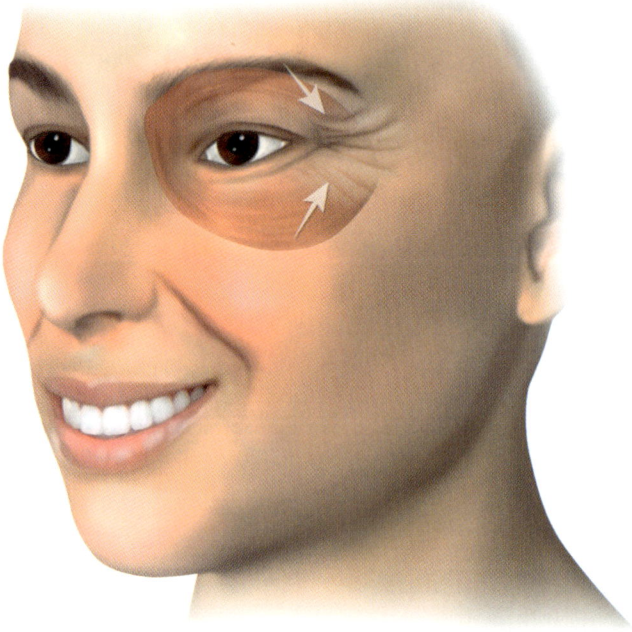

Figure 9 The formation of wrinkles around the eyes

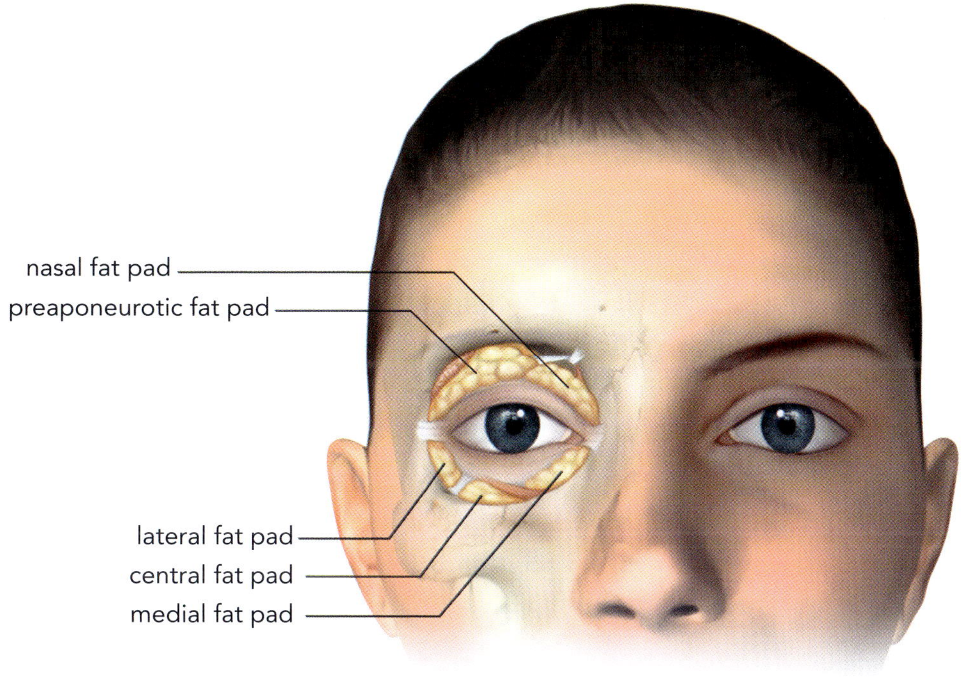

Figure 10 Fat pads

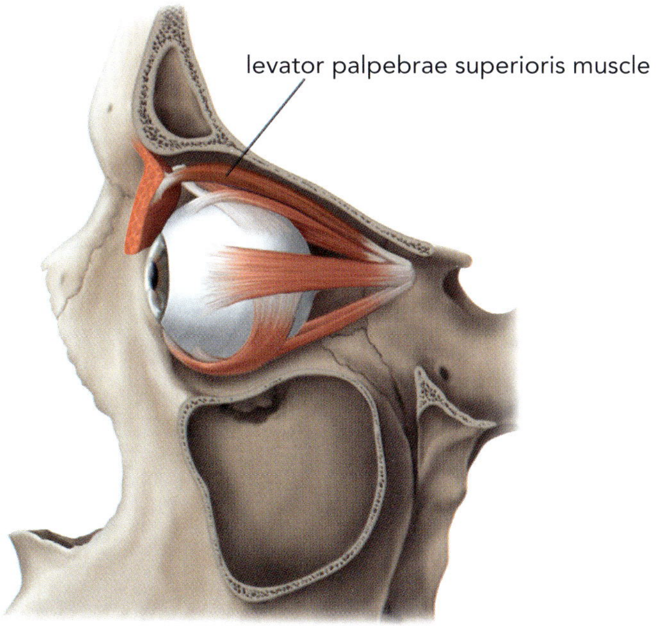

Figure 11 The levator palpebrae superioris muscle

MIDDLE THIRD OF THE FACE

The middle third of the face is the area between two horizontal lines, one passing across the brow arch and the other across the base of the nose (fig. 12). It includes the nose, cheekbones, cheeks and ears. This area contains mimetic muscles and skeletal muscles.

The mimetic muscles are represented by the nasal muscles only, if we exclude the platysma, known in this area as the SMAS, the superficial bundles of which we block with micro-botulinum techniques.

The **masseter muscle**, a skeletal muscle (fig. 13) which runs from the outer surface of the mandibular bone, from the angle up to the zygomatic arch to be precise, is of much more interest. Its muscular bundles are strong when contracted and give the jaw an unattractive square shape, which is commonly associated with the expression of strength or volition. These bundles are particularly developed in those who suffer from bruxism and in Asian people. It should be stressed that it is a deep muscle and must therefore be injected deeply.

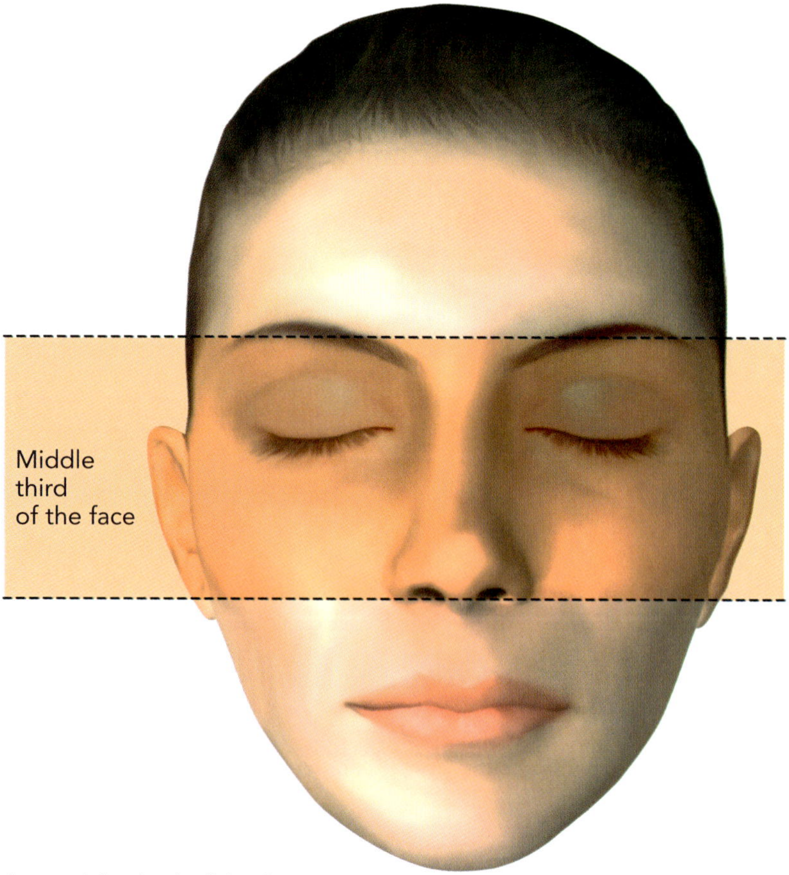

Figure 12 The middle third of the face

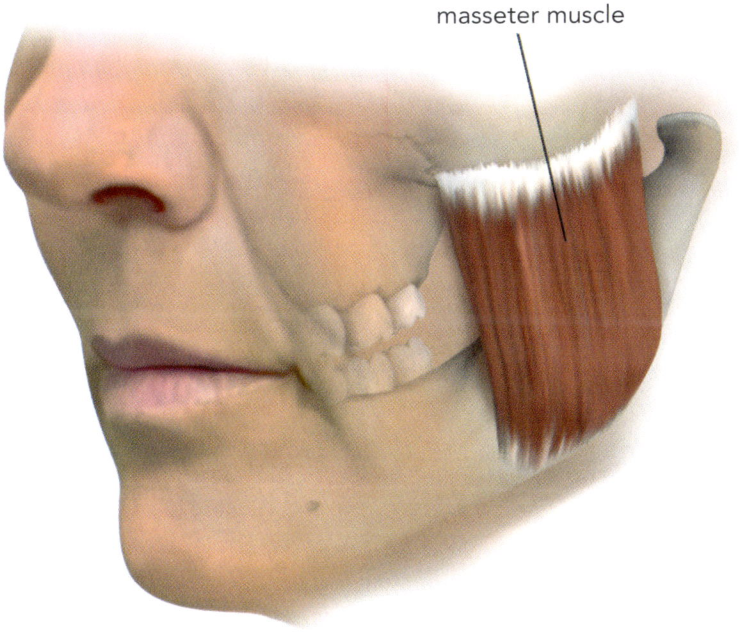

Figure 13 The masseter muscle

LOWER THIRD OF THE FACE

The lower third of the face lies between the subnasal line and a line that touches the lower edge of the chin (menton). It is divided into three subregions: the upper lip region, the lower lip region and the chin region (fig. 14). Consequently, it includes the lips, the chin and the jawline.

The muscles of the upper lip are represented by four matching muscles: the **zygomaticus minor muscle**, which runs from the cheekbone towards the labial commissure, the **quadratus labii superioris**, which is implanted on the upper lip and lifts it, the **caninus muscle and the incisivus muscle**, which are of little importance.

There are three small muscles in the lower lip: the triangulis muscle, also known as the **depressor anguli oris** (DAO) muscle, the quadratus chin muscle and the incisivus inferioris muscle. The depressor anguli oris (DAO) muscle is a triangular muscle that originates in the most superficial layer of the orbicularis oris muscle and the risorius muscle; it originates from the mandible and joins the depressor anguli oris. When it contracts, it works with the **depressor labrii inferioris** (DLI) to lower the lower lip and the buccal rim. This muscle contributes to the formation of what is normally referred to as a "marionette line" (fig. 15). The **zygomaticus major muscle** originates from the anterior part of the zygomatic bone protuberance and, proceeding downwards and medially, meets the orbicularis muscle and ends on the modiolus. The **risorius muscle** is represented by a very thin sheet located no more, but often less, than half a centimetre to the side of the labial commissures, below the horizontal line commonly referred to as the intercheilion (fig. 16). It originates mainly from the SMAS, the masseter fascia and the parotid fascia, extending as far as the modiolus; its action consists in lifting the corners of the mouth when we the smile. It may or may not be infiltrated in the so-called Nefertiti lift. The zygomaticus major muscle, the levator anguli oris (LAO), the depressor anguli oris (DAO) and the risorius are commonly referred to as **lip dilator muscles**.

Without a doubt, however, the **orbicularis oris muscle** (fig. 17) is the most important lip muscle and is a mimetic muscle which forms the muscular part of the lips, on which all the other muscles converge. This, like the orbicularis oculi muscle, is a sphincter muscle, the main function of which is to open and close the lips.

The **buccinator muscle** is a small quadrangular sheet of muscle that converges towards the commissural areas. Its etymology derives from the Latin buccina, which means trumpet and its purpose is to compress the cavities of the vestibule of the mouth to compress air for playing wind instruments and for blowing. Its most important function, however, is to compress the cheeks against the teeth and to move food from the cheeks towards the teeth to be chewed.

The **levator labii superioris** (LLS) is one of the three muscles that start in the upper lip and end in the nasal alar, merging with the zygomaticus minor muscle and the nasal alar elevator (fig. 18). It is important to know of its existence to prevent accidental infiltration, which causes marked asymmetry of the lips, with the drooping of the affected half of the lip.

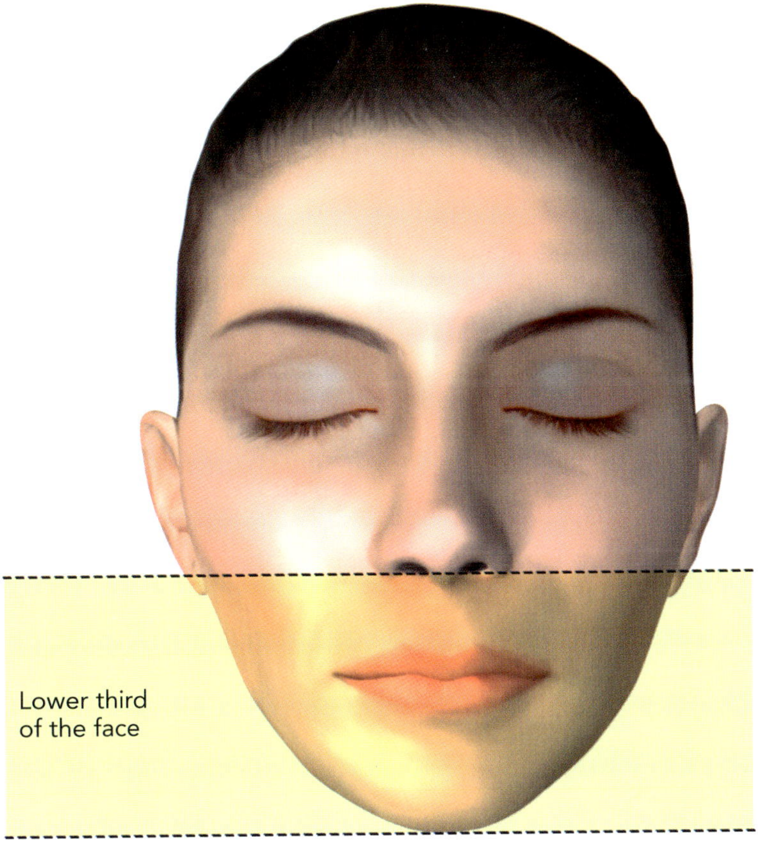

Figure 14 The lower third of the face

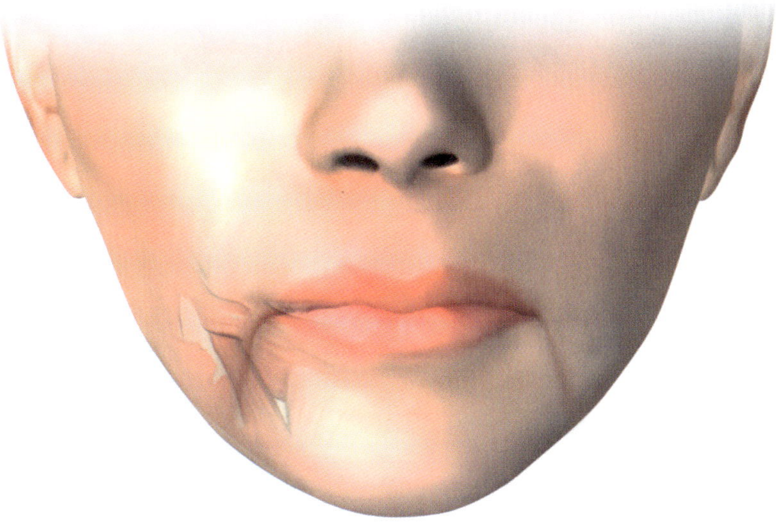

Figure 15 Marionette lines

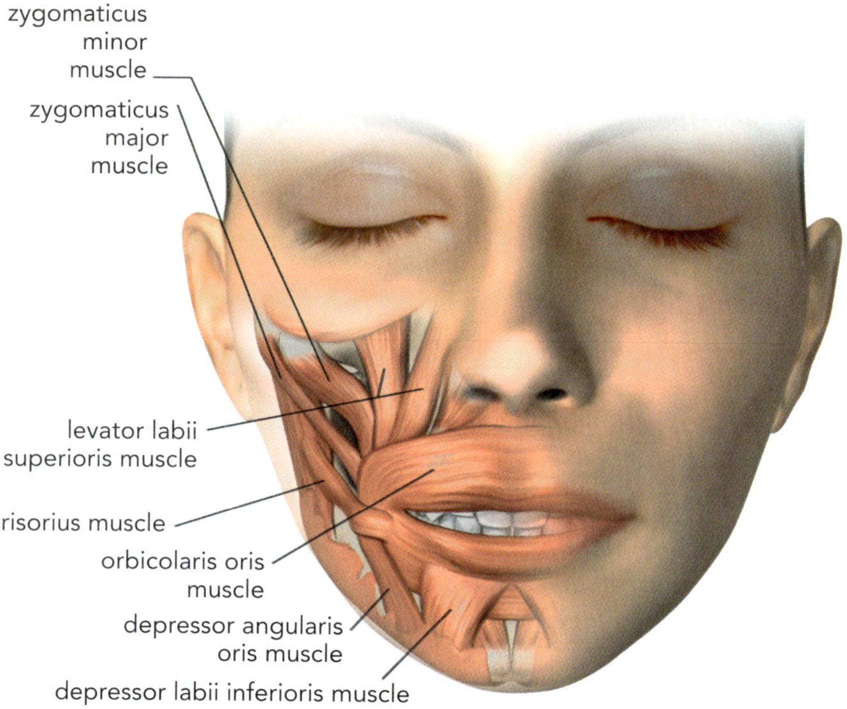

Figure 16 The muscles of the lower third of the face

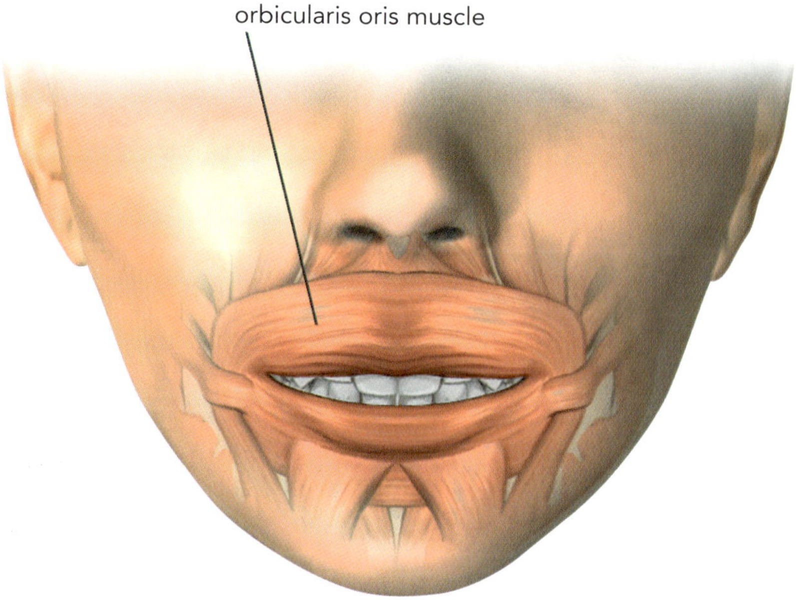

Figure 17 The orbicularis oris muscle

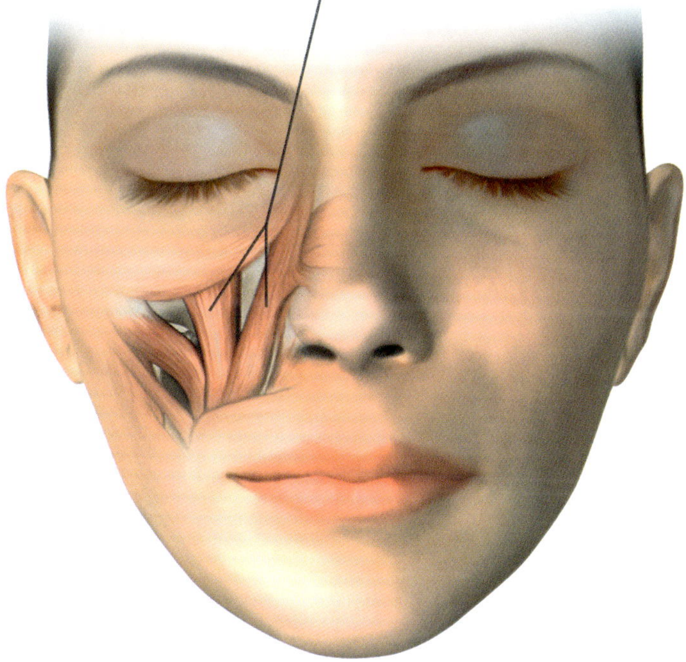

Figure 18 The levator labrii superioris muscle

NECK

The neck region is limited to the area between the cervical-cephalic line which, passing through the lower margin of the mandible, extends backwards to the external occipital protuberance, and a lower line, the cervical-thoracic line, which extends backwards from the jugular incisura to the spinous process of the 7th cervical vertebra (C7), over the margin of the clavicle (fig. 19).

There are numerous neck muscles, but the only muscle of interest in terms of the use of botulinum toxin is the platysma muscle.

The **platysma muscle** (fig. 3), also known as the **superficial neck muscle**, belongs to the group of cutaneous muscles, those which, like the mimetic muscles, do not engage with the skeleton, but run through the thickness of the skin. From the subcutaneous connective tissue and from the aponeurosis which covers the pectoralis major muscle in the chest, approximately level with the second rib, it runs up the clavicle, crosses the side of the neck and ends above the mandible, with anterior fibres running towards the corner of the mouth and with posterior fibres which merge with the aponeurosis covering the parotid gland above the

masseter muscle, which then becomes deep. The platysma has another peculiarity: it can stretch the skin of the neck upwards in oblique folds or, on the contrary, pull the skin of the chin and the corners of the mouth downwards.
The platysma may separate over time, forming two or more very conspicuous fasciae in the anterior region, which can be treated with the toxin.

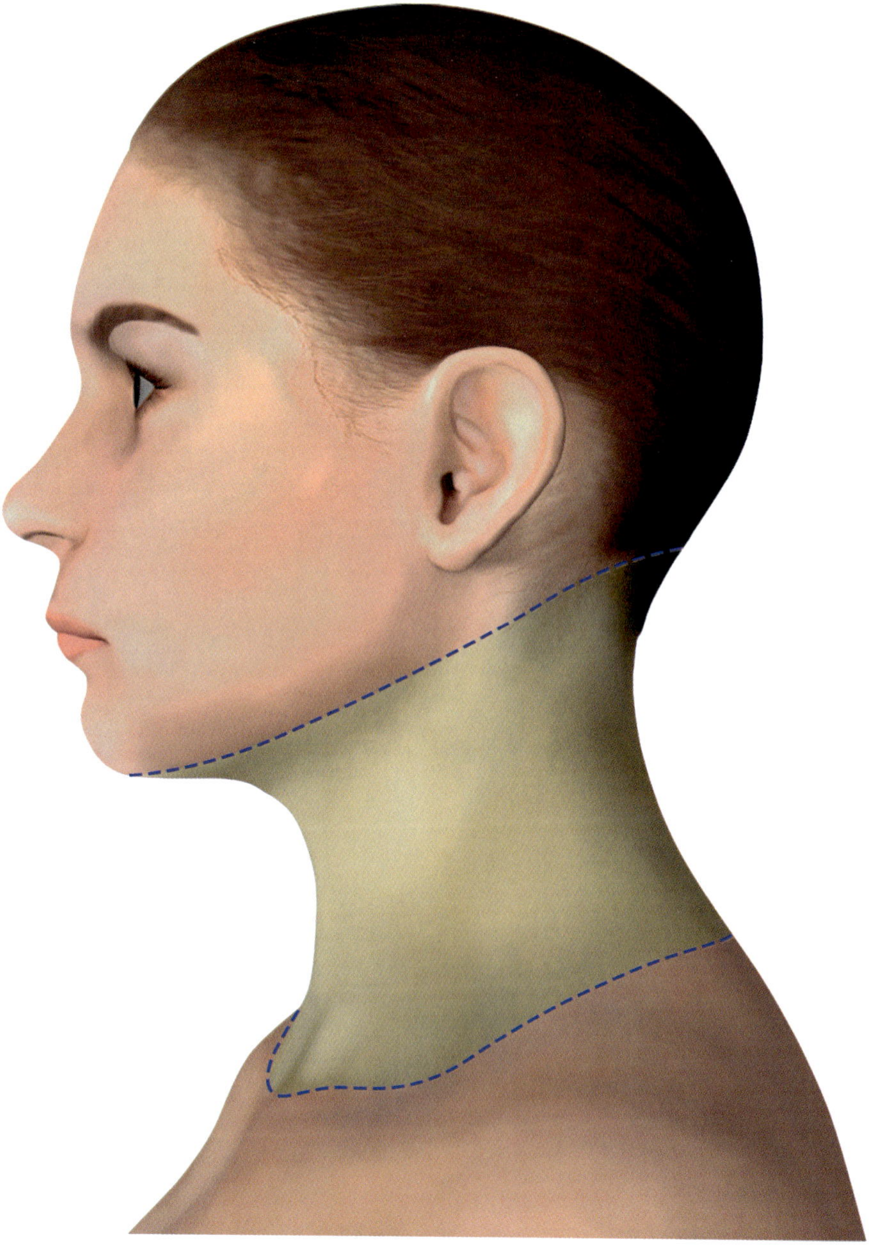

Figure 19 Limits of the neck

PSYCHOLOGICAL ASPECTS OF THE PATIENT WHO APPROACHES BOTULINUM TOXIN

Maria Vittoria Giatti

A request for plastic surgery to change or improve the body often hides important psychological implications. During the initial consultation, it is essential to investigate what the patient really wants and what their needs are, in order to offer the most appropriate treatment.

Treatment with botulinum toxin to correct expression lines is the most widely used non-surgical aesthetic procedure almost all over the world, except in Italy, where it ranks second, despite being extremely safe. The patient can be afraid of approaching this kind of procedure for various reasons, first and foremost the fear of an unnatural or Mephistophelian result (fig. 21) and of being left with a face that looks "frozen" and expressionless. This is compounded by the erroneous association of danger and "death" linked to botulism, which patients mistakenly identify with botulinum toxin in general. In Italy, patients usually ask for a more natural and discreet correction, unlike in the United States, for example, where there is a preference for stereotypical accentuations of facial roundness (with deliberately pronounced cheekbones and lips) and stronger modulations of botulinum toxin. The standards of beauty change not only through the ages but also depending on geographical area, reflecting people's different cultures and fashions.

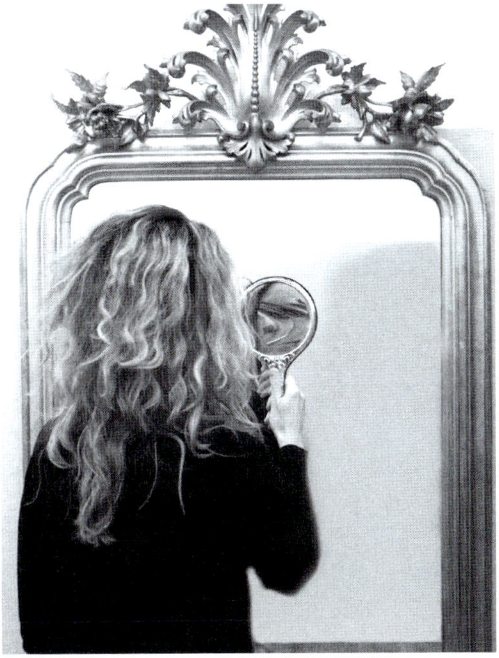

Figure 20 The need for change often hides psychological implications that should not be underestimated

After the summer of 2020, with the events of the Covid-19 pandemic and the need to use protective masks that leave only the upper third of the face uncovered, there was a significant increase in the number of procedures performed with botulinum toxin, due to increased demand for rejuvenation of the eyes and forehead, the only areas visible in public.

Psychological implications

Some patients who request correction with botulinum toxin also mention the fact that their outward appearance, which seems scowling and aggressive (mainly due to a hypertrophy of the

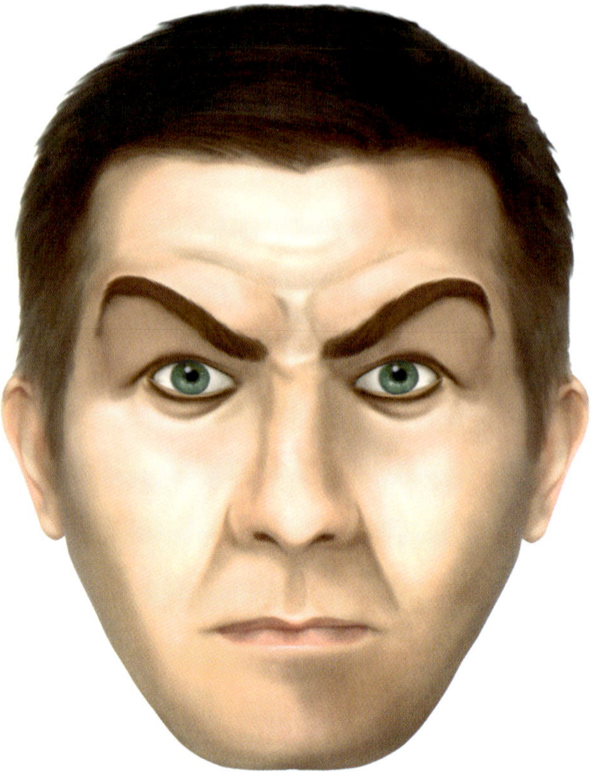

Figure 21 Mephistophelian eyebrow

facial expression muscles and their hypertonia) does not reflect their real nature, which is gentle and calm, sometimes hinting at what is known as Minotaur Syndrome, as described in scientific literature in the field of plastic surgery. This syndrome describes the discrepancy between the individual's true personality and the negative appearance of their face, which often leads to a series of social problems and difficulties in interpersonal relations (fig. 22).

After treatment with botulinum toxin, it has been shown that several psychosocial parameters such as self-esteem, quality of life, confidence and self-perception are improved. It is possible to objectify the results with various assessments, examples being the Global Aesthetic Improvement Scale (Gais), the Sat-p Test, which assesses subjective satisfaction and quality of life, the Face-Q Aesthetics Scale, the Rosenberg Self-Esteem Scale (Ses), and the Whoqol-Bref, which assesses the perception of quality of life. These are very simple tests that can be administered quickly and filled in by the patient before treatment and at subsequent check-ups. A series of questions (with attribution of specific scores to the answers) is used to investigate various parameters linked to self-perception, improvement after treatment, satisfaction, and self-esteem, mostly

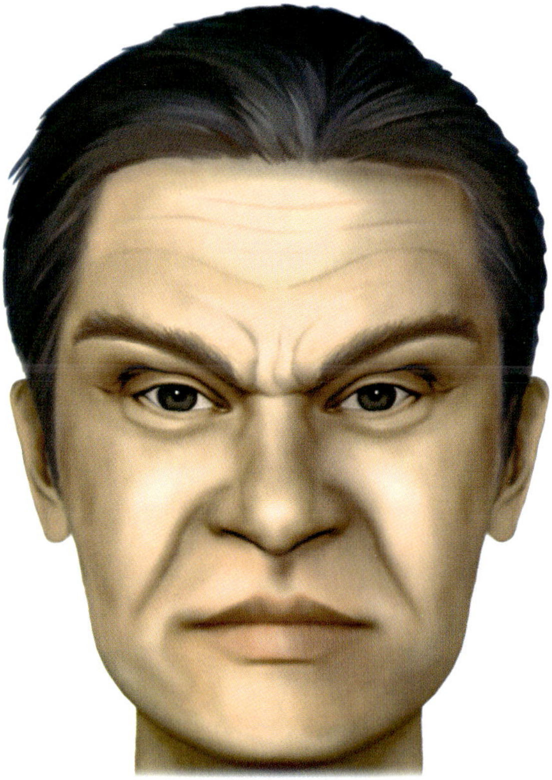

Figure 22 Minotaur syndrome

covering the psychological, physical, psychophysical, professional, and relational areas.
Lastly, the patient should be reassured during the medical examination. This can be achieved by talking about muscle relaxation instead of paralysis, about botulinum protein instead of "poison" (many people associate botulinum toxin with this concept), and about the result of a rested face instead of an expressionless face. Emphasis should be placed on the fact that a correct technique with the right modulation and personalisation on the anatomic-clinical and gender characteristics of the patient, calibrated according to age and degree of ageing, performed by a specialist, offers a guarantee of harmonious and natural results.

Bibliography

History of botulinum

1. Dressler D. Botulinum toxin drugs: brief history and outlook. J Neural Transm (Vienna). 2016 Mar;123(3):277-9.

2. Erbguth FJ, Naumann M. Historical aspects of botulinum toxin: Justinus Kerner (1786-1862) and the "sausage poison". Neurology. 1999;53(8):1850-1853.
3. Erbguth FJ. From poison to remedy: the chequered history of botulinum toxin. J Neural Transm (Vienna). 2008;115(4):559-565.
4. Jabbari B. History of Botulinum Toxin Treatment in Movement Disorders. Tremor Other Hyperkinet Mov (N Y). 2016;6:394.
5. Satila H. The route of botulinum toxin from cause of food poisoning to medical remedy. Duodecim. 2014;130:1523–30.

Botulinum toxin and how it works

6. Eisele KH, Fink K, Vey M, Taylor HV. Studies on the dissociation of botulinum neurotoxin type A complexes. Toxicon. 2011;57(4):555-565.
7. Fernández-Salas E, Wang J, Molina Y, Nelson JB, Jacky BP, Aoki KR. Botulinum neurotoxin serotype A specific cell-based potency assay to replace the mouse bioassay. PLoS One. 2012;7(11):e49516.
8. Kane MA, Gold MH, Coleman WP 3rd, et al. A Randomized, Double-Blind Trial to Investigate the Equivalence of IncobotulinumtoxinA and OnabotulinumtoxinA for Glabellar Frown Lines. Dermatol Surg. 2015;41(11):1310-1319.
9. Muti G, Harrington L. A prospective rater- and subject-blinded study comparing the efficacy of incobotulinumtoxinA and onabotulinumtoxinA to treat crow's feet: a clinical crossover evaluation. Dermatol Surg. 2015;41 Suppl 1:S39-S46.
10. Rossetto O, Pirazzini M, Montecucco C. Botulinum neurotoxins: genetic, structural and mechanistic insights. Nat Rev Microbiol. 2014;12(8):535-549.
11. Schantz EJ, Johnson EA. Properties and use of botulinum toxin and other microbial neurotoxins in medicine. Microbiol Rev. 1992;56(1):80-99.
12. Schiavo G, Rossetto O, Montecucco C. Clostridial neurotoxins as tools to investigate the molecular events of neurotransmitter release. Semin Cell Biol. 1994;5(4):221-229.
13. Scott AB. Botulinum toxin injection of eye muscles to correct strabismus. Trans Am Ophthalmol Soc. 1981;79:734-770.
14. Steinhardt RA, Bi G, Alderton JM. Cell membrane resealing by a vesicular mechanism similar to neurotransmitter release. Science. 1994;263(5145):390-393.

Dilution and diffusion

15. Borodic GE, Ferrante R, Pearce LB, Smith K. Histologic assessment of dose-related diffusion and muscle fiber response after therapeutic botulinum A toxin injections. Mov Disord. 1994 Jan;9(1):31-9.
16. Brin MF, Lyons KE, Doucette J, Adler CH, Caviness JN, Comella CL, Dubinsky RM, Friedman JH, Manyam BV, Matsumoto JY, Pullman SL, Rajput AH, Sethi KD, Tanner C, Koller WC. A randomized, double masked, controlled trial of botulinum toxin type A in essential hand tremor. Neurology. 2001 Jun 12;56(11):1523-8.

17. Brodsky MA, Swope DM, Grimes D. Diffusion of botulinum toxins. Tremor Other Hyperkinet Mov (N Y). 2012;2.
18. Carli L, Montecucco C, Rossetto O. Assay of diffusion of different botulinum neurotoxin type a formulations injected in the mouse leg. Muscle Nerve. 2009 Sep;40(3):374-80.
19. Comella CL, Buchman AS, Tanner CM, Brown-Toms NC, Goetz CG. Botulinum toxin injection for spasmodic torticollis: increased magnitude of benefit with electromyographic assistance. Neurology. 1992 Apr;42(4):878-82.
20. de Almeida AT, De Boulle K. Diffusion characteristics of botulinum neurotoxin products and their clinical significance in cosmetic applications. J Cosmet Laser Ther. 2007;9 Suppl 1:17-22.
21. Dover JS, Monheit G, Greener M, Pickett A. Botulinum Toxin in Aesthetic Medicine: Myths and Realities. Dermatol Surg. 2018 Feb;44(2):249-260.
22. Muti GF, Basso M. Treatment of Lateral Periorbital Lines with Different Dilutions of IncobotulinumtoxinA. J Clin Aesthet Dermatol. 2017 Sep;10(9):27-29.
23. Pickett A, Dodd S, Rzany B. Confusion about diffusion and the art of misinterpreting data when comparing different botulinum toxins used in aesthetic applications. J Cosmet Laser Ther. 2008 Sep;10(3):181-3.
24. Sconfienza LM, Lacelli F, Bruno A, Serafini G. Ultrasound guidance can improve the outcome of botulinum toxin A injection. Eur J Phys Rehabil Med. 2009 Mar;45(1):153.
25. Simpson DM, Gracies JM, Yablon SA, Barbano R, Brashear A; BoNT/TZD Study Team. Botulinum neurotoxin versus tizanidine in upper limb spasticity: a placebo-controlled study. J Neurol Neurosurg Psychiatry. 2009 Apr;80(4):380-5.

Immunogenicity of botulinum toxin

26. Bellows S, Jankovic J. Immunogenicity Associated with Botulinum Toxin Treatment. Toxins (Basel). 2019 Aug 26;11(9):491.
27. Frevert J. Pharmaceutical, biological, and clinical properties of botulinum neurotoxin type A products. Drugs R D. 2015 Mar;15(1):1-9.
28. Benecke R. Clinical relevance of botulinum toxin immunogenicity. BioDrugs. 2012 Apr 1;26(2): e1-9.
29. Dressler D. Clinical presentation and management of antibody-induced failure of botulinum toxin therapy. Mov Disord. 2004 Mar;19 Suppl 8:S92-S100.
30. Hefter H, Hartmann C, et al. Prospective analysis of neutralising antibody titres in secondary non-responders under continuous treatment with a botulinumtoxin type A preparation free of complexing proteins--a single cohort 4-year follow-up study. BMJ Open. 2012 Aug 4;2(4):e000646.
31. Wang L, Sun Y, Yang W, Lindo P, Singh BR. Type A botulinum neurotoxin complex proteins differentially modulate host response of neuronal cells. Toxicon. 2014 May; 82:52-60.
32. Pickett A. Immunogenicity issues related to botulinum toxins in clinical use cannot be answered by speculation about product characteristics.

BioDrugs. 2013 Feb;27(1):83-4.
33. Stengel G, Bee EK. Antibody-induced secondary treatment failure in a patient treated with botulinum toxin type A for glabellar frown lines. Clin Interv Aging. 2011;6:281-4.

Morphodynamic anatomy

34. Mezzogiorno V, Mezzogiorno A. Compendio di anatomia umana, Piccin
35. Testut L, Latarjet A. Anatomia umana, Utet.
36. Testut L., Jacob O. Trattato di anatomia topografica, Edra.
37. Netter Frank H, Standring S. Netter Gray. L'anatomia: Anatomia del Gray-Atlante di anatomia umana di Netter, Edra.
38. VV. AA. Prometheus. Testo atlante di anatomia, Edises.
39. Kim HJ, Seo KK, Lee HK, Kim J. Anatomia clinica del volto per filler e tossina botulinica, Piccin.
40. Kontis TC, Lacombe VG. Iniezioni di tossina botulinica e filler in medicina estetica, Piccin.
41. Grappolini S. Blefaroplastica e tecniche ancillari, Piccin.

Psychological aspects of the patient who approaches botulinum toxin

42. Morselli PG. The Minotaur syndrome: plastic surgery of the facial skeleton. Aesthetic Plast Surg. 1993;17(2):99-102.
43. Dayan SH, Arkins JP, Patel AB, Gal TJ. A double-blind, randomized, placebo-controlled health-outcomes survey of the effect of botulinum toxin type a injections on quality of life and self-esteem. Dermatol Surg. 2010;36 Suppl 4:2088-2097.
44. Molina B, Grangier Y, Mole B, et al. Patient satisfaction after the treatment of glabellar lines with Botulinum toxin type A (Speywood Unit): a multi-centre European observational study. J Eur Acad Dermatol Venereol. 2015;29(7):1382-1388.
45. Tang M, Li W, Ji F, Li X, Zhang Y, Liu P. Impact of botulinum toxin injections on quality of life and self-esteem in patients with blepharospasm. Psychol Health Med. 2019;24(5):513-518.
46. Majani G, Callegari S. TEST SAT-P: soddisfazione soggettiva e qualità della vita. Centro Studi Erickson 1998.

2

TREATMENT

Giovanni Brunelli, Patrizia Piersini, Maria Vittoria Giatti

PATIENT SELECTION

Giovanni Brunelli

Ageing processes are the result of intrinsic (genetic) and extrinsic (environmental, behavioural) factors; the latter include photo-induced skin damage, which plays an important role as it causes the formation of brown marks, dry skin, elastosis and static wrinkles.

At the same time, communication, in all its forms, but especially *de visu*, is an essential part of contemporary life, forming the basis of our interpersonal relationships. It has been proven that we assess the people we meet within just a few seconds of setting eyes on them.

Mimetic muscles are used to express a range of emotions, including joy, surprise, worry, sadness and anger. However, these little muscles sometimes act independently of our will, as is often the case with the muscles we use to furrow our brows, and this can give the person we are talking to the wrong impression.

Virtually any patient can be eligible for treatment with botulinum toxin. In theory - and based on the instructions of the Italian Drug Agency (Aifa) - we should not treat patients over the age of 65, making exceptions only if they are psychologically disturbed by their expression lines.

As we know, however, an increasing proportion of toxin treatments are performed off-label, meaning that they are carried out independently of the indications on the product leaflet and under our direct responsibility. As a result, we can offer patients the possibility of treating other areas of the face and the neck.

It is of course necessary to collect an adequate medical history in order to exclude patients presenting contra-indications to treatment. Examples of these are known allergies to the neurotoxin or to one of the excipients, particularly human albumin, lactose monohydrate and sucrose. Other examples include the presence of neurological diseases, such as myasthenia gravis, Lambert-Eaton syndrome, amyotrophic lateral sclerosis (ALS), peripheral muscle disorders (although sufferers are unlikely to come to our clinics with this type of request), a positive history of dysphagia, inflammation or infection of the injection point, and pregnant or breastfeeding women. Once we have ascertained that there are no contra-indications, we can proceed.

It is a good idea to give patients a mirror and ask them what flaws they see that they would like to correct. They often complain of minor or hard-to-correct flaws, while they tend not to be aware of the presence of asymmetries, which could become apparent later. It should be noted that it may not be possible to fully correct deep static furrows or that their correction may require several sessions and combination with other aesthetic medical techniques.

One of the conditions that should alert us when injecting the frontalis muscle is the coexistence of a drooping eyebrow or an evident blepharochalasis of the upper eyelid. As we know, the frontalis

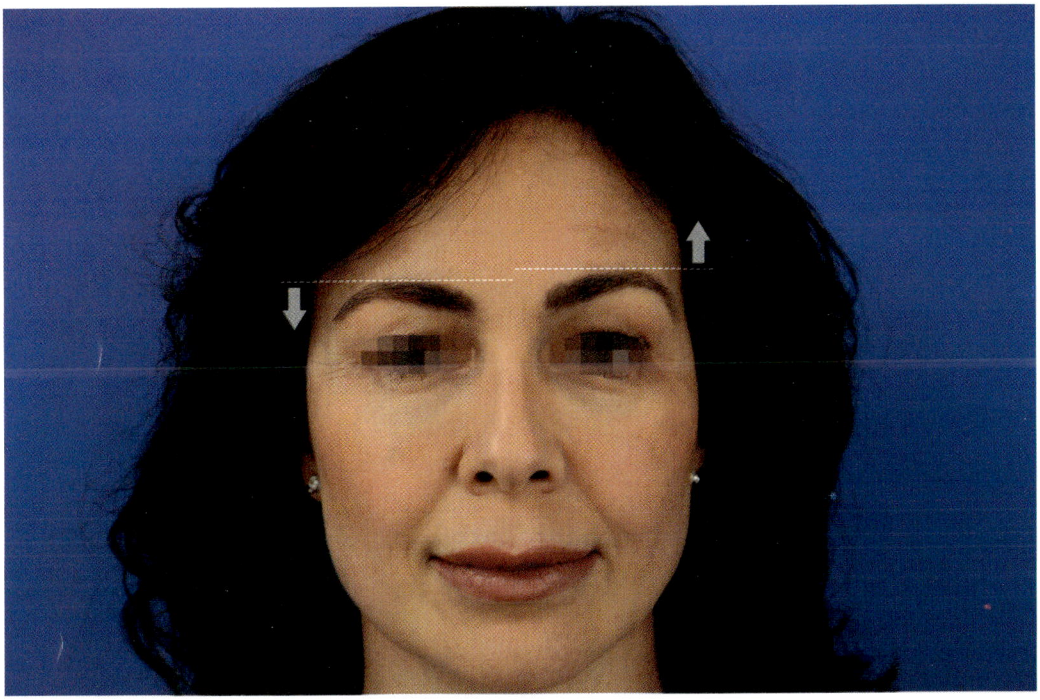

Figure 1 Eyebrow asymmetry: the right eyebrow is about 5 mm lower. Consequently, there is more excess skin on the right upper eyelid than on the left

is the only elevator muscle in this area and, when it contracts, it not only pulls the eyebrow upwards, but also lifts the excess skin of the eyelid (fig. 1).

If there is a lot of excess skin, the frontalis muscle should be treated very conservatively, and patients should be informed of the possibility that, after treatment, they might have the impression that there has been an increase in the excess skin on the eyelid. Of course it is impossible for botulinum toxin to cause an increase in the skin; it is the weakening of the frontalis muscle that makes it impossible to balance this excess. If patients are unwilling to accept this consequence, then perhaps it is better to refuse to perform this treatment and offer blepharoplasty.

It is also worth assessing the tone of the lower eyelid to detect any slackness using the eyelid distraction test or snap test.

If unrealistic demands are made, as in all areas of medicine and surgery, it is better not to perform the treatment.

CONTRAINDICATIONS

Patrizia Piersini

The use of botulinum protein has increased exponentially in recent years, so it is important to have a thorough understanding of the absolute and relative contraindications to its injection and of when not to offer this treatment to patients.

General contraindications

Botulinum protein should not be a therapeutic choice in patients with unrealistic expectations of the results that can be achieved and with psychiatric disorders, such as dysmorphophobia.

Particular attention must also be paid to patients in whom altered facial expressions may have significant consequences for their work, such as actors, politicians or singers, who need to be able to express their emotions fully and are afraid that botulinum may make their faces less expressive. In this case, injections with fillers with a specific rheology, capable of adapting to facial dynamics, could be a good alternative.

As for other injectables used in aesthetic medicine, contraindications include pregnancy and breastfeeding, where no trials exist, as well as immunocompromised patients.

Allergies

Treatment with botulinum is contraindicated if there is a clinical history of allergy to *Clostridium botulinum* type A or the albumin carrier substance, or of intolerance to lactose (Abobotulinum) or sucrose (Incobotulinum).

Infections in the area chosen for injection

Do not inject into treatment areas affected by active dermatitis, such as herpes simplex or psoriasis, or if there is inflammation or infection present in the proposed injection site.

Localised neurological pathologies

Injection is contraindicated in patients suffering from dysphagia or respiratory disorders and should not be used for facial rejuvenation in patients who have pre-existing eyelid ptosis, in patients who have undergone surgery that may have repositioned or weakened the muscles or in patients with Bell's palsy (facial weakness or paralysis caused by dysfunction of the facial nerve or VII cranial nerve).

Systemic neurological pathologies

Patients with neuropathies or neuromuscular diseases such as Lambert-Eaton syndrome, amyotrophic lateral sclerosis (ALS) or myasthenia gravis should not be treated, because even very low doses of the toxin could cause a neuromuscular crisis. In Lambert-Eaton syndrome, antibodies targeting cross-tumour antigens react with the calcium channels involved in acetylcholine release, leading to impaired neuromuscular transmission.

Interaction with other drugs

Some classes of antibiotics interact with

TABLE 1 - DRUGS THAT INTERFERE WITH BOTULINUM TOXIN

DRUGS	INTERACTION
Antibiotics	Potentiate BT
Acetylcholinesterase Inhibitors	Decrease BT
Succinylcholine	Potentiate BT
Curare	Potentiate BT
Magnesium Sulfate	Potentiate BT
Quinine	Potentiate BT
Calcium Channel Blockers	Mechanism not explained
Cyclosporine	Potentiate BT
Pancuronio, Rocuronio, Veruconio, Galamine	Potentiate BT
Penicillamine	Potentiate BT

Source: based on Toxina Botulínica na Dermatolgia. Azulay et al (2016)

botulinum protein and many have a presynaptic action, which decreases the release of acetylcholine, but also a post-synaptic action. The best known include:

- aminoglycoside antibiotics (e.g.: streptomycin, gentamicin, amikacin, tobramycin or neomycin, which are used to treat serious bacterial infections such as those from Gram-negative bacteria), as high doses of aminoglycosides may prevent the release of acetylcholine from the neuromuscular plate and produce a clinical "botulinum-like" syndrome. This effect may be related to a blockage of the calcium channels. Symptoms rapidly regress when the drug is fully catabolised or with the administration of calcium salts; their action may enhance that of botulinum;
- tetracycline, which could increase the risk or severity of complications from botulinum toxin;
- polymyxins, which inhibit acetylcholine release and reduce post-junctional sensitivity. This blockage cannot be reversed with the use of calcium salts.

When botulinum is administered for aesthetic medical treatments or hyperhidrosis, particular attention should be paid to patients taking the following drugs:

- chloroquine and hydroxychloroquine (aminoquinolines), which antagonise the paresis effect of botulinum by acting both on the cell membrane to inhibit binding and internalisation of the toxin, and inside the cell by inhibiting the lysosomal process of the toxin;
- cyclosporine (immunosuppressant), as it has been reported that it can cause neuromuscular blockage characterised by muscle weakness and respiratory failure, and can enhance the effect of botulinum;
- penicillamine (chelating agent and anti-inflammatory drug for rheumatoid arthritis), which binds to acetylcholine receptors and stimulates the synthesis of prostaglandin E-1

by interfering with neuromuscular transmission;
- magnesium sulphate (anticonvulsant), which enhances the action of neuromuscular blockers and consequently of botulinum toxin;
- acetylcholinesterase inhibitors, which act as botulinum antagonists by increasing the production of acetylcholine at the neuromuscular junction;
- calcium channel blockers or calcium antagonist drugs (antihypertensives), which can accentuate the effects of botulinum.

Moreover, Fiacchino et al. reported that botulinum interferes with neuromuscular blockers such as vecuronium (a non-depolarising competitive neuromuscular blocker used as an adjuvant in surgical procedures) and could therefore cause reduced response to the effects of vecuronium, but also to neuromuscular blockers used in anaesthesiology in general.
Lastly, careful monitoring should be carried out in children and adolescents as botulinum may alter cellular functions such as axonal growth.

PRE-INJECTION ASSESSMENT

Giovanni Brunelli

The patient who comes to us for the first time with a request for botulinum toxin treatment should be observed carefully. During the initial consultation it is useful to ask open questions, encouraging the patient to talk for a few minutes and checking for certain clinical data (tab. 2).
This brief chat is useful not only to understand the person sitting in front of us and any health problems they may have. During this short period of time, it is often possible to observe asymmetries, not only of the face, but also, and above all, of the mimetic muscles, which frequently cause wrinkles of varying depths and extensions, especially on the forehead and between the eyebrows.
It is fairly common to find a much deeper glabella lines on one side or more wrinkles on one side of the forehead than the other; sometimes one of the eyebrows is slightly higher than the other.
Many patients with numerous horizontal wrinkles on the forehead show signs of ptosis of the upper eyelid or, at least, of dermatochalasis, which requires compensation by contraction of the frontalis (the only muscle that lifts the eyebrow). We must then ask the patient, at least the first time we treat them, to contract the muscles that we want to treat as much as possible and record these differences on the patient's record form, which each individual can set out according to their own habits and requirements, for reference during subse-

TABLE 2 - INITIAL INTERVIEW

Anamnestic assessment	Allergies Drugs currently being taken Neuromuscular diseases Pregnancy and/or breast feeding
Psychological assessment	Unrealistic desires Dysmorphophobia
Clinical assessment of the region concerned	Asymmetries Ptosis Surgical indications

quent sessions (fig. 2).
It is also important to record the number of units of botulinum injected into each injection site, for future reference. Each patient is different, and it is sometimes necessary to adjust the amount injected, but if we do not keep track of this, it is very hard to remember what has been done.
The next step is to draw on our patients, as shown in video 2.1, which covers the treatment of the upper third. We usually only mark the three main points in the eye area. Sometimes, however, two more external points can be added to cover more of the extension of the orbicularis muscle, as we can see in video 2.1.
In video 2.2 we can appreciate the dynamic results two weeks after treatment.
As we know, the indications for treatment with botulinum toxin have increased dramatically in recent years, and patients no longer require treatment of the upper third of the face alone. For some time now, there has been talk of treatment of the whole face, neck and decolletage, as well as the treatment of axillary, palmar and plantar hyperhidrosis, not to mention indications relating to other non-aesthetic medical fields.
Botulinum may be used for various dermatological problems, such as the treatment of oily skin, erythrosis or scars. Therefore, all our patients' requests should be listened to and assessed before proceeding with injection treatment.
Younger colleagues, who have recently begun (or are about to begin) practicing botulinum treatments, should begin with the upper third of the face, where the anatomy of the mimetic muscles is easy to learn and the results are reproducible, before venturing into the middle and lower thirds of the face, where anatomical variations are more common and some inconvenience may be incurred.

CLINICAL CASES

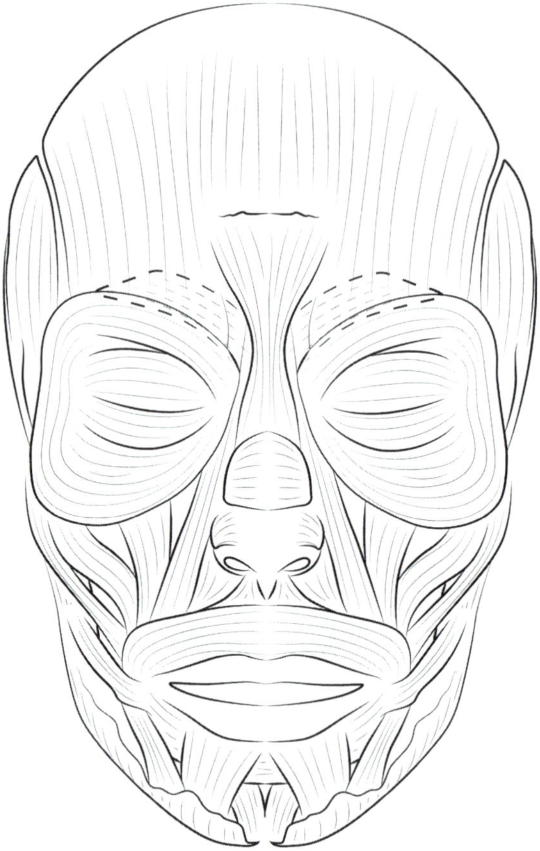

Figure 2 Patient records

VIDEO 2.1

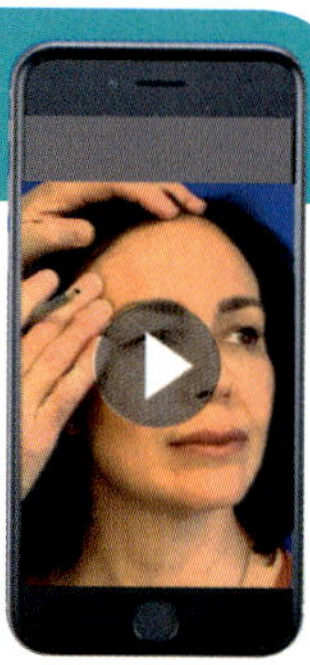

Upper third: drawing before treatment

VIDEO 2.2

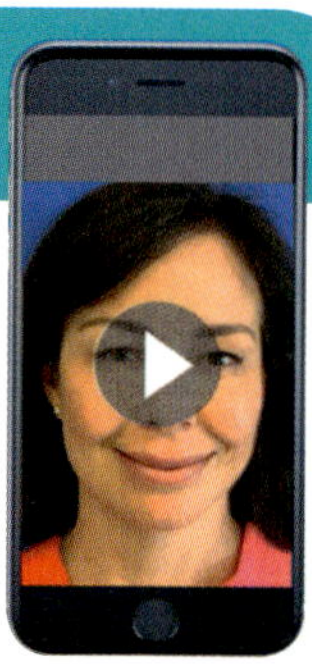

Upper third: result 15 days after injection

CLINICAL CASES

CLINICAL CASE 1

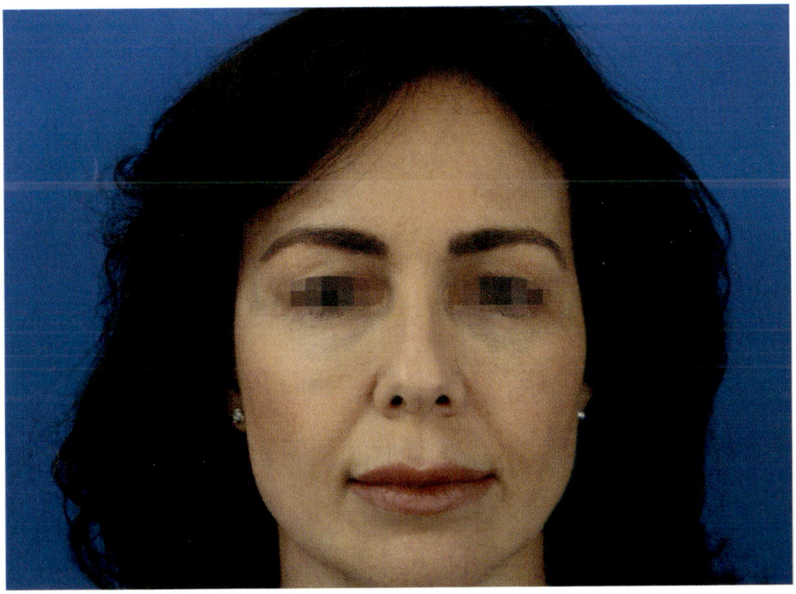

BEFORE
<

AFTER
>

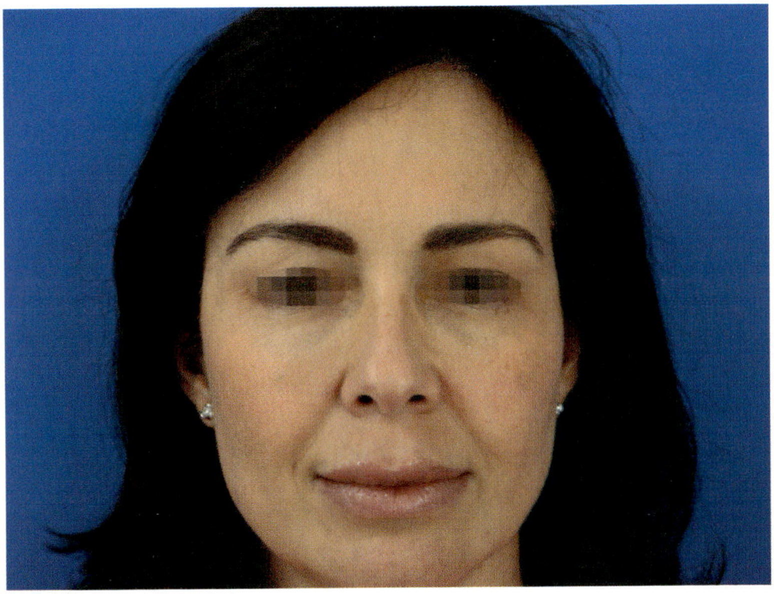

Figure 3 Basal status before treatment and basal status 15 days after treatment with botulinum toxin

CLINICAL CASES

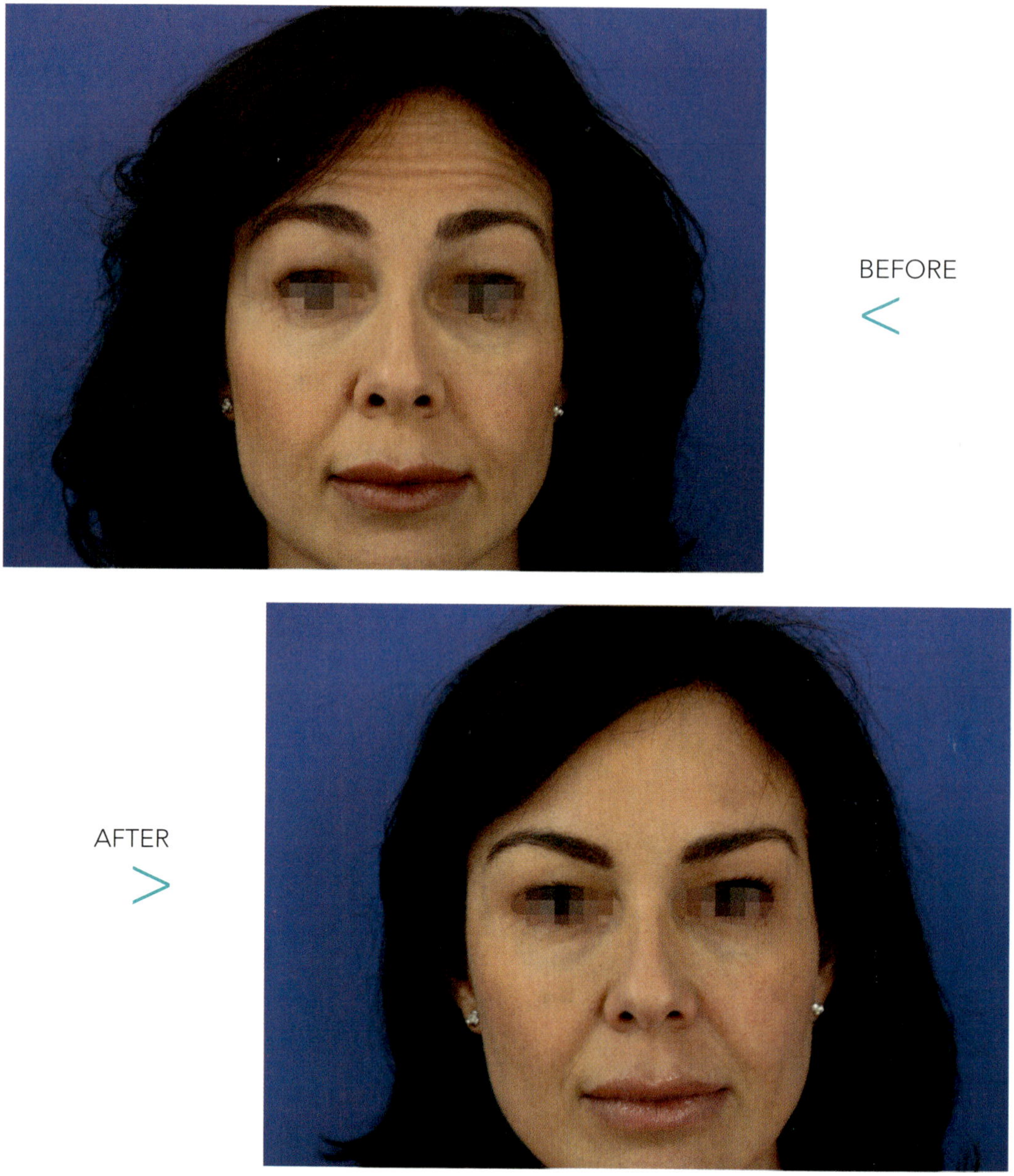

Figure 4 Maximum contraction of the frontalis muscle before treatment and 15 days after treatment with botulinum toxin

CLINICAL CASES

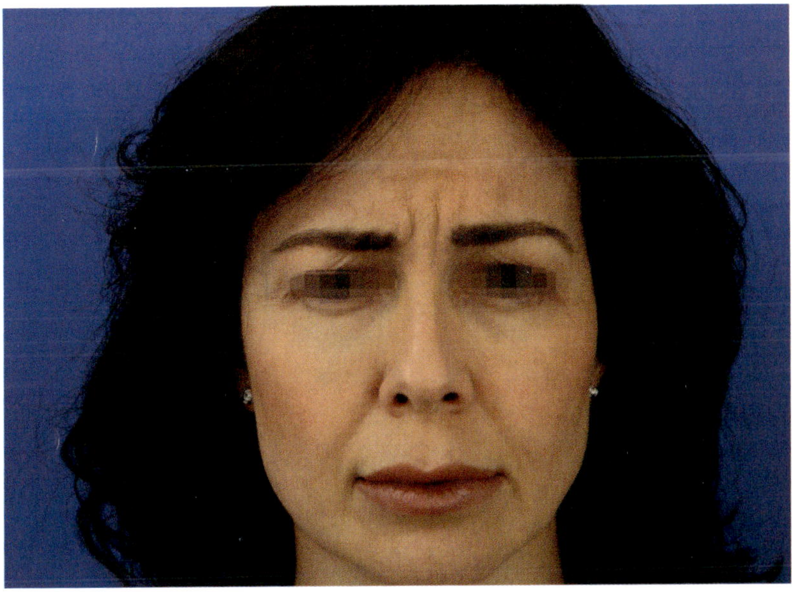

BEFORE

<

AFTER

>

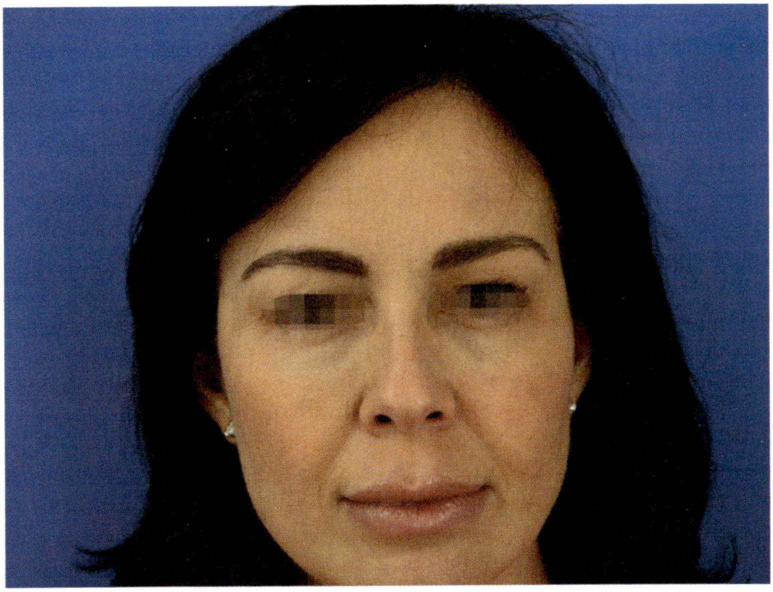

Figure 5 Maximum contraction of the corrugator muscles before treatment and 15 days after treatment with botulinum toxin

CLINICAL CASES

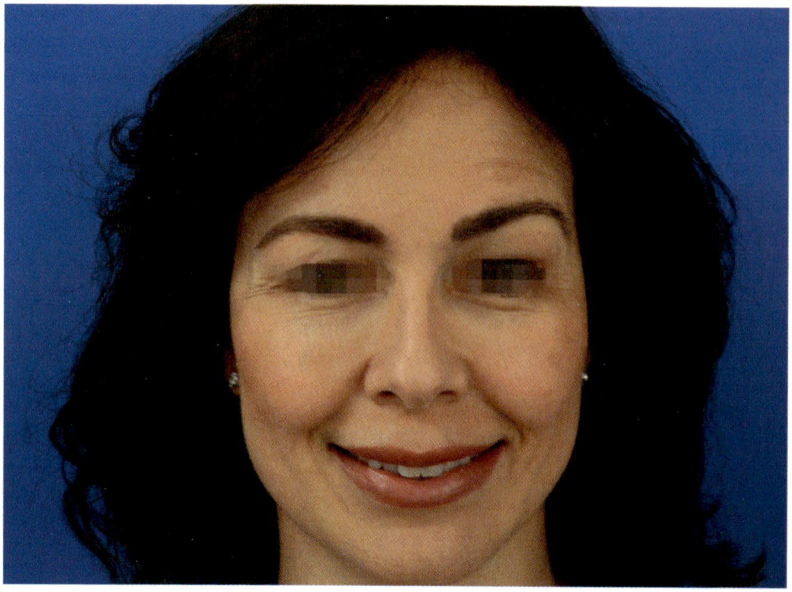

BEFORE

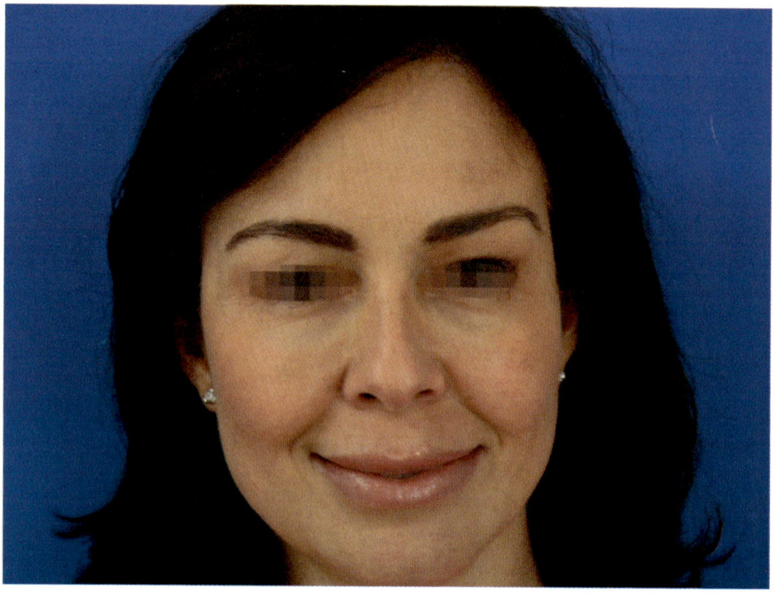

AFTER

Figure 6 Maximum contraction of the orbicularis muscle before treatment and 15 days after treatment with botulinum toxin

THE HYPERKINETIC AND HYPERTONIC PATIENT

Giovanni Brunelli

Alterations to the upper third of the face are mainly due to actinic damage caused by chronic exposure to ultraviolet rays, gravitational alterations caused by loss of skin elasticity and, of course, the action of the mimetic muscles.

The upper third of the face is constantly subject to dynamic stress caused by the contraction of the frontalis muscle, the corrugator and the procerus. These muscles are continuously activated during facial expressions and can convey scowling, frowning, surprised, quizzical, curious expressions, and many others, depending largely on the position of the head and tail of the eyebrow.

It is easy to observe a diversity of attitudes in the patients who come to our studio, each of whom requires a different therapeutic approach.

There are patients who can be defined as "normokinetic", in whom we find a correspondence between their emotional state and facial expressions. In these subjects there is a perfect synchrony between muscle movement and expression. They usually have almost no expression lines when at rest and treatment with botulinum toxin is long lasting. These patients are the best candidates for treatment with botulinum toxin.

In the hyperkinetic patient, on the other hand, there is no concordance between the emotions they wish to express and the muscular contraction. The mimetic muscles move frequently and apparently inappropriately, even when a certain expression is not required. This often results in the formation of numerous wrinkles, which respond well to treatment with botulinum toxin, although the duration of correction is often shorter than usual. Patients should be made aware of this and are happy to return a little more frequently to maintain a good level of muscle relaxation (fig. 7).

In the hypertonic patient, there is a permanent contraction, especially of the procerus muscle and the corrugator supercilii. Basically, these patients are unable to adopt a relaxed expression and it may look as though they are frowning or aggressive, even in perfectly calm conditions, which can interfere with normal interpersonal relationships. The duration of the effects of botulinum in this group of patients is short, sometimes even less than three months (figs. 8a-8b). Treatment of hypertonic patients often requires combination with fillers, injected about a fortnight after botulinum (fig. 8c). This can result in a better correction of the aesthetic defect. It is important to stress that the filler should only be injected after the botulinum because otherwise it could be displaced by the contraction of these small but powerful muscles and would also be reabsorbed more quickly. Over time, after some treatment with botulinum toxin, the hypertonic patient will be able to switch to the hyperkinetic category (and then to the normokinetic category) and be treated with botulinum toxin alone.

The speed of transition from one category to another is not defined but depends on the depth of the wrinkles and the regularity with which patients return to the doctor for treatment.

CLINICAL CASES

CLINICAL CASE 2

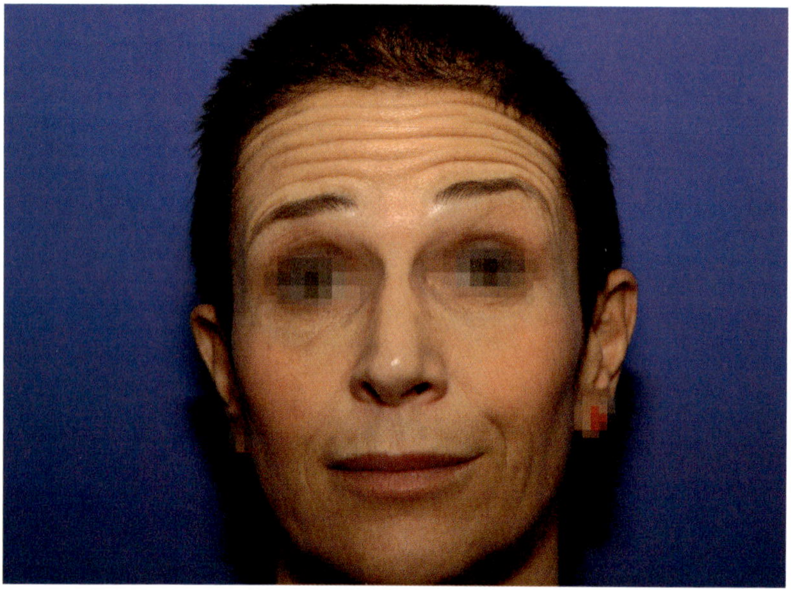

BEFORE

AFTER

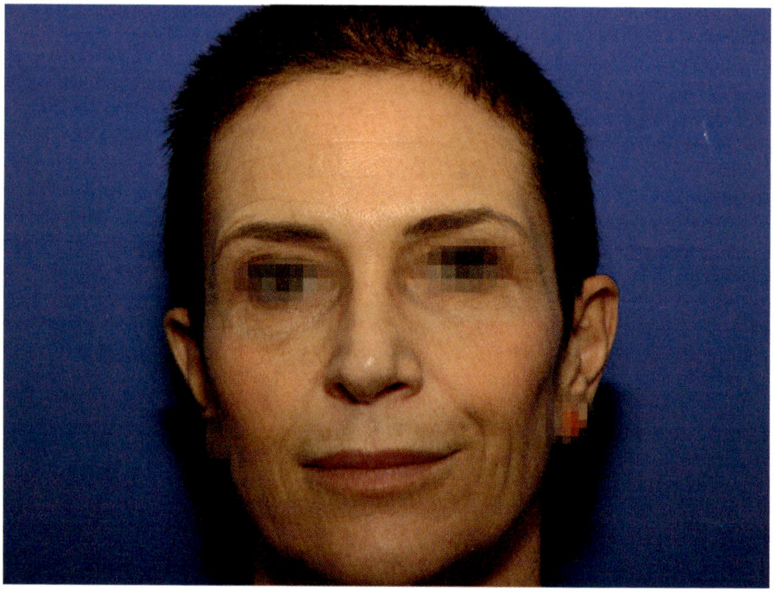

Figure 7 Example of a hyperkinetic patient in contraction. Note the formation of numerous horizontal wrinkles. In the 15-day follow-up note the permanence of a small compensation line positioned slightly cranially to the right eyebrow and the "memory" of a deep horizontal wrinkle

CLINICAL CASES

CLINICAL CASE 3

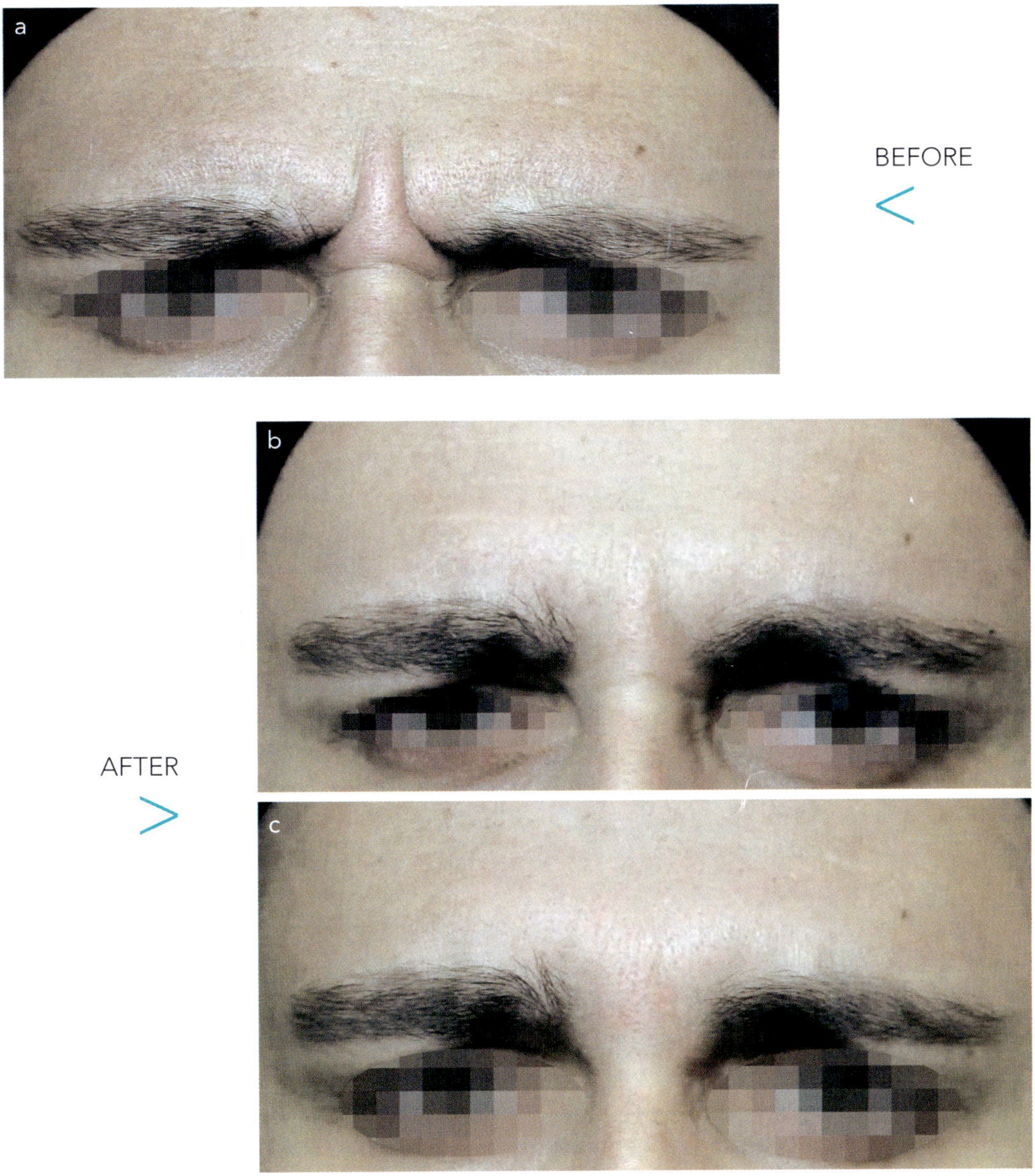

Figure 8 Example of a hypertonic patient. Permanent contraction of the corrugator muscles, conveying a frown or angry expression (a). In the 15-day follow-up (b) note the marked improvement in the glabella lines, however still visible. In (c), the same patient after correction of the glabella lines with filler, with good resolution of the aesthetic flaw

PHOTOGRAPHY

Giovanni Brunelli

As with all aesthetic medical and surgical treatments, patients undergoing treatment with botulinum toxin must be carefully photographed.
The photo is a useful communication tool to show our patients the results achieved by treatment, especially in the rare event that our work is challenged.
Pictures are also used to prepare scientific work or communications for presentation at conferences.
The quality of our shots is crucial. We often see poor photographs during presentations at conferences which prevent us from assessing the quality of the result for various reasons: blurred images, uneven backgrounds, the presence of objects or people in the background which generate confusion and distract our attention, different lighting and undesirable shadows, unsuitable focal length, images which are too light or too dark.
The numerous indications for botulinum toxin require different types of images. The vast majority of our treatments are aimed at reducing wrinkles caused by the mimetic muscles, modulating the strength of contraction of these muscles. In these cases, it is necessary to take photographs of our patients in a static position (which highlights wrinkles that are also present when at rest, those that are usually harder to eliminate) and, immediately afterwards, during maximum contraction of the muscles concerned. The pictures should also feature the drawings on our patients' skin, possibly indicating the number of units used in each injection point; this could be useful for quick reference during subsequent sessions.
The same shots should be repeated a couple of weeks later, when the botulinum has achieved its maximum result, but this is not often easy to do. Patients who have botulinum injections usually return only after four or five months, as the results are almost always highly satisfactory and long-lasting. It is hard to get them to come back to us sooner just to take pictures. Consequently, follow-up pictures are usually taken during appointments made for other types of treatment. A good trick is to offer a check-up 15 days later for a possible "retouch", in which case patients are usually more inclined to return.
Pictures are of little use when treating hyperhidrosis, unless the Minor test, which can prove a reduction in perspiration, is performed. They can be of value when treating scars or dermatological conditions and in all cases where pre- and post-treatment differences are significant.
Here are ten tips for getting the most out of your photos.

PHOTOGRAPHY GUIDELINES

1. Set up a suitable background: the best colours to achieve a good contrast are light grey and light blue.
2. Lighting, of course, is crucial. You need to create white light or natural light (3,300/3,500 degrees Kelvin). You can use spotlights with adequate light output or circular LED lights inside which to place your mobile phone or camera in order to obtain more uniform lighting. These lights are inexpensive and easy to find.
3. Another important element is light diffusion. Direct light must be avoided, it is better to diffuse it by reflecting it on white panels, so that it falls on the subject as softly as possible. This will prevent the formation of annoying shadows or areas that are too bright or even burnt by direct light.
4. There are lots of digital cameras on the market, but to achieve satisfactory results it would be best to take the photos in manual mode (even the latest mobile phones have this facility).
5. If you are using a camera, it is advisable to use a zoom lens, so that you can change the frame as required. The standard zoom lens is usually an 18/55, which is basically a standard lens that can enlarge the frame.
6. Camera settings:
- Exposure time: 1/125 of a second
- f8 aperture (aperture of the lens)

Once these settings have been adjusted, set the sensitivity (ISO) so that the exposure meter is centred (---0--- correct exposure).
7. For maximum image quality, the RAW setting would be ideal, but this takes up a lot of memory space, so if the photos are not going to undergo extreme processing or exaggerated enlargement, shooting in JPEG will suffice.
8. It is advisable to take the photos so that they can be adapted to various needs, such as archiving or publication in magazines, on social media, etc., so bear in mind that the picture may be forced into particular formats, as happens on Instagram and in some professional publications, for example.
9. When taking the picture, you need to hold the camera still. The pressure exerted often makes the picture crooked, but this problem can be overcome by using a tripod or by resting the elbows on a stable surface.
10. The pictures taken should be downloaded as soon as possible and not just kept in the camera. This will prevent the risk of losing them forever; a hard disk, stored in a secure, dry place, can be a good "safe", however it is better to have another hard disk to use as a backup.

PRE-TREATMENT MATERIALS AND PREPARATION OF THE PATIENT

Giovanni Brunelli

No special or hard to find materials are required for treatment with botulinum toxin. It is a good idea to have a sterile cloth on which to place the necessary items, which of course must be changed after every patient.

Once the consent form has been signed and the preliminary interview has been completed, it is time for action.

A series of procedures must be carried out, as follows.

1. Carefully the patient. Patients often arrive covered in layers of cosmetics, which are as useful for covering their imperfections as they are annoying for the doctor to remove. This step is important because, if the patient is not thoroughly cleansed, our needle may transport a series of foreign substances deep into the skin and ultimately cause foreign body tattoos.

2. Disinfect the area to be injected, as usual.

3. Photograph the patient in various positions, both statically and dynamically, also after mapping, to remember where we injected the toxin the previous time.

4. Draw the area to be treated with a dermographic pencil, either in a standing or seated position. Remember that gravity alters the facial features when the patient is lying down, so if we mark the points in this position, they may not be correct.

5. Have the patient relax on the couch; I personally keep the backrest inclined by at least 45° for the comfort of both the patient and the doctor.

6. After putting on gloves, open a vial of sterile saline solution (available in 2 ml vials, which are more than sufficient for standard single-patient use).

7. Draw off the necessary amount of saline solution.

8. Open the packaging of the botulinum, remove the plastic cover, disinfect the rubber stopper and then slowly hydrate the powder with the saline solution, holding the plunger gently and turning the needle towards the wall of the vial, ensuring that the syringe empties itself due to the vacuum inside the vial. If this does not happen, this means that, for some reason, the vacuum has not been maintained, the botulinum has been exposed to oxygen and the vial needs replacing. Remember that *Clostridium botulinum* is an obligate anaerobic bacillus and that it is inactivated by air.

9. After reconstitution, the solution must be checked visually before use: only transparent, colourless, particle-free solutions should be used.

10. Gently rotate the vial to allow optimal hydration of all the powder contained.

11. Draw off the required amount of liquid into an insulin syringe, removing any small air bubbles, and proceed with injection, using a small needle (33G x 4 or 33G x 13). This will make the experience much less painful for the patient and more precise for the doctor, as the liquid will be harder to

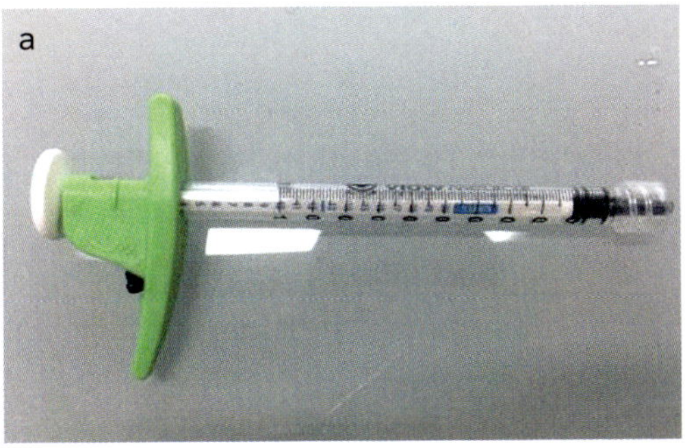

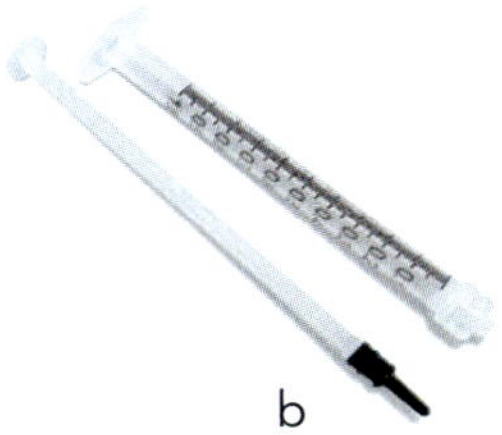

b

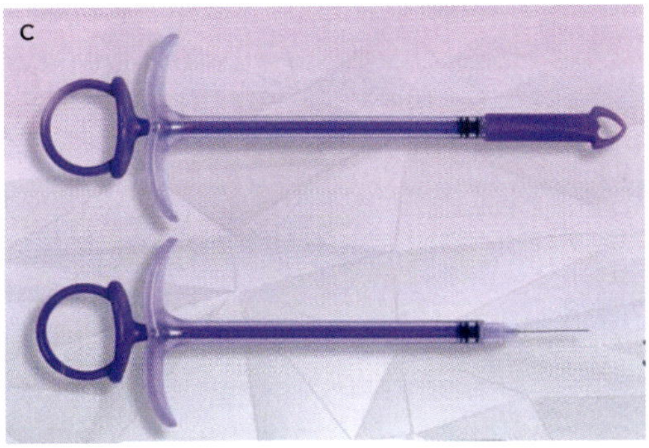

Figure 9 Kits with state-of-the-art adapters and syringes designed specifically for botulinum treatment. Example of Dutch syringes with click by TSK (a), Bont Kit marketed by Seltec (b) and French syringes with Loveliness heart cap by Aesthetic Group with special adapters (c)

dispense and we will have more control over the amount injected. Practical purpose-built kits, adapters and state-of-the-art syringes are also available for botulinum treatment (fig. 9). Some are ergonomic and others come with pre-marked injection lines that can make the doctor's job easier and reduce product waste: they have an automatic locking mechanism so that only the dose selected can be injected (easily audible with a click during injection), increasing the uniformity and naturalness of treatment.

12. Compress each injection site for a few seconds to avoid even the slightest bleeding.

13. After treatment, disinfect the injected area again.

Now all you have to do is check that the patients are well and say goodbye, recommending that they wait at least two weeks before coming back for a possible check-up. Then be prepared to provide a thorough explanation when, two or three days later, the same old question comes up: "Doctor, how come I still can't see anything?".

MAPPING

Maria Vittoria Giatti

In plastic surgery and aesthetic medicine, it is not only useful but always essential to carry out an accurate pre-operative or pre-treatment drawing, which is the basis for the correct planning and implementation of treatment and enables more effective results, as well as the prevention of complications.

This is also the case when performing botulinum toxin treatment, particularly for aesthetic purposes in the treatment of rhytidosis.

We always start by cleansing the skin to remove any make-up, impurities, oiliness and sebum. Preference is given to bio-affine cleansers without surfactants that respect the skin's physiological pH and do not irritate, containing non-aggressive soothing and bacteriostatic agents. You can use cleansing wipes or professional medical make-up removal solutions, which are very practical as they require no rinsing, making them quick and convenient to use in the surgery.

The patient is made to sit with their back straight.

In order to carry out a correct mapping, it is necessary to observe the patient both in static and in dynamic situations, in order to highlight the wrinkles present when resting and those that are accentuated by muscular activity, as well as any asymmetries that may not always be visible in the absence of movement.

We must remember that the expression lines we correct with botulinum tend to develop perpendicular to the vector of tension (contraction) of the muscles and the direction of their fibres (fig. 10).

When mapping the upper third of the face, for example, it is essential to carry out a careful preliminary analysis of the fronto-orbital balance (fig. 11), meaning the functionality of the muscles that raise the eyebrow (mainly the frontalis muscle) and the muscles that lower the eyebrow (procerus, corrugators, orbicularis oculi, depressor superciliis), as well as an assessment of any eyelid ptosis. A simple test to highlight eyelid ptosis is to ask the patient to look straight ahead, placing one hand on the forehead in such a way as to block the frontalis muscle, and then ask them to look up. This eliminates the forehead component and assesses the actual function of the eyelid-elevator muscle (fig. 12). A good method for assessing brow ptosis or asymmetry is to use the Ocular Asymmetry Measuring Device (fig. 13), which particularly highlights unilateral brow ptosis. This instrument can easily be replaced by a T-shaped stick, placed in line with the vertical median axis of the patient's face, thereby assessing the height of the two eyebrows (or any difference in height between the two) (fig. 14).

The patient is then asked to perform certain movements to highlight muscle activity and accentuate the appearance of wrinkles, which are then marked with a light linear drawing. The patient is then asked to perform the same ma-

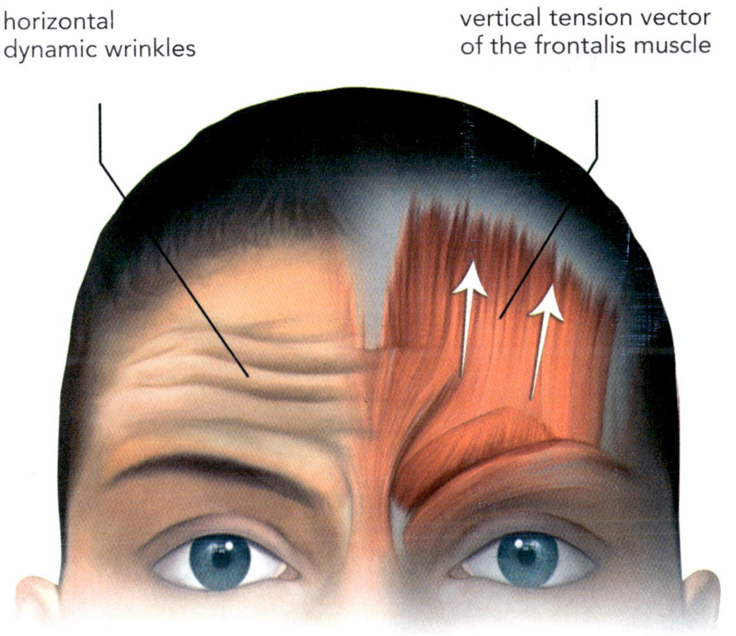

Figure 10 Dynamic wrinkles perpendicular to the tension vector of the frontalis muscle

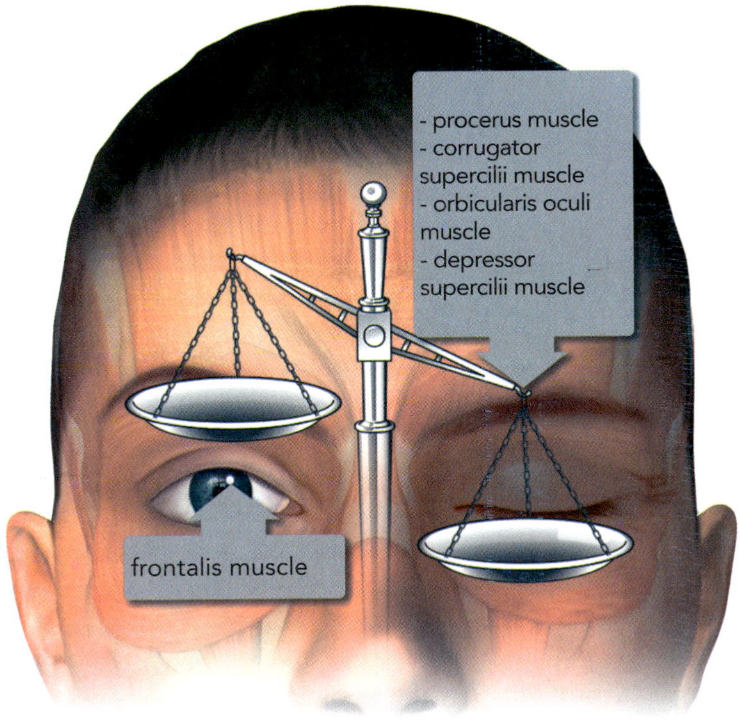

Figure 11 The fronto-orbital balance

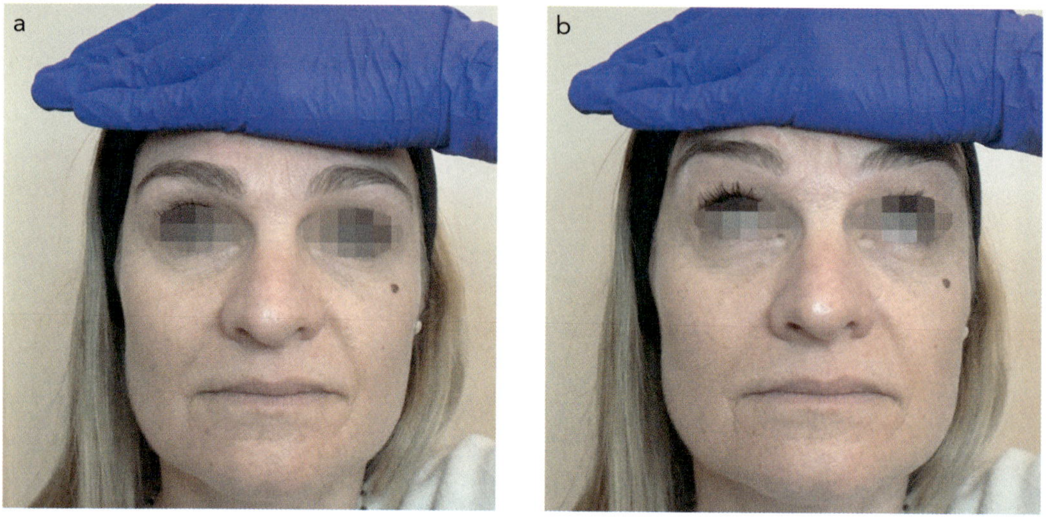

Figure 12 Frontalis muscle blocking manoeuvre: block the frontalis muscle with one hand (a), ask the patient look up (b)

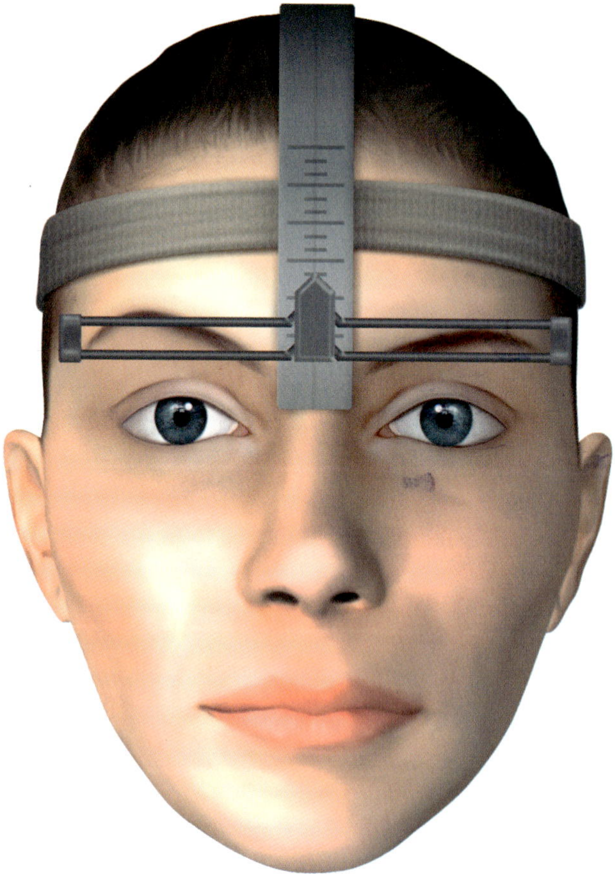

Figure 13 Ocular Asymmetry Measuring Device

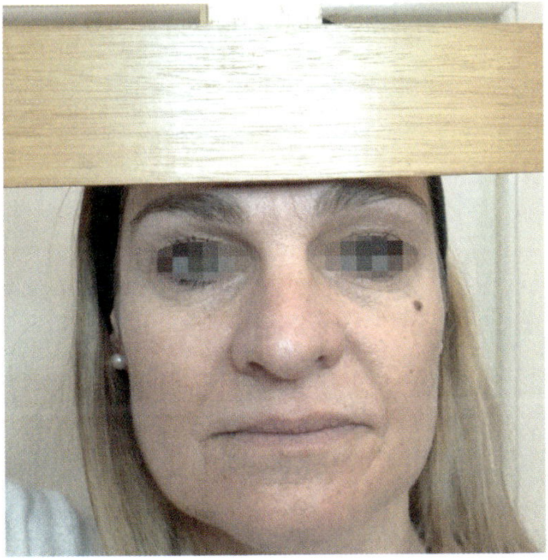

Figure 14 T-stick assessment of eyebrows on a patient's face

noeuvres and the injection points are mapped.
The movements most frequently used during mapping include (fig. 15):
- corrugating the brows;
- raising the brows;
- squinting;
- forcing a smile;
- looking up;
- puckering the lips;
- grinding the teeth;

Figure 15 Facial movements

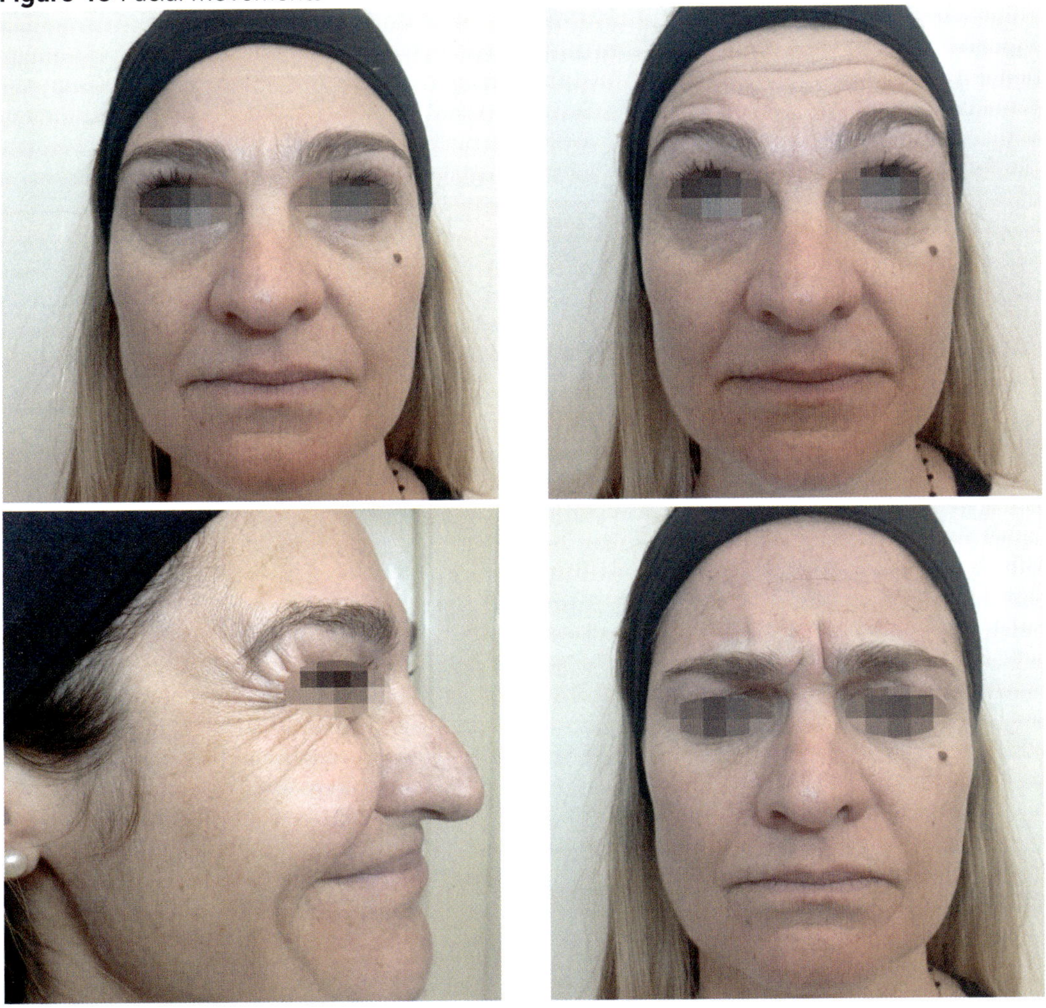

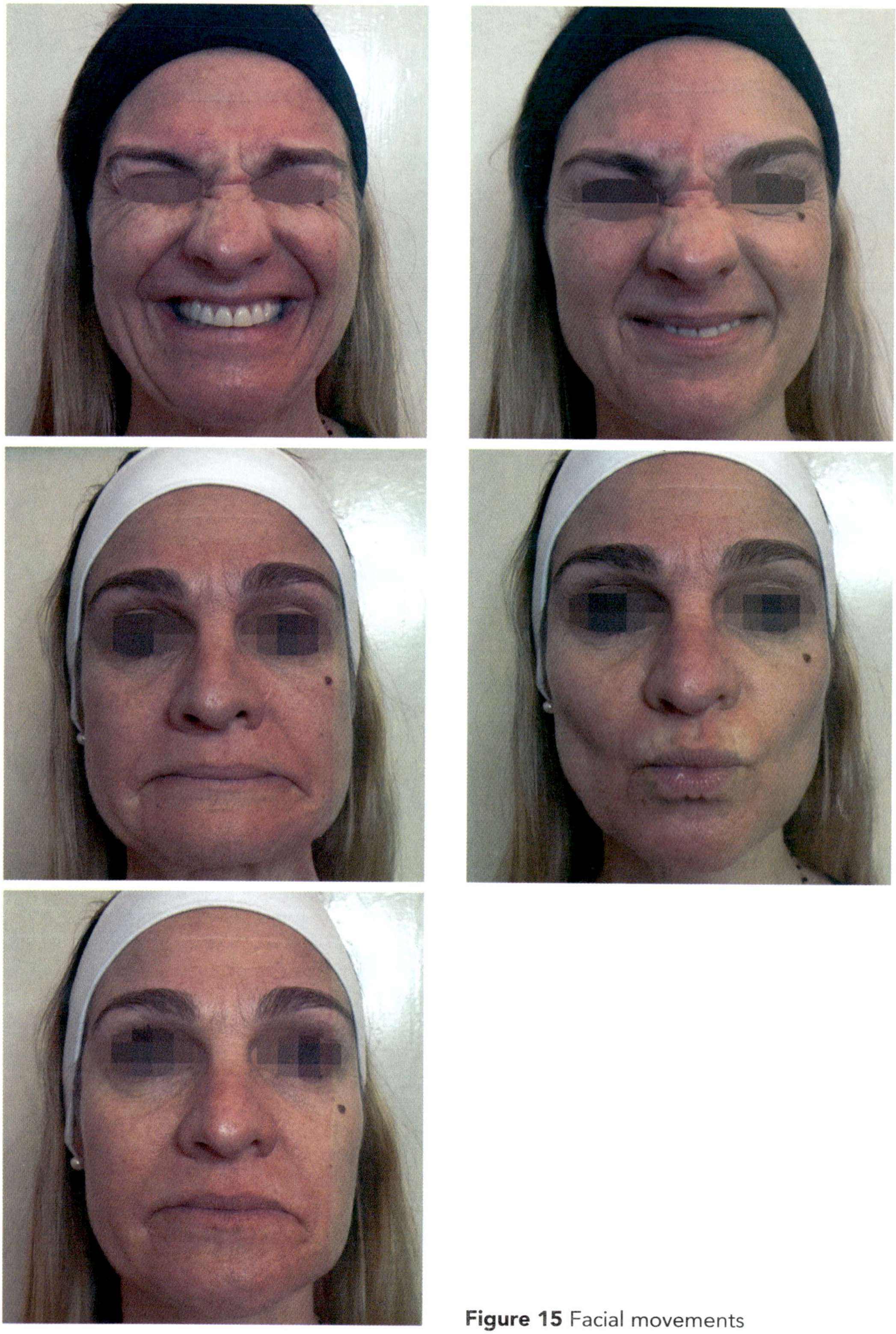

Figure 15 Facial movements

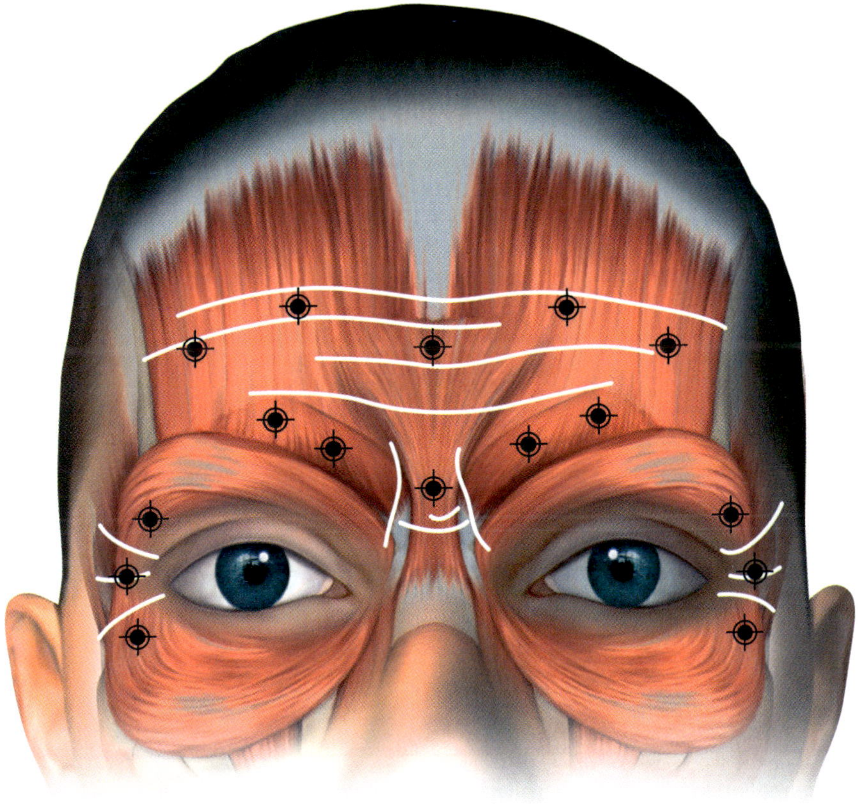

Figure 16 Mapping

- contracting the chin;
- wrinkling the nose.

It is advisable to use a dermographic pencil (possibly in two different colours to highlight wrinkles and injection points); it is best to avoid using a dermographic pen, which would be harder to erase after treatment and would involve rubbing, which is inappropriate immediately after injections (fig. 16).

The amount of botulinum toxin to be injected can also be marked, so that when the patient is photographed, the treatment plan can be quickly viewed in the files and the amount of toxin can be confirmed or varied during checks and subsequent treatments (figs. 17-20). These doses will then be recorded in the patient's medical records, which will be kept at the surgery, and in the medical report/card/booklet given to the patient to bring with them whenever they return to the surgery. Careful personalised mapping must be carried out for each area to be treated, considering any anatomical variability, gender characterisation (man, woman), asymmetries and anatomical structures to be avoided (ar-

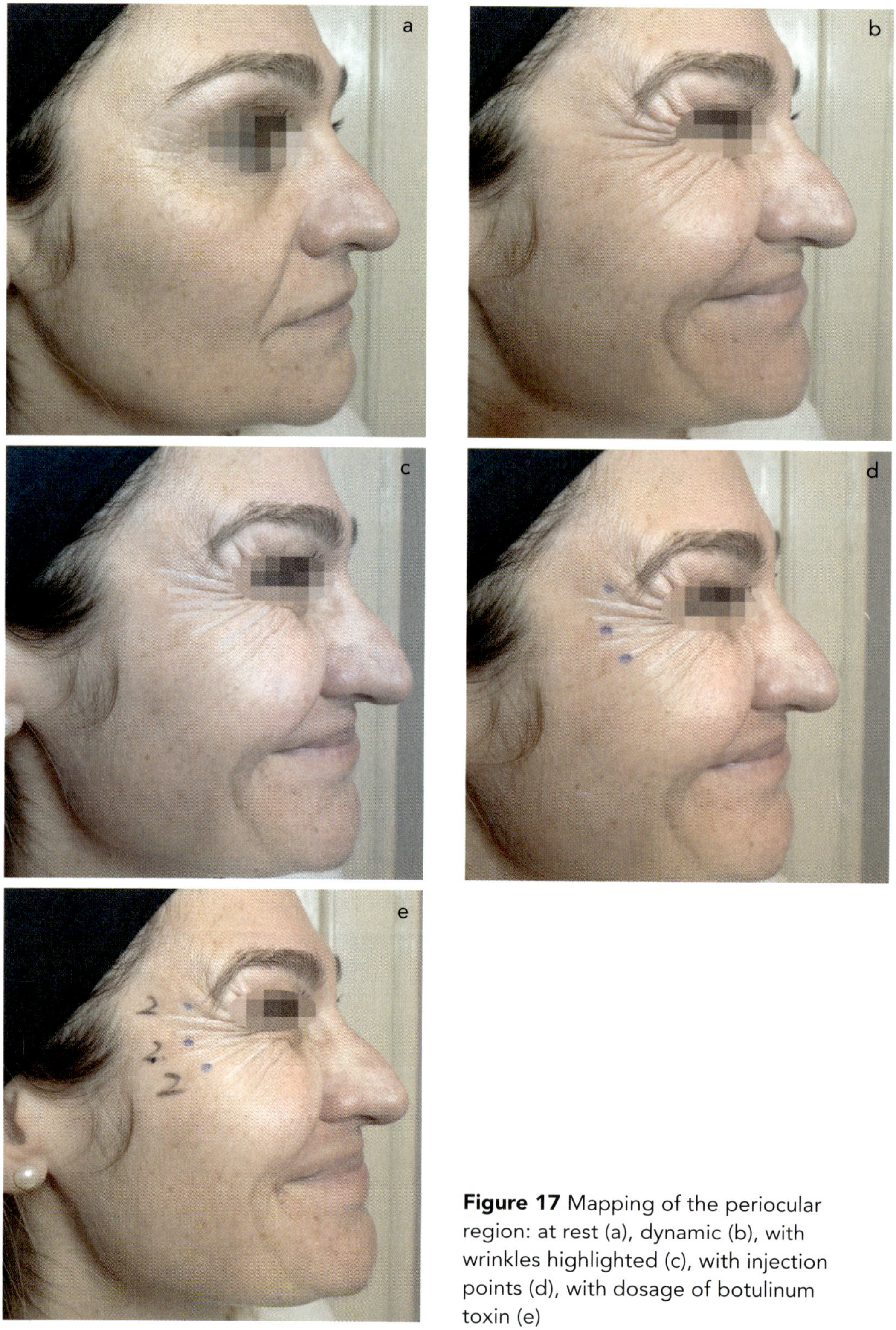

Figure 17 Mapping of the periocular region: at rest (a), dynamic (b), with wrinkles highlighted (c), with injection points (d), with dosage of botulinum toxin (e)

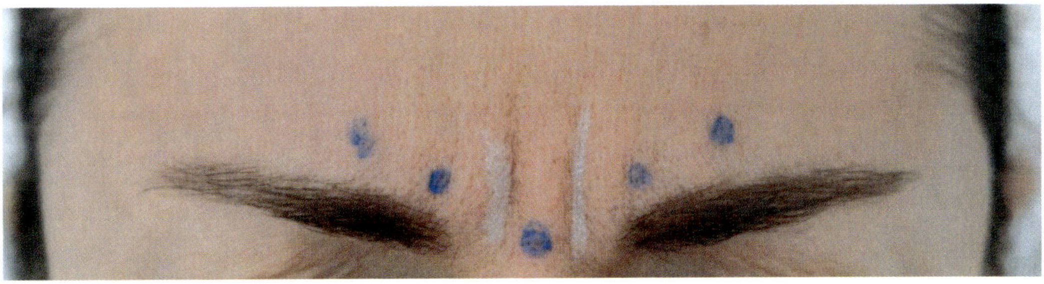

Figure 18 Glabella region mapping

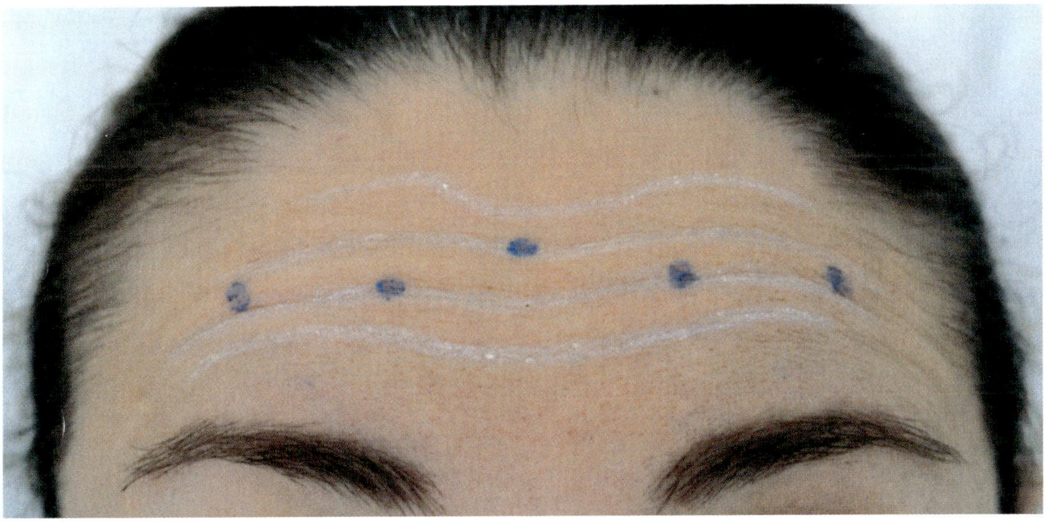

Figure 19 Frontalis region mapping

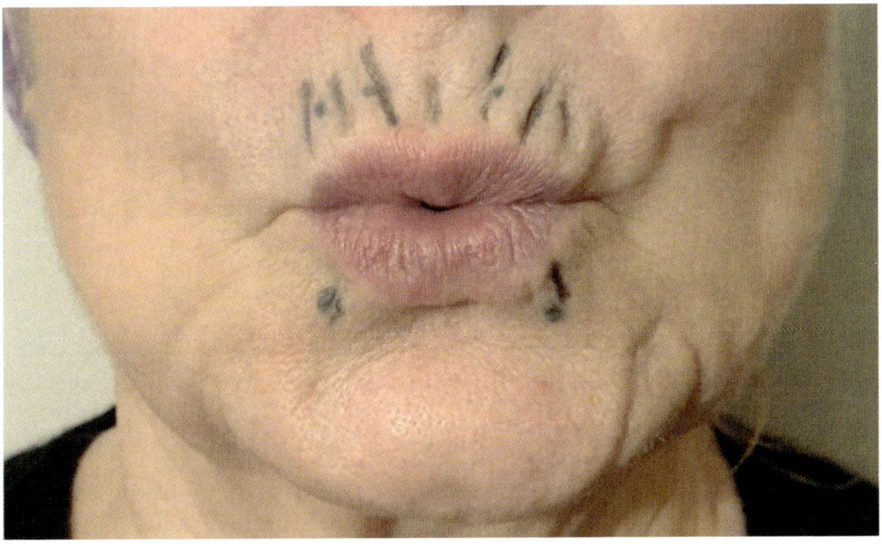

Figure 20 Crow's feet mapping

teries, nerves, veins, etc.). For the specific mapping of each anatomical area, please see the pertinent sections in the chapter on treatment areas.
After correct mapping, the skin can be disinfected (taking care not to erase the drawing) and the treatment can be carried out. Care should be taken to inject close to the point drawn, and not on top of it, to avoid tattooing the pigment of the dermographic pencil with the needle (a rare but possible occurrence).

To recap, correct mapping is accomplished by performing the following steps:
- cleansing the skin;
- observing the patient in static and dynamic situations;
- performing specific manoeuvres to accentuate lines and highlight asymmetries;
- drawing the wrinkles caused by underlying muscle activity;
- mapping the injection points, with possible indication of doses.

INTRAMUSCULAR, SUBCUTANEOUS OR INTRADERMAL INJECTION?

Giovanni Brunelli

As we know, botulinum is a toxin produced by *Clostridium botulinum*, an obligate anaerobic bacterium which causes flaccid paralysis of striated muscles by inhibiting the release of acetylcholine at the neuromuscular junction.
This paralysis is only temporary, because chemotactic recall of the denervated muscle will cause the formation of new axonal buds after a while. These will emerge and form new points of contact with the muscles.
Botulinum toxin is normally used to reduce the strength of contraction of the mimetic muscles and thereby diminish the depth of expression lines, in some cases succeeding in eliminating them; for several years it was used on the upper third of the face only, which is the on-label indication for this drug.
Ongoing research, however, has shown that botulinum can be used in a large number of off-label applications, not officially declared on the product leaflet but still available under the doctor's direct responsibility. In recent years, the number of articles published on the various uses of botulinum has multiplied and includes neurological, ophthalmological and other commonly observed medical indications.
As far as aesthetics is concerned, off-label indications include the correction of various flaws which require classic intramuscular injection. Examples include gummy smile, the weakening of muscles such as the Depressor Anguli Oris (DAO), which causes marionette lines, or the masseter, which is responsible for nocturnal bruxism and which, when hypertrophic, alters the jawline. There are others too, along with certain treatments that require very shallow injection, such as the treatment of hyperseborrhea, hyperhidrosis and facial redness, the improvement of skin texture and small surface wrinkles or the treatment of hypertrophic or keloid scars.
Ideally, the needle should always be positioned in the muscle, as this is always the target of the toxin, but in practice, it is not always possible to understand exactly where the tip of our needle is positioned. It can be particularly difficult to know whether we are in the muscle or in the subcutaneous tissue. The subcutis has practically no nerve endings, so if injection takes place in this area, the doctor may not realise that they are not in the right plane. However, subcutaneous injection seems to be just as effective as intramuscular injection in terms of the quality of the end result, particularly if the injection is followed by the application of pressure, which allows the substance to reach the target muscles through contiguity, given the thinness of the fasciae.
The intramuscular injection technique requires no particular explanation. The needle that comes with the insulin syringe (usually a 25 G) is normally replaced with a finer one, such as a 33 G/13 mm or 33 G/4 mm. This makes the tre-

atment much less uncomfortable for patients, who are more likely to return for repeat applications. Some muscles, such as the corrugators, which have a pseudo-cylindrical shape, can be pinched between the thumb and forefinger of the non-dominant hand before being injected; for others, such as the frontalis, which is a flat muscle, it is sufficient to introduce the needle deeply, almost in contact with the periosteum, and inject the desired amount of drug.
The intradermal technique is also simple, but slightly different.
A scientific paper published in 2015 shows that the average thickness of the dermis on the forehead varies from a maximum of 1252 μm in the upper and lateral regions to a minimum of 1172 μm in the lower and lateral regions. We then have to add the epidermis, which is actually very thin, at a maximum of about 46 μm. Consequently, the total thickness of the epidermis and dermis on the forehead reaches a maximum of 1297 μm and a minimum of 1212 μm. In the anterior region of the neck, the maximum thickness of the epidermis and dermis is almost 1300 μm, while in the lateral region an average thickness of 1473 μm can be reached.
It is therefore possible to carry out intradermal injections, with a few little tweaks. Using a 33 G needle, which has a thickness of 0.24 mm, and inserting only the tip, almost tangentially to the skin, it is possible to create the characteristic bump, which indicates the intradermal position (video 2.3). A certain amount of resistance must be encountered during injection, quite different from that experienced during intramuscular injection. If the injection proceeds without encountering this resistance, it means that we are injecting a little too deeply, at least into the subcutaneous tissue.
The 33 G needle allows the delivery of the botulinum solution, which has the same density as saline solution. It is much better to use insulin syringes with a luer-lock coupling to prevent the syringe from disconnecting when the plunger is pushed, resulting in massive spillage and loss of the precious substance.
As we can see in video 2.3, the part of the forehead between the eyebrows and the two cm safety margin is only injected intradermally. This makes it possible to eliminate the so-called "compensation wrinkles" caused by the contraction of the most distal portion of the frontalis muscle, but without causing the feared lowering of the eyebrow.
Intradermal injection, which is more common in the so-called microbotulinum technique, is more painful than

VIDEO 2.3

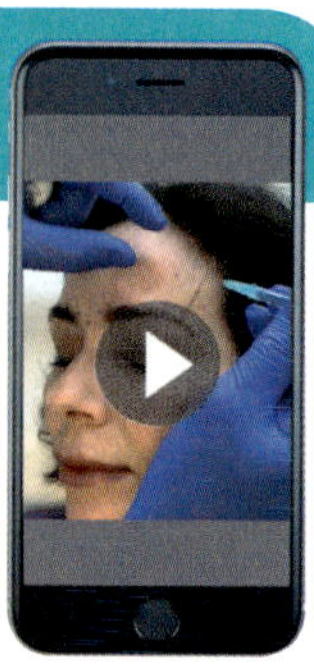

Intramuscular and intradermal injection

VIDEO 2.4

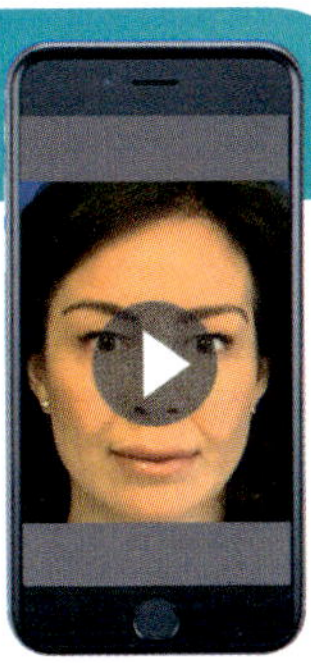

Intramuscular and intradermal result

VIDEO 2.5

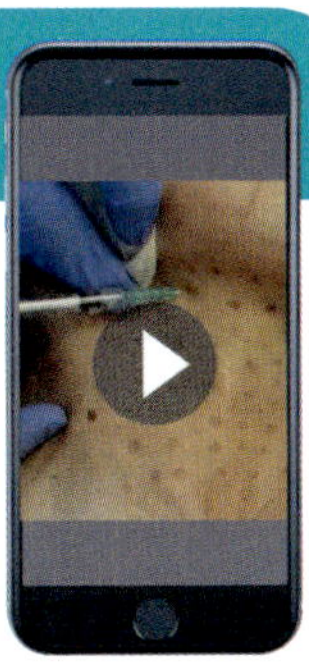

Intradermal microbotulinum in the neck

intramuscular injection, as the dermis is rich in nociceptive nerve endings which are stimulated by dilation. It is best to warn patients that this slight additional pain will be rewarded by a better result, also in terms of skin quality (video 2.4).

The intradermal technique is particularly useful in the lower two-thirds of the face, where it is often desirable to improve the quality of the skin without undesirable effects on the underlying muscles, and in the neck, which is usually treated with the microbotulinum technique (video 2.5).

We can therefore say that the intramuscular and intradermal techniques can be safely combined to give our treatments superior quality and synergistic results.

POST-TREATMENT RECOMMENDATIONS

Maria Vittoria Giatti

After treatment with botulinum toxin, the patient should be given a list of recommendations to follow in order to avoid side effects and to optimise the end result. In addition to explaining everything verbally, of course, in simple and clear words, it is also preferable to issue all the recommendations in written form, so that the patient can read them again at home. This also creates a documented record (useful also for medical and legal reasons) that the correct information has been provided after the performance of the medical procedure. We can include it in our specialist report or create specific protocols for each treatment and annex them to it.

Thorough recommendations post treatment with botulinum (especially after treatment for dynamic facial wrinkles) should include the following:

- avoid touching and rubbing the areas treated for the first 24 hours;
- avoid exposure to sunlight and UV lamps immediately after treatment (if small bruises are present, use a sunscreen with an SPF of 50+ until they disappear completely);
- in the case of bruising, apply specific creams (containing escin, arnica, lactoferrin) to speed up its resolution);
- avoid prolonged exposure to extreme heat (sauna, Turkish bath, steam from cooking or ironing) for 3-7 days;
- avoid make-up for the first few hours after treatment (or use specific soothing and photoprotective medical make-up);
- in the event of a severe headache (which very occasionally occurs after treatment of the upper third of the face), take paracetamol (if there are no anamnestic contraindications);

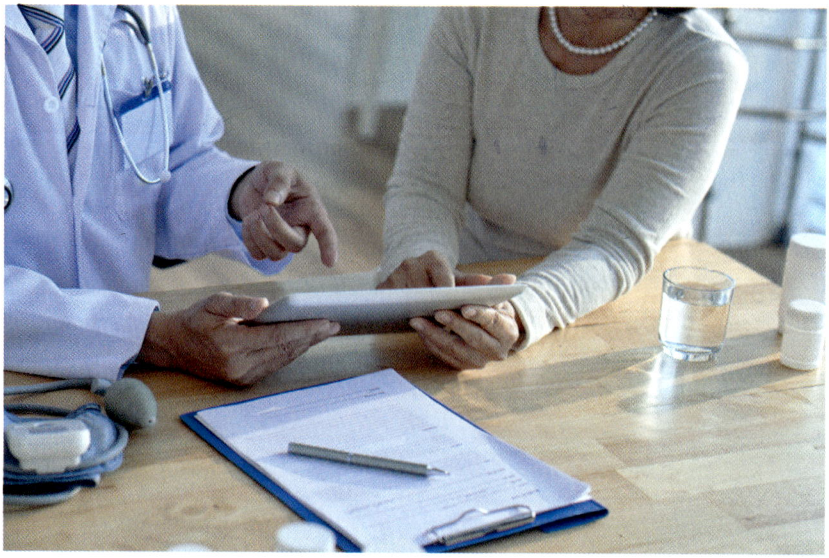

Figure 21 Post-treatment recommendations

- do not take drugs without medical advice (some antibiotics, antidepressants, muscle relaxants, anticonvulsants and anticoagulants may cause problems after treatment);
- if possible, avoid wearing overly compressive motorbike helmets, tennis-style headbands or tight headgear for 24 hours;
- reassure the patient that the effect may not be visible until 3 to 7 days after treatment and in some rare cases it may take up to 14 days for it to become fully effective;
- invite the patient to correct expressive attitudes and flaws that lead to repeated activity of the muscles being treated (e.g.: squinting if suitable lenses are not used to correct sight impairment, frowning and screwing up the face, failure to wear protective sunglasses in bright sunlight, etc.);
- report any adverse event or problem promptly to the doctor who performed the treatment;
- schedule a check-up after two to three weeks (for possible touch-ups or symmetries) and/or a new botulinum toxin treatment after four to six months;

It is also advisable to issue an appropriate dermocosmetic and nutraceutical prescription, to synchronise with the medical treatment carried out and accompany our patients with specific skin care until the next treatment, for a global and complete anti-ageing approach.

The choice of dermo-cosmetic should be tailored to the area being treated (e.g.: an eye serum if the eye area has been corrected, or an anti-ageing lip cream if the lip area has been treated), but also to the specific requirements of the individual patient's skin (photo-ageing, chrono-ageing, etc.). Preference should be given to dermocosmetics containing redensifying, firming, anti-ageing, anti-oxidant formulations, skin-restructuring complexes (e.g.: hyaluronic acid, coenzyme Q10, glutathione, N-acetylglucosamine, alphalipoic acid, vitamin C, vitamin E, etc.), micro-contracting botulinum-like substances (e.g.: gamma-aminobutyric acid) or biomimetic peptides with a myorelaxant effect (acetyl hexapeptide-8, acetyl hexapeptide-3, palmitoyl hexapeptide-19, etc.), or biomimetic peptides that stimulate the production of hyaluronic acid and collagen (palmitoyl pentapeptide-3, palmitoyl pentapeptide-4, palmitoyl tripeptide-28, methylglucoside-6-phosphate, etc.). Biomimetic peptides, synthetic substances made up of amino acid sequences, "mimic" the action of the natural protein they resemble by binding in a highly specific way to receptors in cells that regulate particular biological processes. There are also specific mask formulations, to be used a couple of times a week to complement the botulinum toxin treatment. These are very practical and popular with patients.

A combined nutraceutical consisting of substances that contribute to normal skin function from within can also be recommended. These can have a regenerating, restructuring and anti-ageing action (resveratrol, coenzyme Q10, N-acetyl cysteine, N-acetyl glucosamine, folic acid, vitamin C, vitamin E, vitamin A, collagen, vitamin B1-B2-B12, etc.).

Patient Name *Mario Rossi*

Treatment date *10/05/2021*

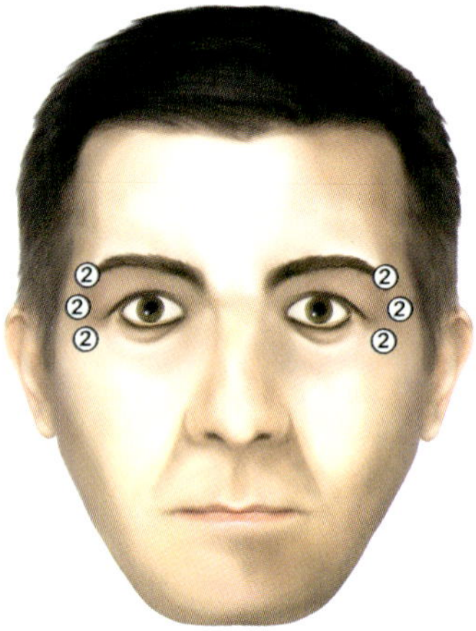

Area treated	Product	Quantity
Eye area	*X X X*	*2+2+2 per side*

Figure 22 Patient records

Together with the post-treatment report and recommendations, the patient should be given a card indicating the type of botulinum toxin used (accompanied by the product label and the batch number on the packaging, if possible), the injection sites and dosages. This card should be brought to future appointments. This information should also be filed in the patient's medical records kept at the surgery (fig. 22).

Bibliography

Patient selection

1. Baker TJ. Patient selection and psychological evaluation. Clin Plast Surg. 1978;5(1):3-14.
2. Crerand CE, Menard W, Phillips KA. Surgical and minimally invasive cosmetic procedures among persons with body dysmorphic disorder. Ann Plast Surg. 2010;65(1):11-16.
3. Sundaram H, Signorini M, Liew S, et al. Global Aesthetics Consensus: Botulinum Toxin Type A--Evidence-Based Review, Emerging Concepts, and Consensus Recommendations

for Aesthetic Use, Including Updates on Complications. Plast Reconstr Surg. 2016;137(3):518e-529e.

Contraindications

4. Klein AW. Contraindications and complications with the use of botulinum toxin. Clin Dermatol. 2004;22(1):66-75.
5. Wollina U, Konrad H. Managing adverse events associated with botulinum toxin type A: a focus on cosmetic procedures. Am J Clin Dermatol. 2005;6(3):141-150.
6. Guassi Mannina C, Levy Nunes E. Drug Interaction with Botulinum toxin. Journal of Oral Care and Dentistry. Volume 2 Issue 1 – Jul 2020.
7. Huang W, Foster JA, Rogachefsky AS. Pharmacology of botulinum toxin. J Am Acad Dermatol. 2000;43(2 Pt 1):249-259.
8. Azulay MM, Cavalcante R, Cirino P. (2016). Toxina Botulínica na Dermatolgia. 1ED: 136-141.
9. Fiacchino F, Grandi L, Soliveri P, Carella F, Bricchi M. Sensitivity to vecuronium after botulinum toxin administration. J Neurosurg Anesthesiol. 1997;9(2):149-153.
10. Ascher B, Talarico S, Cassuto D, et al. International consensus recommendations on the aesthetic usage of botulinum toxin type A (Speywood Unit)--Part I: Upper facial wrinkles. J Eur Acad Dermatol Venereol. 2010;24(11):1278-1284.

Mapping

11. Faigin G. The Artist's Complete Guide to Facial Expression.Watson-Guptill Publications, New York 1990.

Intramuscular, subcutaneous or intradermal injection?

12. Chopra K, Calva D, Sosin M, et al. A comprehensive examination of topographic thickness of skin in the human face. Aesthet Surg J. 2015;35(8):1007-1013.
13. Ha RY, Nojima K, Adams WP Jr, Brown SA. Analysis of facial skin thickness: defining the relative thickness index. Plast Reconstr Surg. 2005;115(6):1769-1773.
14. Wu WTL. Microbotox of the Lower Face and Neck: Evolution of a Personal Technique and Its Clinical Effects. Plast Reconstr Surg. 2015;136(5 Suppl):92S-100S.
15. Kim YJ, Lim OK, Choi WJ. Are There Differences Between Intradermal and Intramuscular Injections of Botulinum Toxin on the Forehead? Dermatol Surg. 2020;46(12):e126-e131.
16. Gordin EA, Luginbuhl AL, Ortlip T, Heffelfinger RN, Krein H. Subcutaneous vs intramuscular botulinum toxin: split-face randomized study. JAMA Facial Plast Surg. 2014;16(3):193-198.
17. Zhu J, Ji X, Xu Y, et al. The efficacy of intradermal injection of type A botulinum toxin for facial rejuvenation. Dermatol Ther. 2017; Jan;30(1) 1-4.

Post-treatment recommendations

18. Schuh FD. Patient care after Botox injections. Plast Surg Nurs. 1999;19(4):218.
19. Blanes-Mira C, Clemente J, Jodas G, et al. A synthetic hexapeptide (Argireline) with antiwrinkle activity. Int J Cosmet Sci. 2002;24(5):303-310.

3

TREATMENT AREAS

Patrizia Piersini, Alberto Diaspro, Gabriele Muti, Giovanni Brunelli

UPPER THIRD

FOREHEAD

Patrizia Piersini

As the face ages, the upper third develops linear wrinkles on the forehead, due both to the contraction of the anterior portion of the occipitofrontalis muscle (which we will call the frontalis muscle), and to the reduction in the thickness of the dermis and of the subcutaneous fatty tissue, which is already scarce and therefore lacks the necessary support for the skin. While a smooth forehead is undoubtedly a sign of youth, pronounced horizontal forehead wrinkles make the face look tired and sad.

Treatment of the forehead with botulinum can make horizontal wrinkles less noticeable and lengthen the forehead due to relaxation of the muscle. This is recommended when the height of the forehead, from the hairline to the pupil, is less than 6 cm in men and 5.5 cm in women. Raising the forehead, making it higher, can improve the proportion of the three thirds of the face [1].

Anatomy

The occipitofrontalis muscle is a mimetic muscle, consisting of a sheet of fibrous muscle extending from the nape of the neck to the eyebrows. It is made up of two occipital and two frontal parts. The two frontal parts, which are wider, adhere to the overlying subcutaneous tissue, particularly at the eyebrows, and are not connected to any bones. They are connected to the aponeurotic galea above, under the coronal suture, while, below, the medial muscle bundles continue with those of the procerus muscle, the intermediate bundles continue with the corrugator supercilia muscle, and both the intermediate and lateral bundles continue with the orbicularis oculi muscle. The medial muscle bundles diverge at the aponeurotic galea (although not in all patients, figs. 1-2) while they converge at the level of the bridge of the nose. Laterally, the margins of the muscle generally end or taper at the temporal line, but in some patients they extend beyond it (fig. 3) [2].

Being a vertically oriented muscle, its contraction has an "accordion" effect which, by shortening the muscle fibres, raises the eyebrows and brings the scalp forward [3]. The occipital parts, on the other hand, move the scalp backwards, acting as antagonists to the frontalis muscle fibres.

If the frontalis muscle is between the two temporal lines, the wrinkles formed during its contraction are horizontal and parallel to the eyebrows, whereas if it extends laterally to the temporal line, the wrinkles tend to be wavy [4].

Injection technique

When treating the frontalis muscle to reduce horizontal forehead wrinkles,

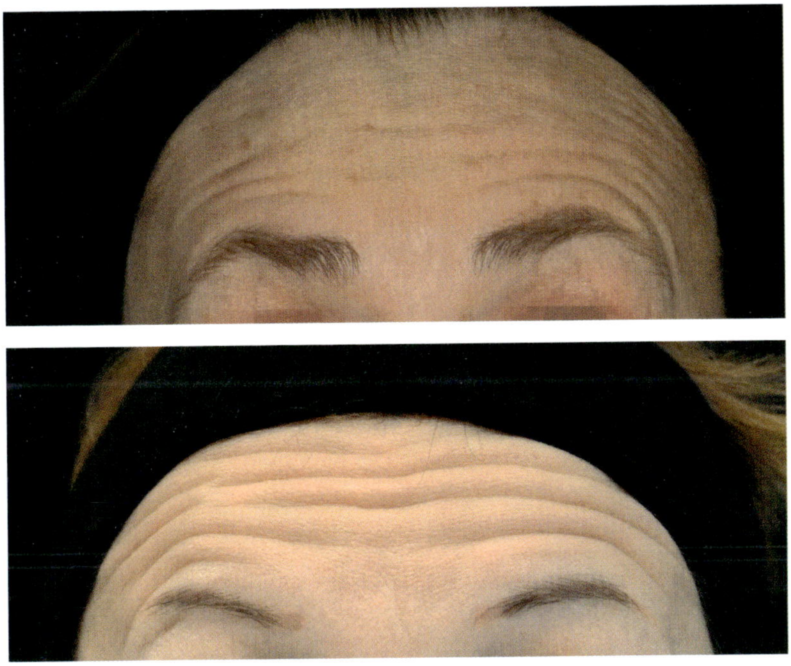

Figure 1 Forehead wrinkles in a patient with frontal parts diverging at the aponeurotic galea (above) and in a patient with non-diverging frontal parts (below)

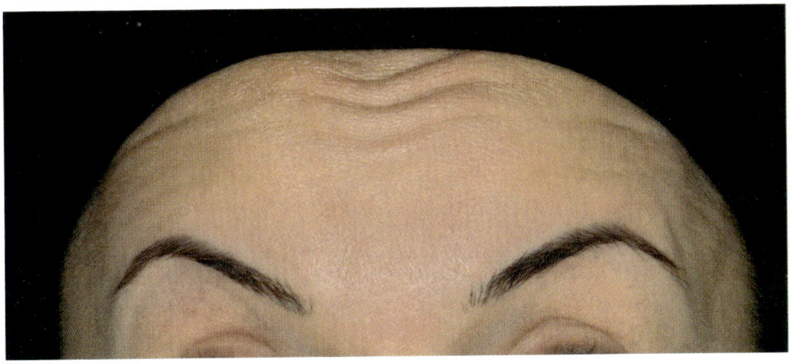

Figure 2 Forehead wrinkles in a patient with frontal parts that corrugate mainly at the galea aponeurotica

it is important to consider that this muscle is the only one that raises the eyebrows. Consequently, it is advisable to treat the muscles of the glabella complex and the superior and canthal points of the eye muscles, which, with their medial approach and brow depressor action, act as antagonists of the frontalis muscle, at the same time as the forehead. Failure to consider this factor can result in an eyebrow ptosis effect, due to the action of the botulinum, giving the patient a sad frown. Despite this consideration, excessive

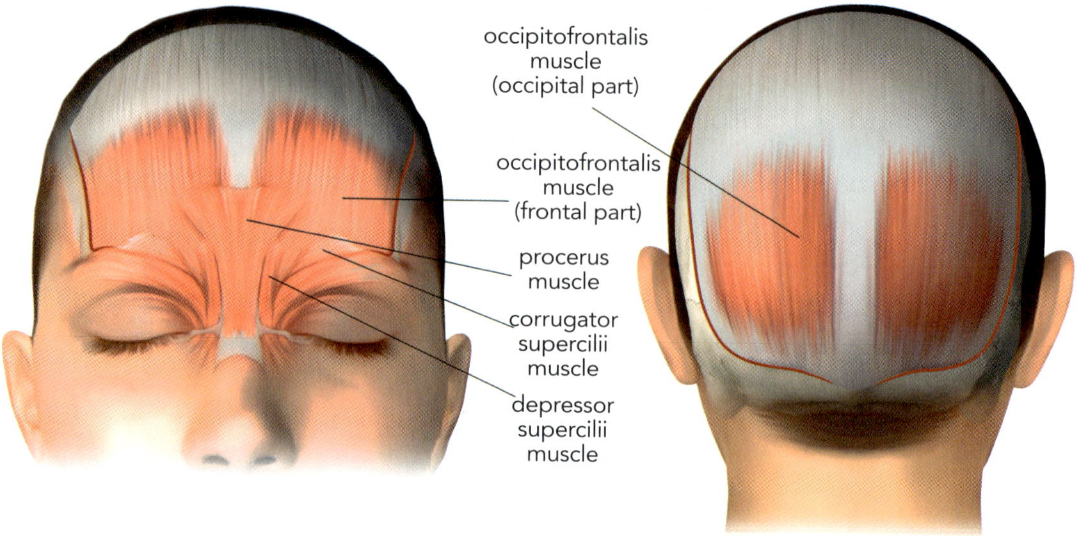

Figure 3 Anatomy of the occipitofrontalis muscle consisting of two occipital and two frontal parts

injection of the forehead can lead to this complication, so it is important to assess the patient before injection.

A very simple test to assess the function of the frontalis muscle before botulinum treatment, involves asking the seated patient to close their eyes and relax their forehead. Massage the patient's forehead to relax the skin and ask them to open their eyes. Immediate contraction of the frontalis muscle means that they use this muscle a lot to raise the eyebrows and adjust their vision, so treatment with botulinum could cause eyebrow ptosis.

The aim of the treatment is never to completely block the frontalis but to make its contraction less effective, leaving a residual movement in the portion immediately above the eyebrows (figs. 5-7) also to preserve the movement of the eyebrow and allow the patient to retain a satisfactory level of facial expression [5].

When injecting botulinum into the forehead, it is important to inject into the upper part of the frontalis muscle. A horizontal line is drawn two cm above the upper orbital rim and injection below this line should be avoided [3]. The remaining part is divided in two halves and the injections should be made only into the cranial portion of the muscle (video 3.1), while it is advisable for experienced injectors to perform more superficial injections with a higher dilution in the more caudal portion (see chapter on microbotulinum) (figs. 3-8).

Video 3.1 shows standard injection technique for the treatment of forehead wrinkles using a 33 G/9 mm needle and botulinum diluted to 1.2 ml, with intramuscular injection.

Video 3.2 shows drawing and injection technique for the treatment of forehead wrinkles using a 33 G/9 mm needle. Intramuscular injection of botulinum at a dilution of 1.2 ml into the cranial por-

VIDEO 3.1

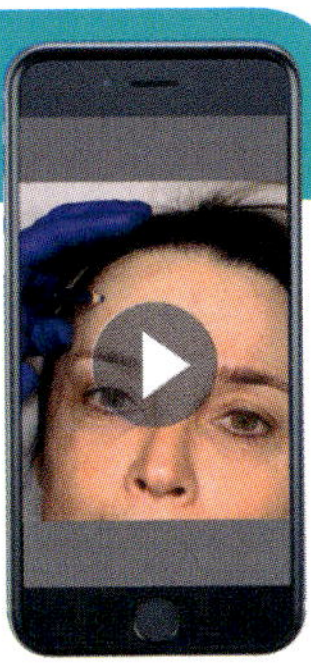

Treatment of forehead wrinkles: drawing and standard injection technique

VIDEO 3.2

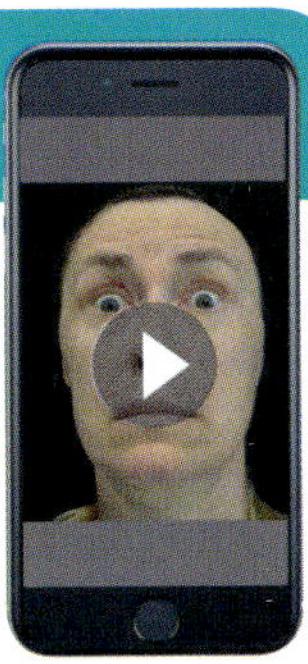

Treatment of forehead wrinkles: drawing and injection technique using a 33 G/9 mm needle

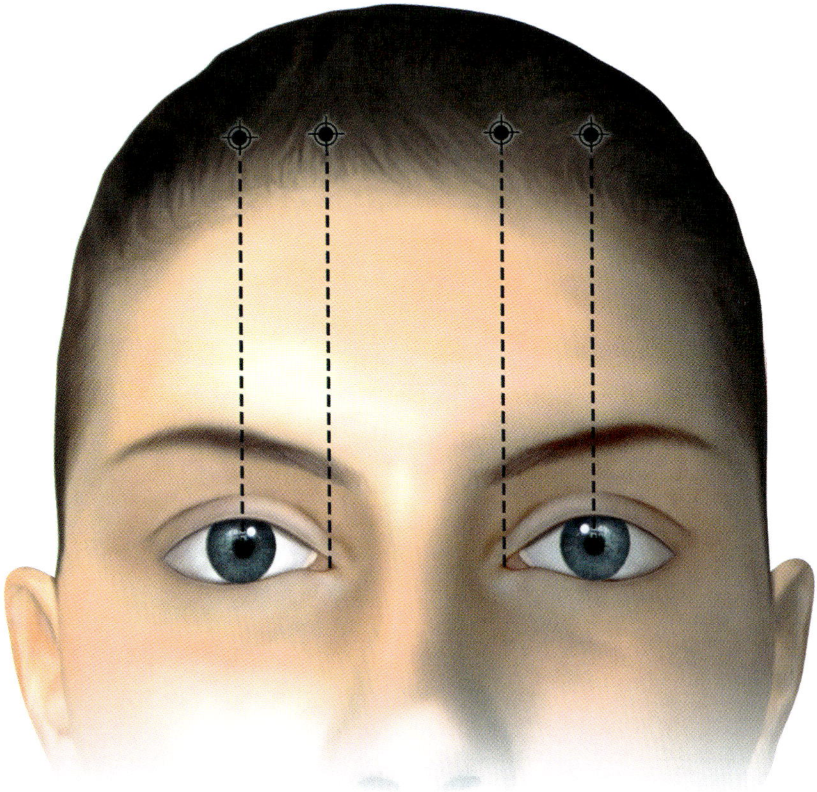

Figure 4 Injection points to obtain a forehead lift

tion (blue dots in the drawing), intradermal injection of microbotulinum into the caudal portion (red dots in the drawing). If the wrinkles are between the two temporal lines, 4-5 points are injected in a zigzag pattern, using 10-15 U Botox or 20-30 U Speywood (video 3.1).
If the wrinkles also extend laterally to the temporal lines, in order to avoid "Mephistophelian eyebrow" (also known as "Spock's eyebrow", after the Vulcan character in Star Trek, with a laterally overexaggerated eyebrow shape, or "Quizzical look") it is necessary to inject another 2-4 U Botox (or 4-8 U Speywood) laterally to the temporal lines. A good way to prevent Mephistophelian eyebrows is to firmly press the glabella at rest with two fingers, simulating the action of the toxin, and then ask the patient to raise their forehead exaggeratedly. If the Mephistophelian effect occurs when the forehead is raised, this must be taken into account when injecting the points of highest elevation. Otherwise, it is possible to proceed as described.
To obtain a forehead lift [1], before performing the treatment, we ask the patient to bring the scalp forward as much as possible, as if the hairline were touching the eyebrows: if the forehead shortens, this is an indication for treatment. After treating the glabella muscles and the frontal portion of the occipitofrontalis muscle, four more points are injected, two for each half of the forehead, 1-1.5 cm inside the hairline, with about 4-5 U Botox each (or 8-10 U Speywood). The first point corresponds to the mid-pupil line, while the second corresponds to the vertical line that touches the inner canthus of the eye (fig. 4) [1].

CLINICAL CASES

CLINICAL CASE 1

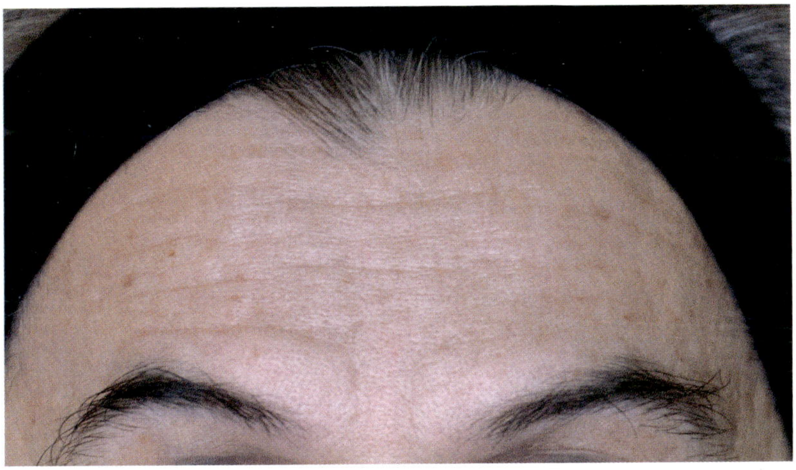

BEFORE

AFTER

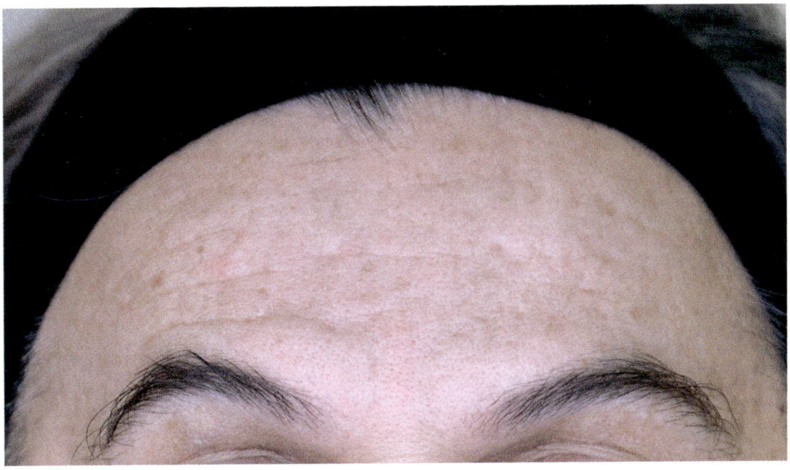

Figure 5 49 year-old patient before and thirty days after treatment with botulinum for forehead wrinkles and glabella lines, with residual movement in the portion immediately above the eyebrows

CLINICAL CASES

CLINICAL CASE 2

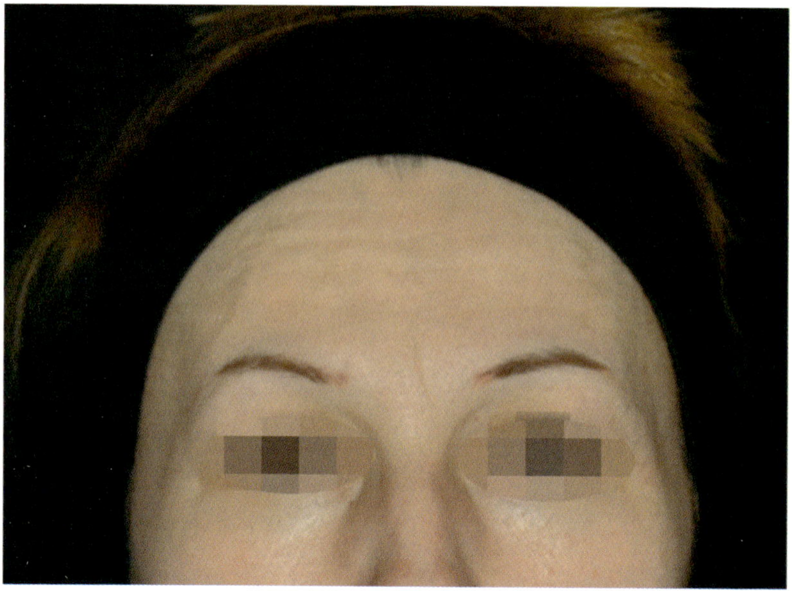

BEFORE

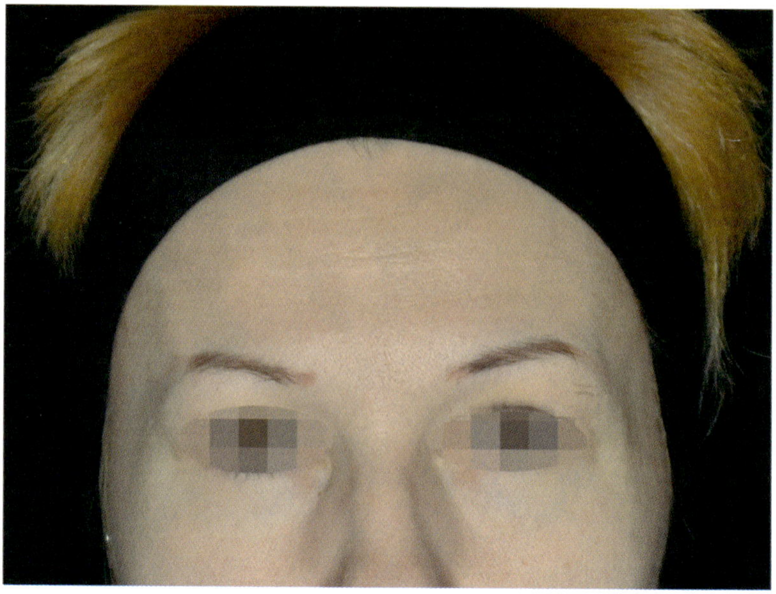

AFTER

Figure 6 48 year-old patient before and thirty days after treatment with botulinum for forehead wrinkles and glabella lines (static)

CLINICAL CASES

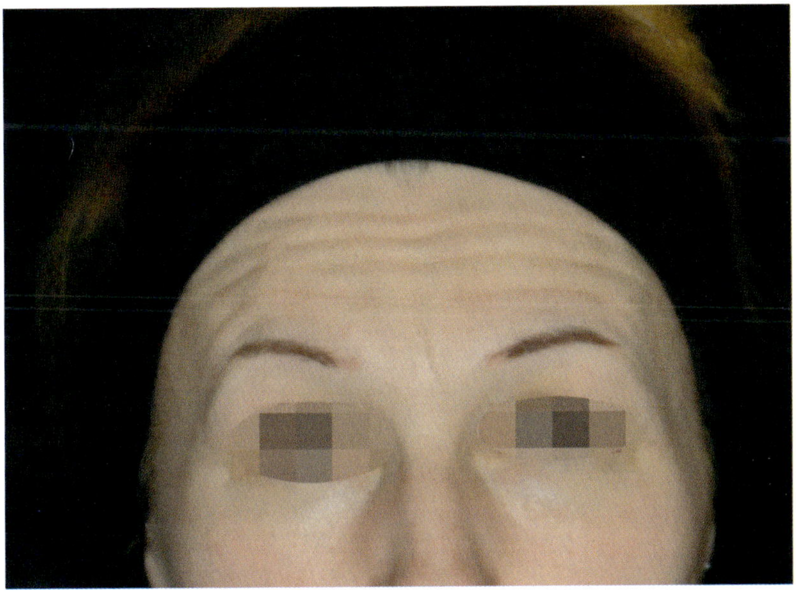

BEFORE

AFTER

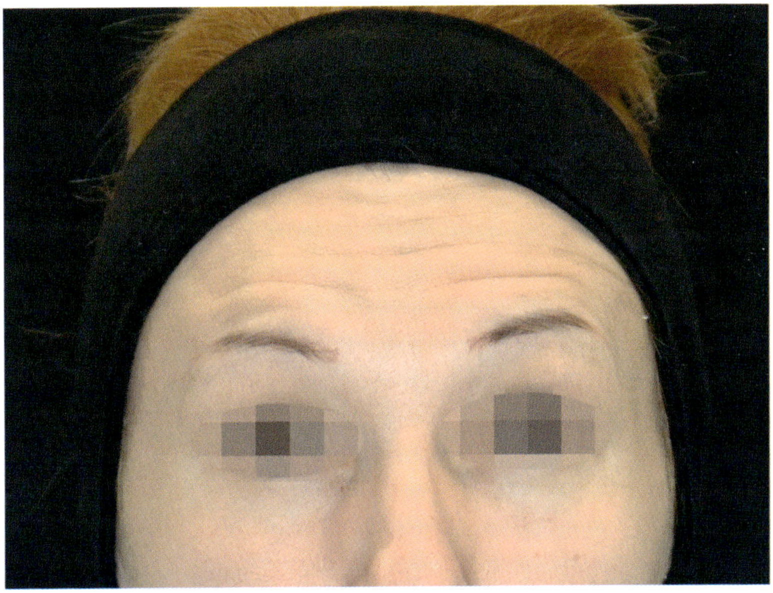

Figure 7 Same patient before and thirty days after treatment with botulinum for forehead wrinkles and glabella lines (dynamic), with residual movement in the portion immediately above the eyebrows

CLINICAL CASES

CLINICAL CASE 3

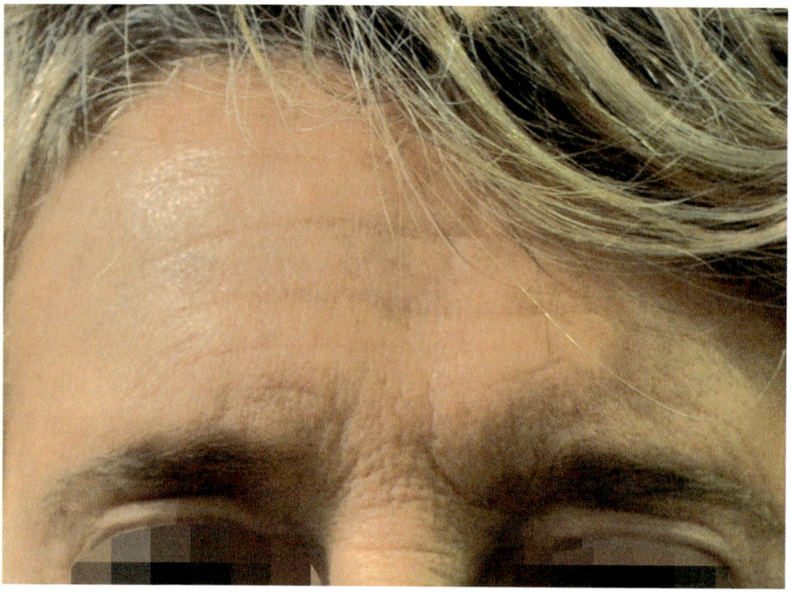

BEFORE

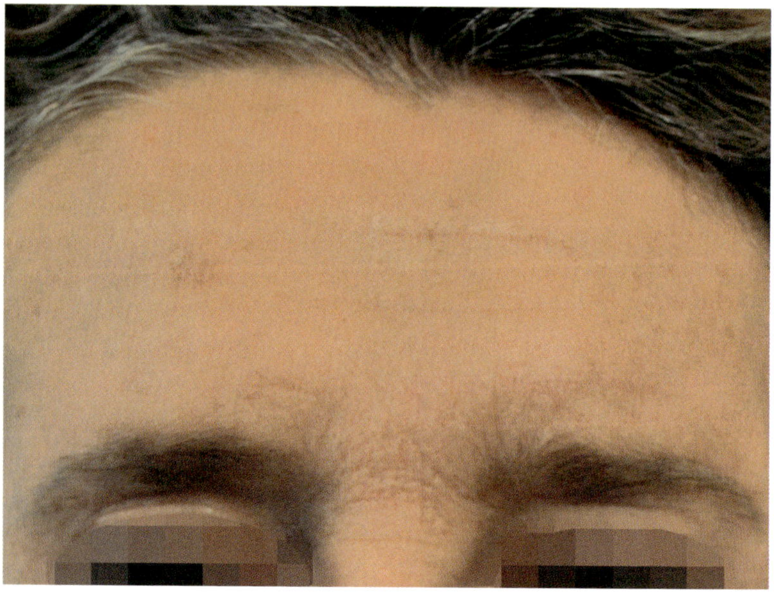

AFTER

Figure 8 59 year-old patient before and thirty days after treatment with botulinum for forehead wrinkles and glabella lines and with microbotulinum in the caudal portion of the frontalis muscle

GLABELLA

Patrizia Piersini

More and more patients are asking for ways to look less tired in a natural way. The most important elements that accentuate facial fatigue are undoubtedly vertical lines, such as nasolabial lines and glabella lines. Glabella lines, also known as "frown lines" or "11 lines", are mimetic lines caused by the contraction of muscles (corrugator supercilii, procerus, depressor supercilii) that bring the eyebrows down and inwards. These lines are associated with facial expressions that have a negative impact on the observer, giving the impression of agitation, sadness, fatigue and anxiety, which is why they should definitely be considered in aesthetic medical treatments for facial rejuvenation [6]. It would also appear that the smoothing or disappearance of these lines has a real influence on mood, providing not only an improvement in self-perception but also really helping to fight depression (see chapter on depression).

Although widely used, fillers are definitely not the treatment of choice for correcting glabella wrinkles because of the risk involved in injecting gels into this area, which is full of blood vessels and anastomoses with the ophthalmic artery. The most feared complication is clearly embolia cutis medicamentosa, due to injection of filler into the infraorbital artery which connects with the retinal artery. Consequently, treatment with botulinum toxin becomes of particular significance and is the first choice in the various treatment options.

The use of botulinum toxin for the treatment of glabella wrinkles dates back to 1987, when it was first proposed by Jean and Alastair Carruthers.

Anatomy

Three main muscles can be identified in the anatomical analysis of the glabella: the corrugator supercilii, the depressor supercilii and the procerus. When analysing the dynamics of this area, the intersection of these muscles with the frontalis muscle and the orbicularis oculi is also important (fig. 9) [7].

The corrugator supercilii muscle, also known as the "frown muscle", is a pyramid shaped muscle positioned at the medial end of the eyebrow. It is located under the frontalis muscle and under the orbicularis oculi at a depth of approximately 4-6 mm [8]. It originates at the medial end of the eyebrow arch and extends laterally for about 25-30 mm to the central part of the supraorbital margin, penetrating the skin. The thickest point, with a thickness of 2-3 mm, is usually between the intersection of two vertical lines, the inner canthus of the eye and the mid-pupillary line, and a horizontal line passing through the centre of the eyebrow (fig. 10).

This muscle draws the eyebrow down and medially and is used to frown and squint.

The depressor supercilii muscle is considered by some anatomists to

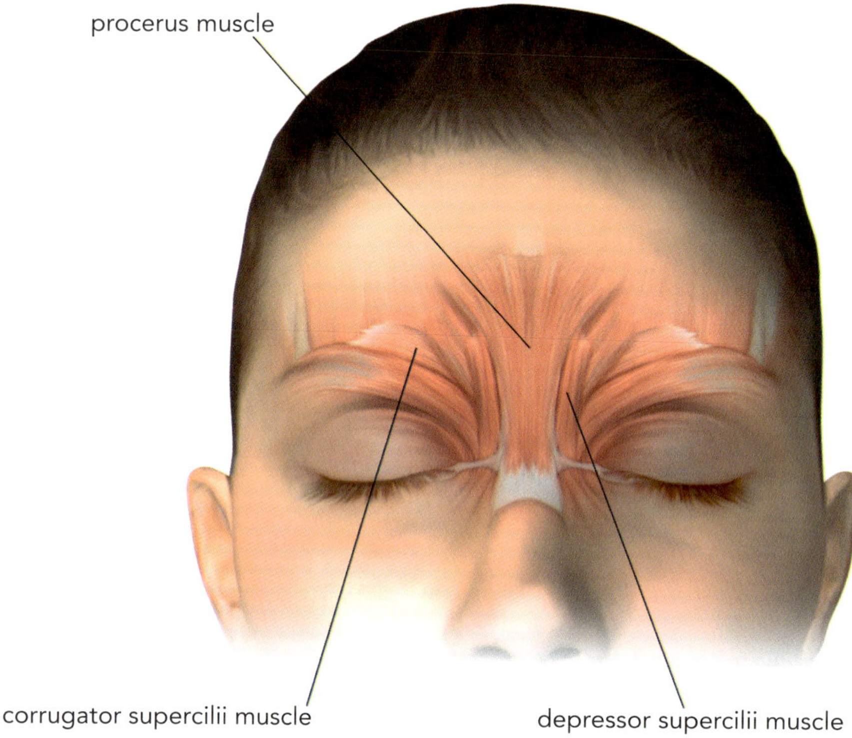

Figure 9 Anatomy of the glabella region

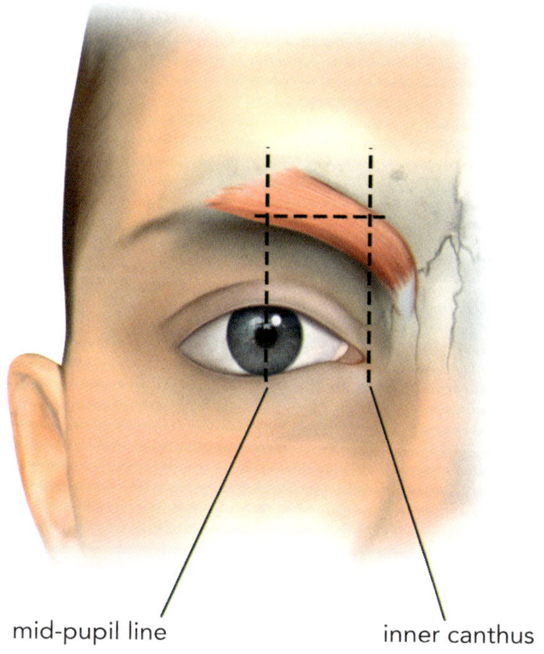

Figure 10 Corrugator supercilii muscle: the part in which the muscle is thicker is between the line of the inner canthus of the eye and the mid-pupil line

be part of the orbicularis oculi, while others see it as a separate muscle with a well-defined effect on the eyebrow [9]. It runs parallel to the fibres of the procerus muscle and originates from the frontal process of the jaw, travelling upwards to about 15 mm from the skin of the eyebrow. It lowers the medial part of the eyebrow, contributing to the action of frowning [7].

The procerus muscle is a thin, pyramid-shaped muscle that originates from the aponeurosis of the fascia that covers the lower part of the nasal bone and the upper part of the lateral nasal cartilage, penetrating the skin of the glabella. Its action is to lower the medial part of the eyebrow and its contraction forms the transverse wrinkles present at the bridge of the nose. These three muscles interact with the orbicularis oculi, which helps lower the eyebrow and also contributes, with its orbital portion, to the formation of the horizontal wrinkles on the bridge of the nose.

Injection technique

In order to achieve the most natural and satisfactory result possible, this area must be assessed individually, carefully considering the patient's contraction pattern, and not using standardised techniques.

According to the study by De Almeida et al. [10] five different types of contraction have been identified and these generally include the most frequent anatomical-functional conditions to be treated, used as the basis for a personalised treatment.

"U" contraction

This mainly involves the procerus muscle and the corrugators. The eyebrows are drawn closer together and lowered, and the movement creates the shape of the letter U. This is the most frequent type of contraction in women (around 32%), while it is only the third pattern in men. There are five injection points to be identified (figs. 11, 16 and 17, video 3.3):

- the first in the procerus at the intersection of two lines which unite the most medial part of the eyebrow to the inner canthus of the contralateral eye, injecting superficially (at a depth of no more than 4 mm) from 5 to 10 U Botox (10-20 U Speywood);
- the second and third points are injected into the thickest part of the corrugator supercilii muscle, injecting 3 U Botox (7 U Speywood) deeply;
- the fourth and fifth points are always injected into the corrugator supercilii muscle, but further to the side, with a

VIDEO 3.3

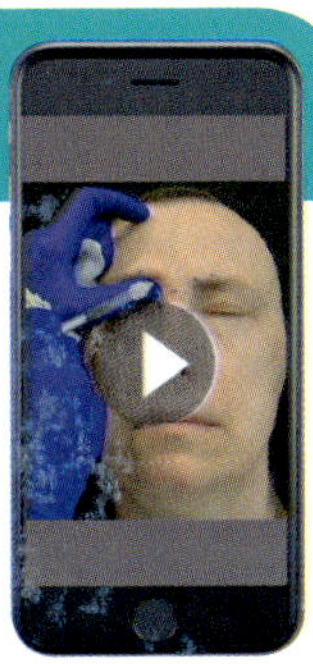

Standard injection technique for the treatment of glabella lines (U contraction)

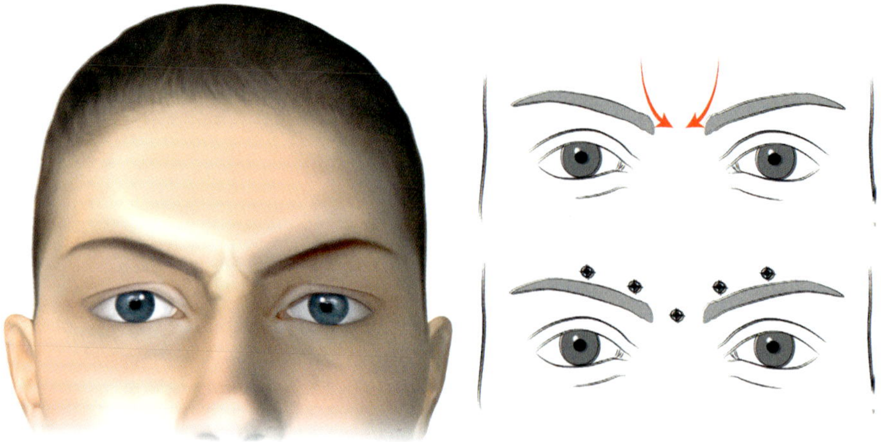

Figure 11 The U contraction mainly involves the procerus and corrugators (Source: based on Almeida et al.)

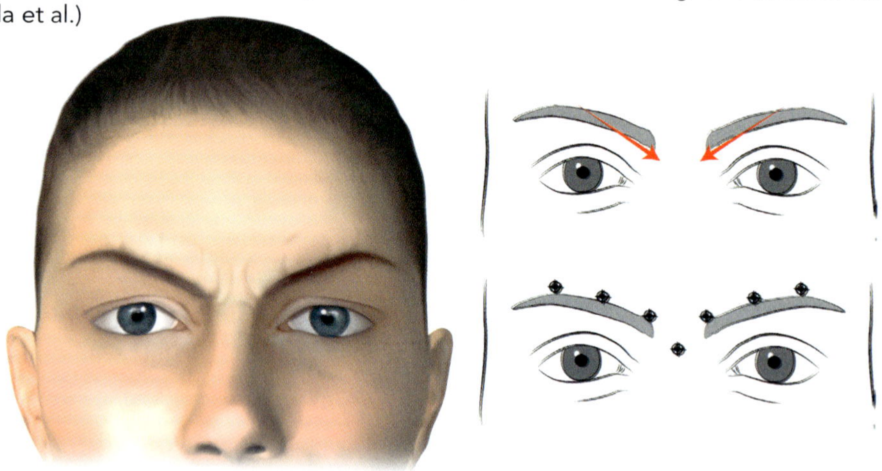

Figure 12 The V contraction involves the procerus, corrugators and medial portion of the orbicularis oculi

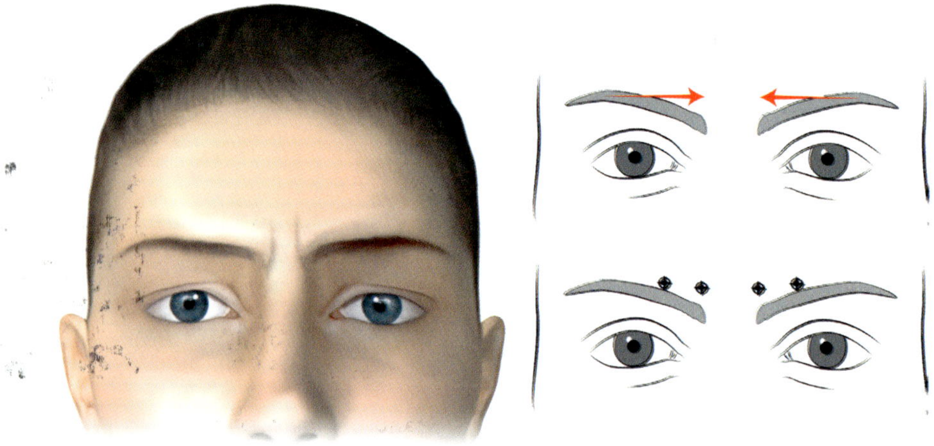

Figure 13 The converging arrow contraction involves the corrugators and the medial portion of the orbicularis oculi

VIDEO 3.4

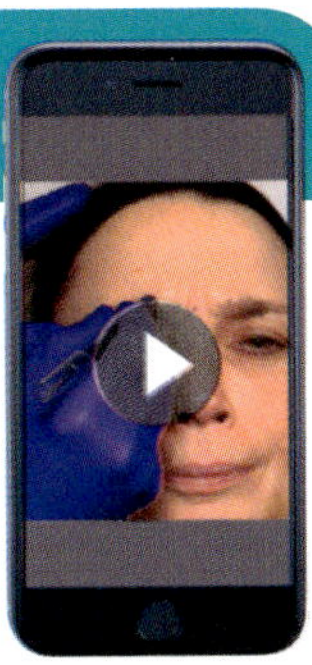

Drawing for the treatment of glabella lines (V contraction)

VIDEO 3.5

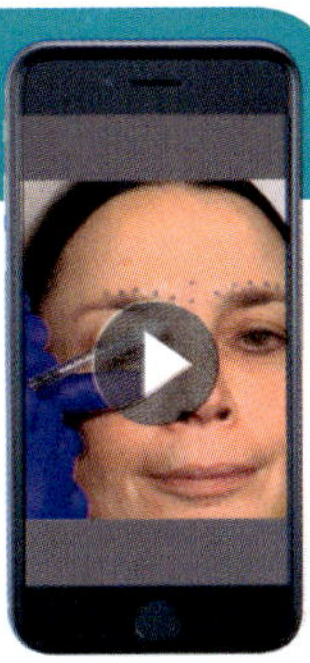

Injection technique for the treatment of glabella lines (V contraction)

shallower injection and a lower dosage (1-3 U Botox or 3-7 U Speywood).

"V" contraction

In this type of contraction, the eyebrows are drawn closer together and even lower than in the previous group and, while at rest, the eyebrows are lower and more horizontal. It involves not only the procerus and corrugator muscles, but also the medial portion of the orbicularis oculi muscle. The "V" contraction is the second most common type of contraction in women and the most frequent in men. These patients require a higher dose of botulinum into the procerus and corrugator supercilii and have seven injection points (figs. 12, 18 and 19, videos 3.4 and 3.5):

- the first in the procerus at the intersection of two lines that unite the most medial part of the eyebrow to the inner canthus of the contralateral eye by superficially injecting, at a depth of no more than 4 mm, 10 U Botox (20 U Speywood);
- the second and third points are identified by pinching the thickest point of the corrugator supercilii muscle between the index finger and thumb of the non-dominant hand and injecting 2-3 U Botox (or 5-7 U Speywood);
- the other four points follow the course of the corrugator supercilii more laterally and superiorly, always remembering to inject superficially.

"Converging arrow" contraction

This consists of drawing the medial part of the eyebrows closer together without or with only slight lowering. The corrugators and the medial portion of the orbicularis muscle are involved. This type of contraction is the third most frequent in women and the second most frequent in men. In the treatment, injections are made horizontally, with little or no treatment of the procerus muscle (1-2 U Botox or 2-4 U Speywood) while treating the corrugators with 1 U Botox (2-3

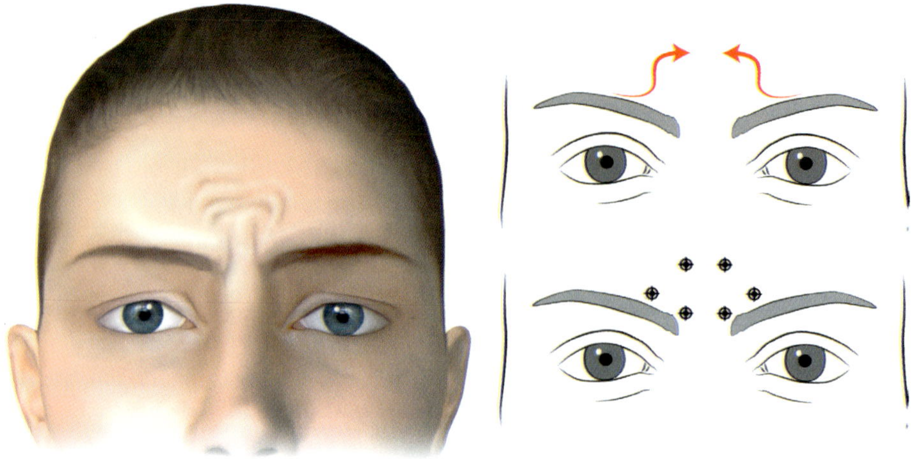

Figure 14 The muscles involved in the Omega contraction are the corrugators, the medial portion of the orbicularis oculi and the frontalis

U Speywood) and the medial portion of the orbicularis with 1 U Botox (2 U Speywood) (fig. 13).

"Omega" contraction

This contraction is due to the drawing together and raising of the glabella region. The procerus muscle is not involved in this case, but the corrugator muscles, the medial portion of the orbicularis and the frontalis muscle are. This is the fourth type of contraction in both men and women. In this case, six points are injected (fig. 14):

- two points, using the index finger and thumb of the non-dominant hand to pinch the thickest point of the corrugator supercilii muscle and injecting 2-4 U Botox (or 5-7 U Speywood);
- two points slightly higher and laterally on the more medial portion of the corrugators (1 U Botox or 2-3 U Speywood);
- two points on the frontalis muscle in the highest part of the contraction of the frontalis.

"Inverted Omega" contraction

In this case, the contraction occurs more downwards than medially. The muscles involved are the procerus, the depressor supercilii, the medial part of the orbicularis muscle and probably also the transverse portion of the nasal muscle. This type of contraction is the least common in both women and men. In this case injections should be made (fig. 15):

- into the procerus at the intersection of two lines that unite the most medial part of the eyebrow to the inner canthus of the contralateral eye by superficially injecting, at a depth of no more than 4 mm, 5-10 U Botox (10-20 U Speywood);
- into the depressor supercilli, 1 U Botox or 2-3 U Speywood;
- a further two points in the transverse part of the nasal muscle and in the

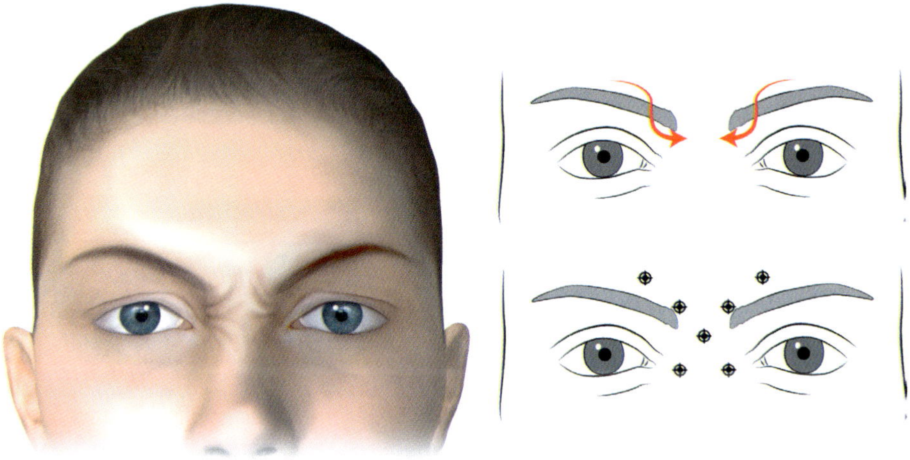

Figure 15 The muscles involved in the inverted Omega contraction are the procerus, the depressor supercilii, the medial portion of the orbiculus oculi and the nasal transverse

medial part of the orbicularis oculi, even though it is not part of the glabella muscle complex.

There are two negative aesthetic effects to be avoided when treating the glabella: a Mephistophelian eyebrow, with depression of the central part of the eyebrow and elevation of the lateral part, or excessive elevation of the medial portion of the eyebrow.

CLINICAL CASES

CLINICAL CASE 4

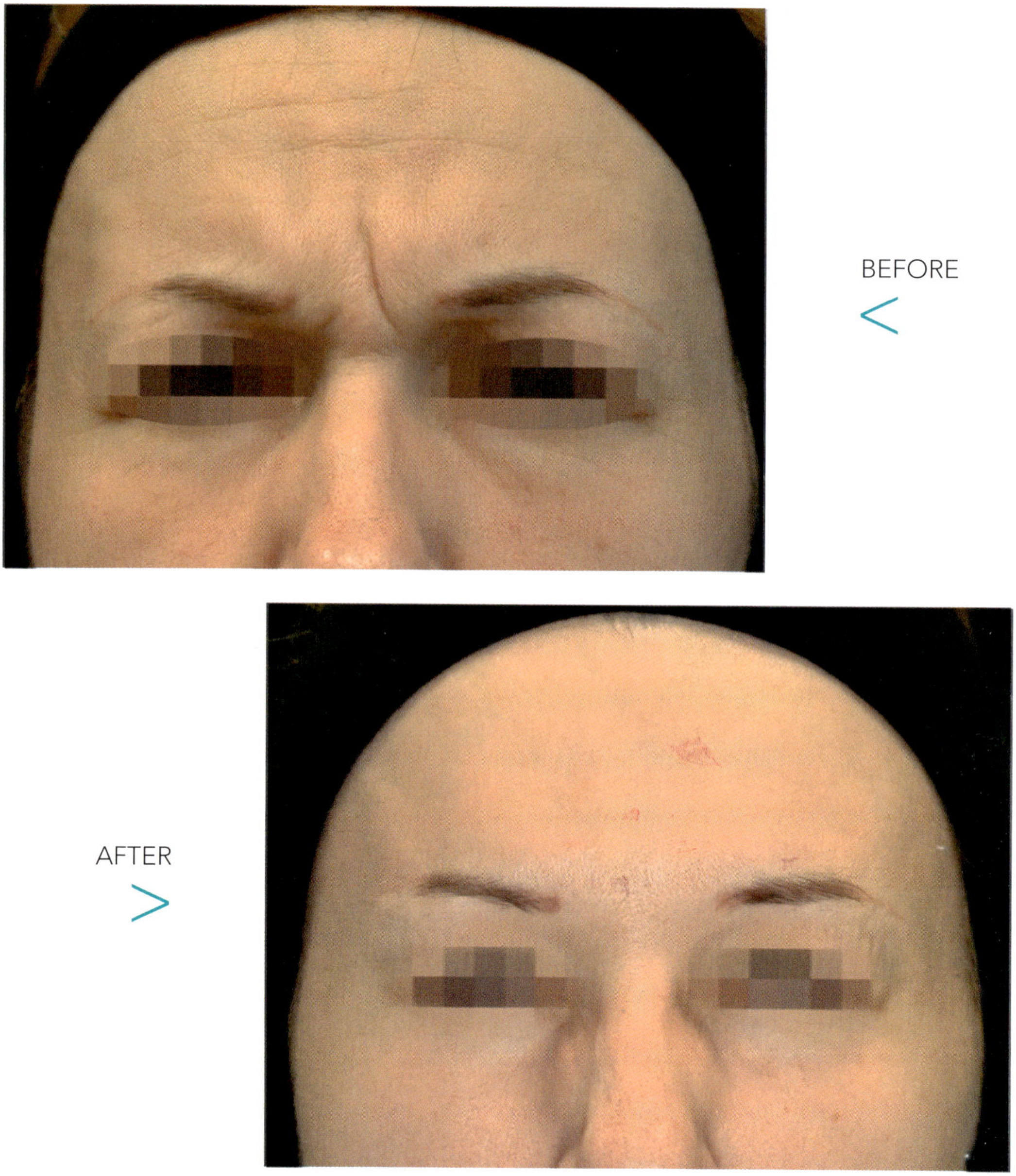

Figure 16 U contraction: 48 year-old patient before and thirty days after treatment with botulinum toxin (dynamic)

CLINICAL CASES

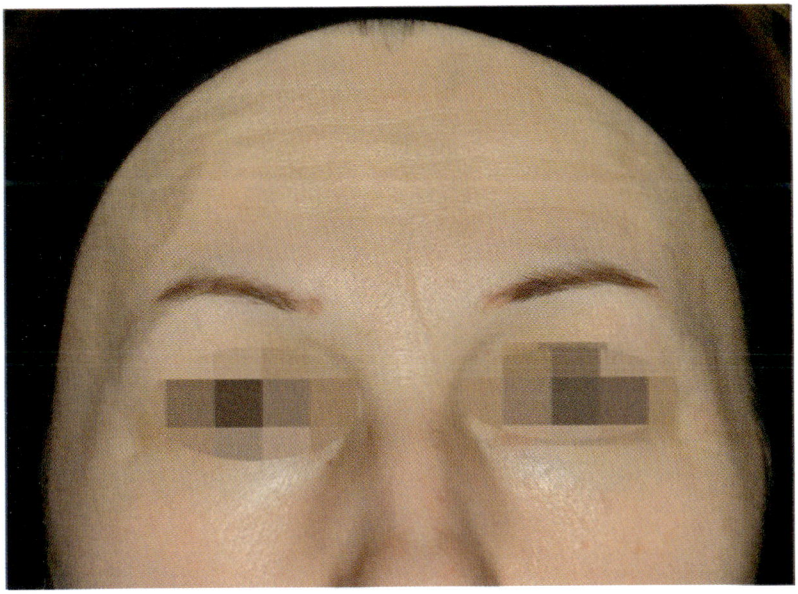

BEFORE

<

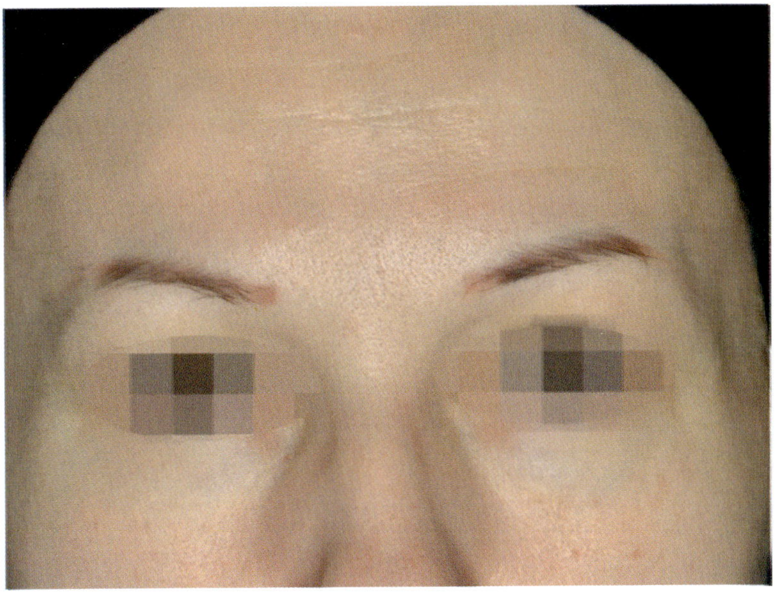

AFTER

>

Figure 17 U contraction: 48 year-old patient before and thirty days after treatment with botulinum toxin (static)

CLINICAL CASES

CLINICAL CASE 5

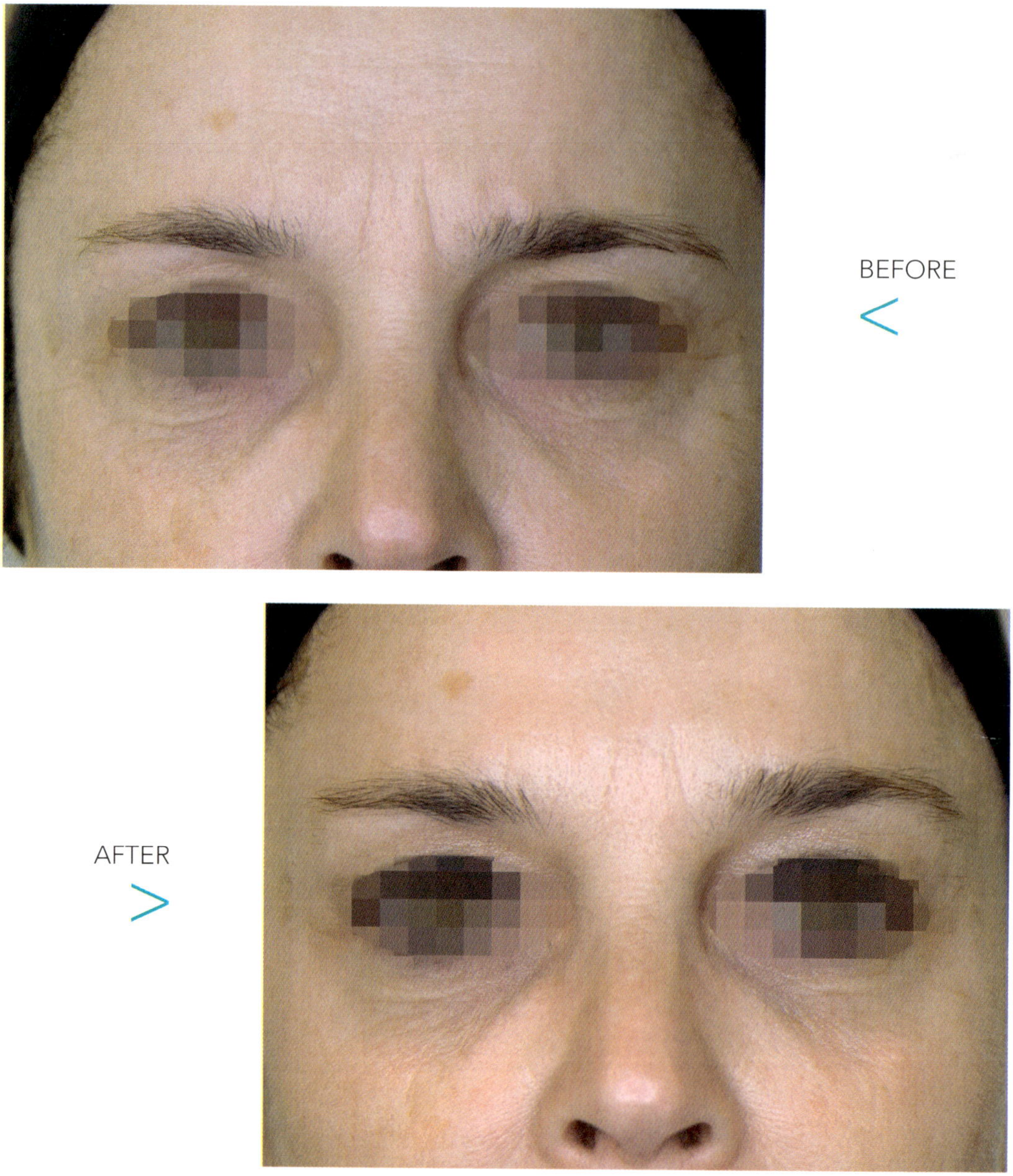

Figure 18 V contraction: 52 year-old patient before and thirty days after treatment of the glabella lines with botulinum toxin (dynamic)

CLINICAL CASES

CLINICAL CASE 6

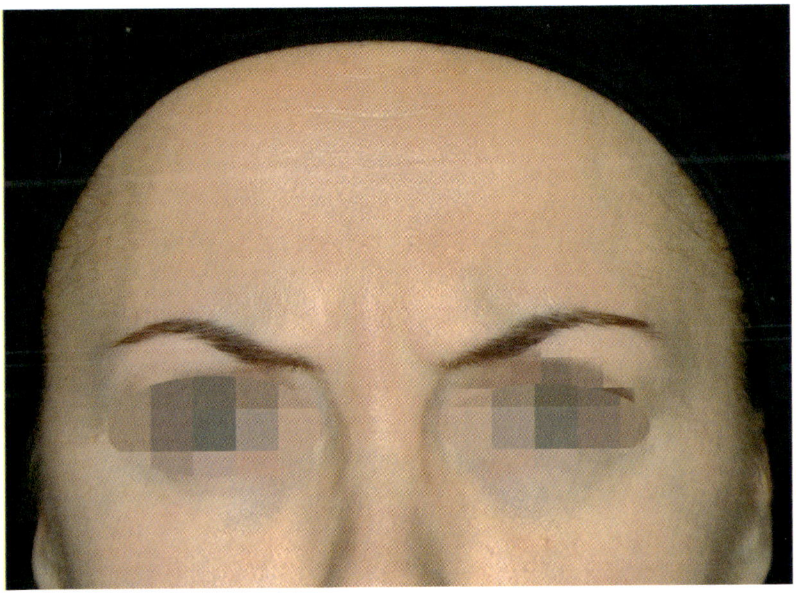

BEFORE
<

AFTER
>

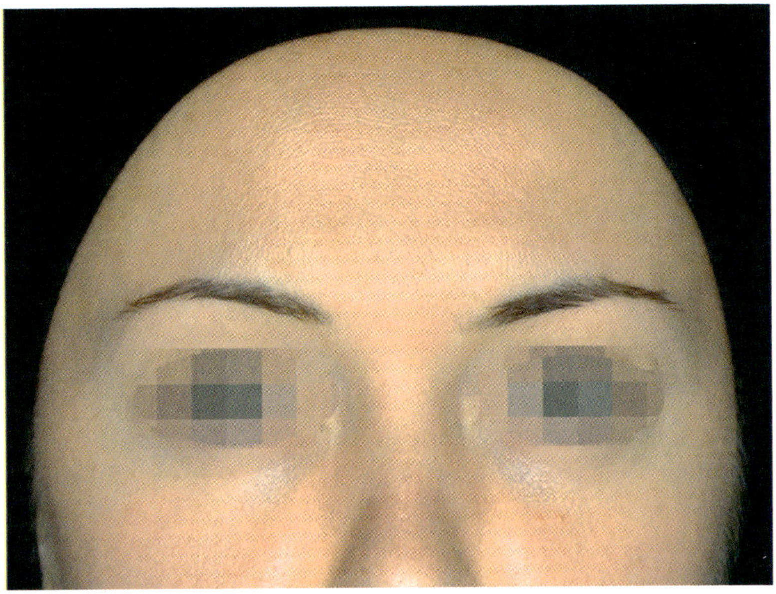

Figure 19 V contraction: 39 year-old patient before and thirty days after treatment of the glabella lines with botulinum toxin (dynamic)

CROW'S FEET

Patrizia Piersini

The eyes are a focal, attractive element of facial aesthetics, and the ageing of this area plays a key role in the appearance of the face.
The correction of wrinkles around the eyes, also known as crow's feet, is an important element for patients who want to rejuvenate the periocular region.
Occasionally, fine and thin lines are also present under the eyes; these are generally caused by the exaggerated contraction of the zygomaticus major muscle, which lifts the zygomatic area and the labial commissure when we smile, and they are usually more visible in a fake smile (fig. 20).
The crow's feet that form around the eyes, making them look old, become evident as the skin ages, due to the loss of structure and to thinning caused by chronological ageing, the thickening of the skin caused by photo-ageing, which makes the wrinkles deeper, and the skin's inability to respond adequately to facial expression and then return to its resting position.
On both the forehead and in the lateral canthus region of the eye, the dermis is thinner along the course of the wrinkle than in areas where wrinkles are not present. The dermis beneath the wrinkle becomes thinner and thinner as the wrinkle deepens, until it reaches about half its original thickness. At this point, the wrinkle continues to deepen, folding the dermis into the subcutaneous tissue [11]. Contet-Andonneau et al. found that the levels of type IV and type VII collagen, chondroitin sulphate and oxytalan fibres, small elastic fibres present in the papillary dermis, are considerably lower in the skin of the face with wrinkles than in skin without wrinkles or the skin of areas of the body that have not been exposed to the sun (e.g.: the abdomen). [12].

Anatomy

The orbicularis oculi muscle is a large, flat sphincter muscle, consisting of an elliptical part, an orbital part, which surrounds the circumference of the orbit, and a palpebral part. It extends to the anterior temporal region, the cheek and the superciliary region. The orbital part of the orbicularis muscle originates from the nasal part of the frontal bone, the frontal process of the maxillary bone and the medial palpebral ligament. The superior fibres intertwine with the fibres of the frontalis, corrugator supercilii and depressor supercilii muscles. The inferior fibres, on the other hand, partly unite with the Levator labii superioris alaeque nasalis (LLSAN), the Levator labii superioris (LLS) and the zygomaticus minor muscles and medially reach the procerus muscle.
The palpebral part, divided into a preseptal and a pretarsal part, is thinner than the orbital part and originates from the medial palpebral ligament.
The fibres run into the eyelids and when they reach the lateral canthus of the eye, they entwine to form the lateral palpebral raphe (fig. 21).

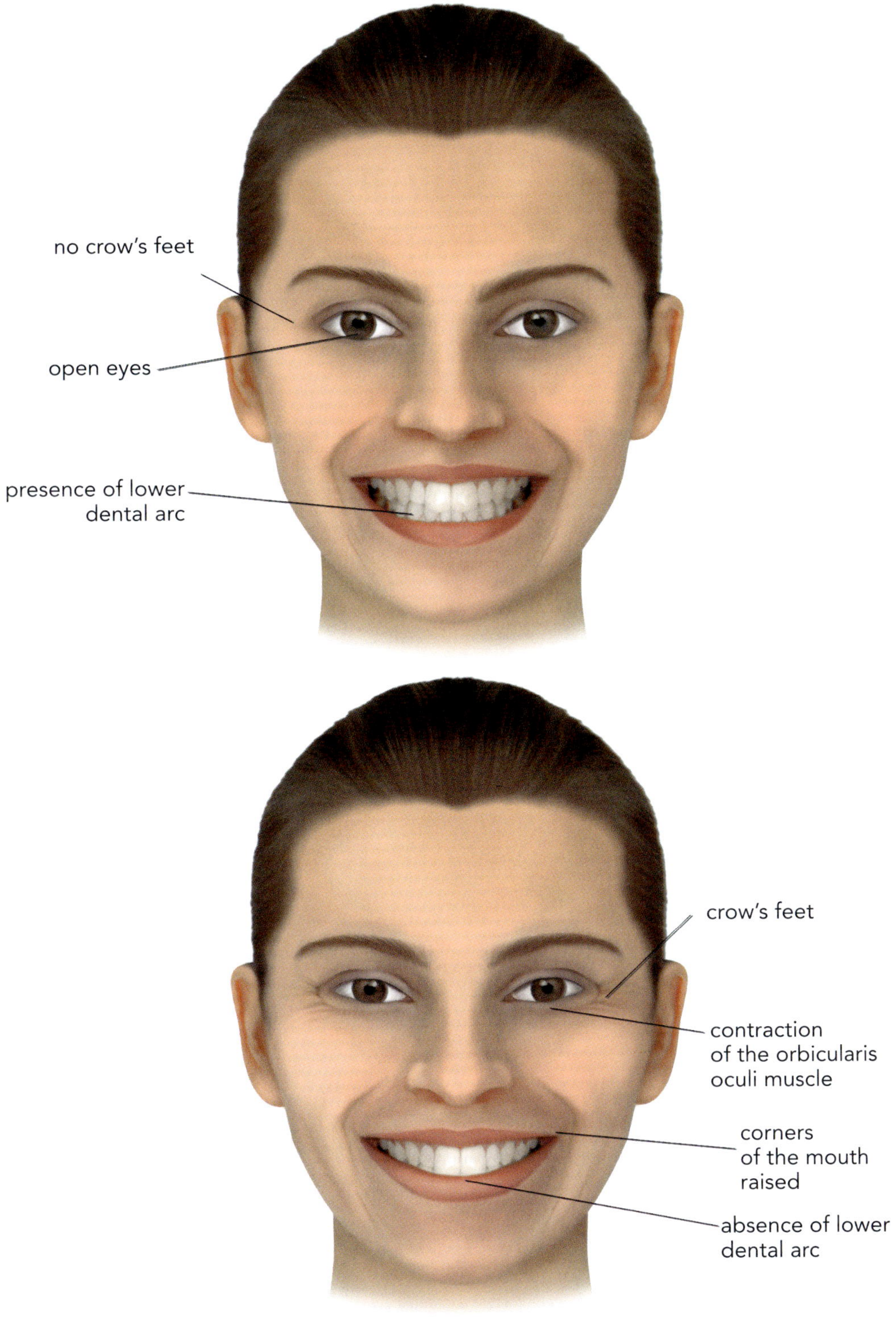

Figure 20 Difference between a fake smile (Pan American) and a genuine smile (Duchenne)

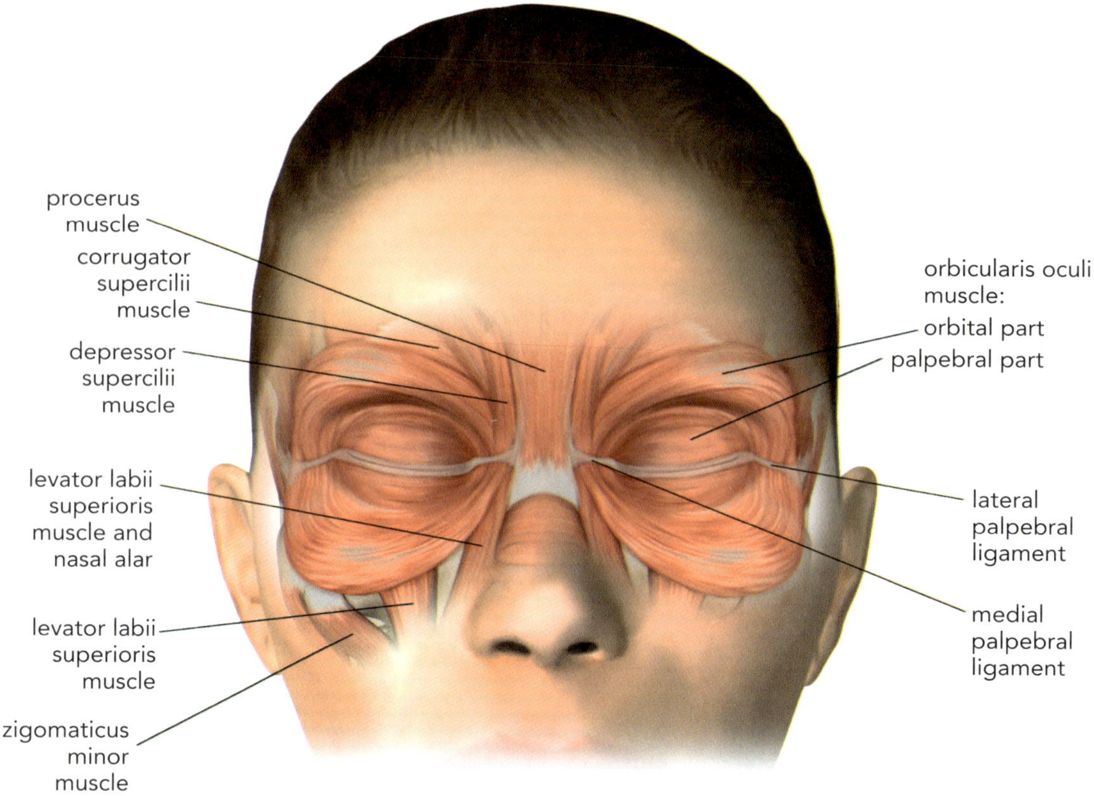

Figure 21 Anatomy of the eye region

The orbicularis muscle is innervated by the temporal and zygomatic ramifications of the facial nerve (7th pair of cranial nerves).

The fibres of the orbital component of the orbicularis muscle open and close the eyelids during voluntary movements, such as blinking or forcibly closing the eye, and those of the lateral part of the orbital portion, the target of botulinum protein therapy, lower the eyebrow and form what we call crow's feet.

The palpebral part of the muscle, on the other hand, when contracted, facilitates the drainage of tears by dilating the lachrymal sac and, with its preseptal portion, is involved in the voluntary, non-forced closure of the eyelids. Both this and the preseptal portion control blinking and keep the eye closed during sleep [13]. Contraction of the preseptal part causes vertical wrinkles of the medial canthus. The lateral portion of the orbicularis oculi muscle also contributes partly to the lowering of the medial and lateral portions of the eyebrow.

Due to this complex spatial orientation, the muscle fibres of the orbicularis, at the outer canthus of the eye, despite being vertically aligned, form horizontal wrinkles, while the horizontal fibres form and favour the occurrence of vertical wrinkles, on the inner rim.

Injection technique

Crow's feet are caused by the vertically aligned fibres of the orbital part of the orbicularis oculi muscle and partly by the zygomatic and risorius muscles [16], which are not the target of botulinum therapy. The treatment of this area aims to relax the lateral part of the orbicularis to smooth the wrinkles, without excessively blocking the muscle. It is important to carry out a pre-injection mapping, accurately identifying the contraction pattern, to identify any asymmetries.

The initial injection site is located at least one cm away from the orbital margin, in order to inject into the orbital portion of the orbicularis muscle and to prevent side effects such as migration to the retractor muscles of the eyelid or the extrinsic muscles of the eye, which could cause diplopia. Two further points are then injected, one more cranial and one more caudal, following the circumferential arc of the orbital rim. It is advisable to inject 2 U Onabotulinum (4 U Speywood) at each point, or 3 U Onabotulinum (6 U Speywood) if the wrinkles are very pronounced, with a total of 6/9 U Onabotulinum (12-18 U Speywood) per side. Injections should be performed superficially, intradermally, without contracting the muscle, creating a visible bump in the areas injected, to minimise the appearance of bruising and to achieve a more pronounced improvement in skin texture thanks to increased collagen production [14].

Video 3.6 shows treatment of crow's feet (standard technique) with a 33 G/9 mm needle and botulinum diluted to 1.2 ml, with superficial injection.

VIDEO 3.6

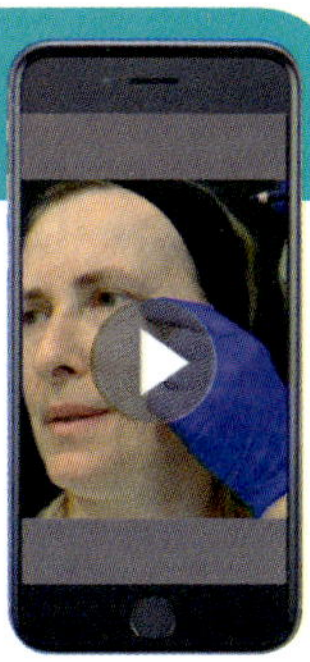

Treatment of crow's feet: standard technique

Even if the wrinkles extend downwards beyond the orbital rim, the most caudal injection should be considered carefully so as not to interfere with the action of the zygomaticus major muscle, which lifts the corner of the mouth upwards and sideways and pushes up the malar fat sac. This can lead to a lack of cheek and lip elevation in the smile, with a very unnatural appearance. These wrinkles can be corrected with fillers or using the microbotulinum technique (figg. 22-26).

Patients with deep crow's feet, including static wrinkles, should be informed that it is often necessary to combine botulinum toxin treatment with other treatments, such as the injection of a hyaluronic acid-based filler specifically for dynamic wrinkles or fractional laser sessions, to achieve an optimal result.

Attention should also be paid to patients with very slack skin on the lower eyelid, as an excessively medial injection may interfere with eyelid function and cause protrusion of the palpebral bags due to weakening of the muscular retention of the septum [15].

For the treatment of undereye lines, reserved for expert operators, a maximum of 1 U Onabotulinum (2 U Speywood) is injected into one or two points in the horizontal lines running parallel to the lower eyelid lash line, remaining as close as possible to the surface to avoid ectropion.

Another possibility for experienced injectors of botulinum toxin in the eye area is to use it to decrease pretarsal hypertrophy and achieve downward displacement of the lower ciliary muscle. When we smile, the eyelid opening narrows and, in patients with pretarsal hypertrophy of the lower eyelid, we notice an increase in the volume of the tarsus, which creates a tired, sagging expression. This has been well described by Jean and Alaistair Carruthers [16], who recommend injecting 2-4 U Onabotulinum (4-7 U Speywood) into the lower pretarsal portion of the orbicularis, 3 mm below the lower lash margin on the mid-pupil line. If the lateral orbital fibres are injected at the same time, to treat wrinkles on the lateral canthus of the eye, a highly satisfactory aesthetic result is achieved.

Patients who did not have a good result in the snap test before injection, who have poor lachrymal secretion or who have had lower blepharoplasty without canthopexy should not be treated with this technique because of the risk of lagophthalmos or ectropion, with consequent scleral exposure (round eye, or scleral show).

CLINICAL CASES

CLINICAL CASE 7

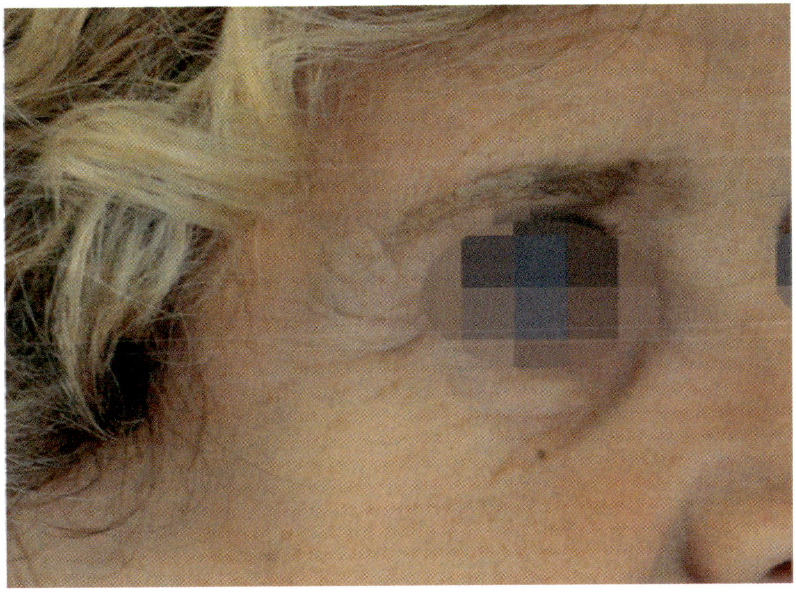

BEFORE
<

AFTER
>

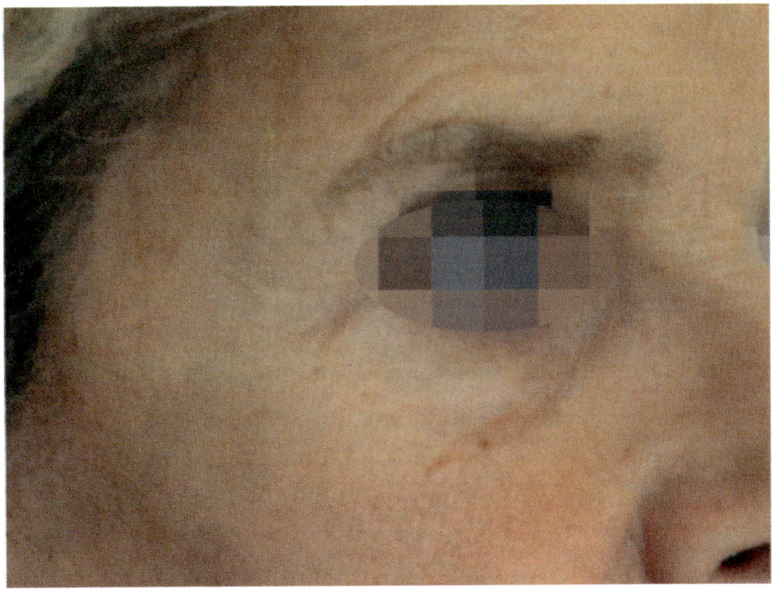

Figure 22 59 year-old patient, static, before and thirty days after treatment of crow's feet with botulinum

CLINICAL CASES

CLINICAL CASE 8

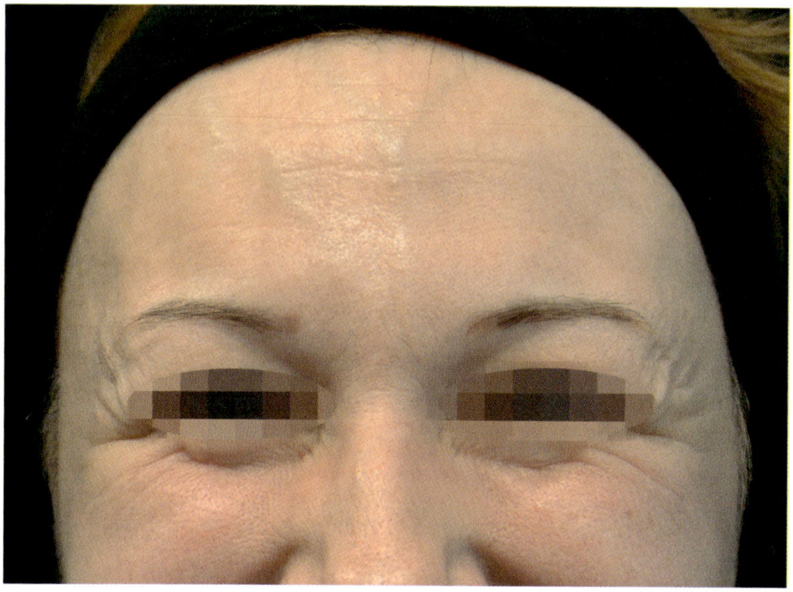

BEFORE

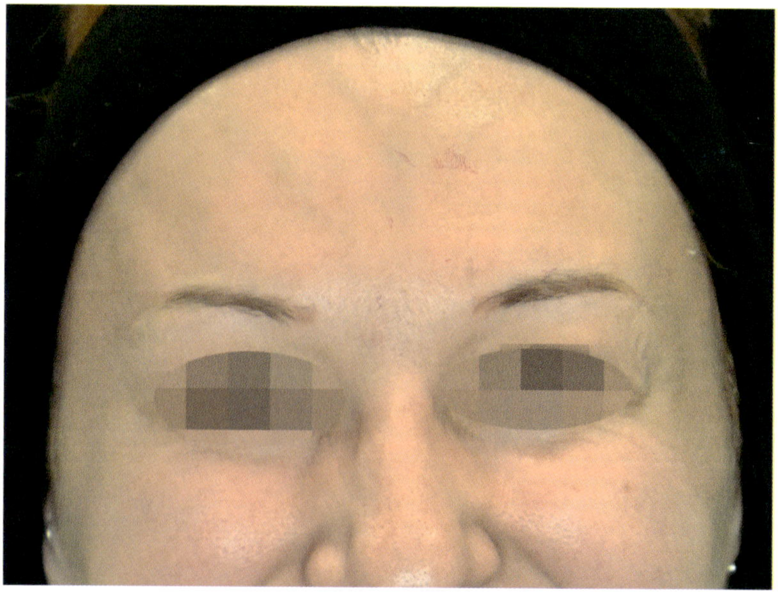

AFTER

Figure 23 48 year-old patient, dynamic, before and thirty days after treatment of crow's feet with botulinum

CLINICAL CASES

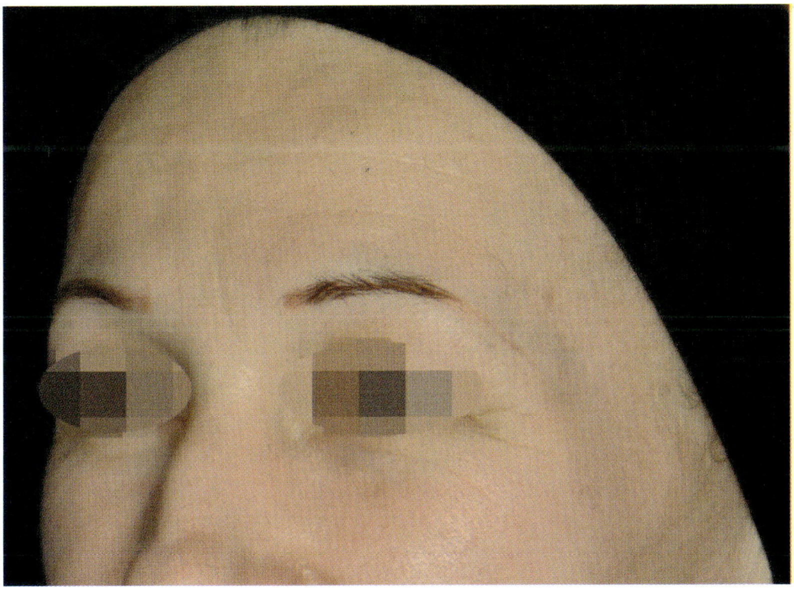

BEFORE <

AFTER >

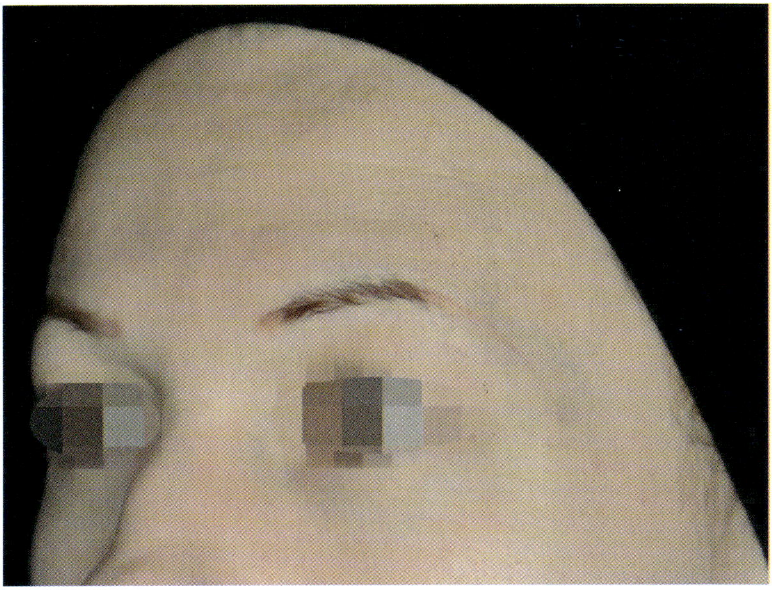

Figure 24 Same patient, static, before and thirty days after treatment of crow's feet with botulinum (left side)

CLINICAL CASES

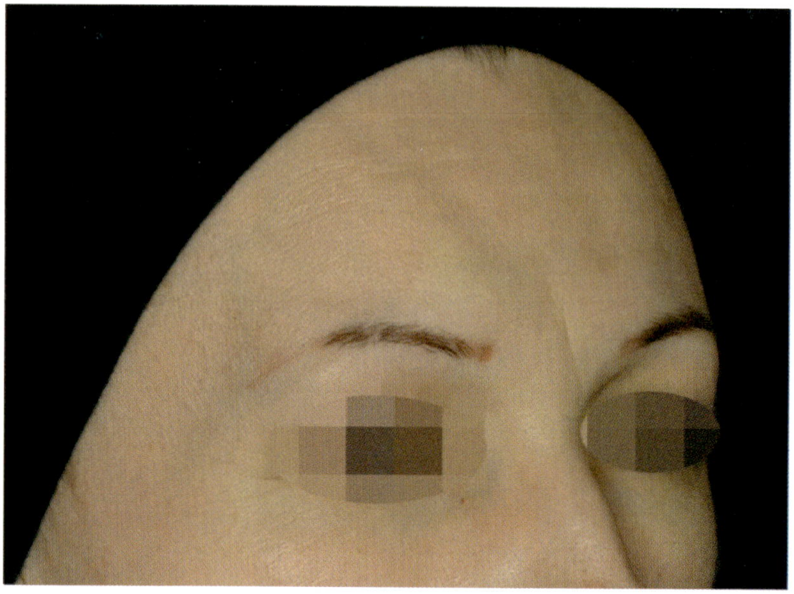

BEFORE

<

AFTER

>

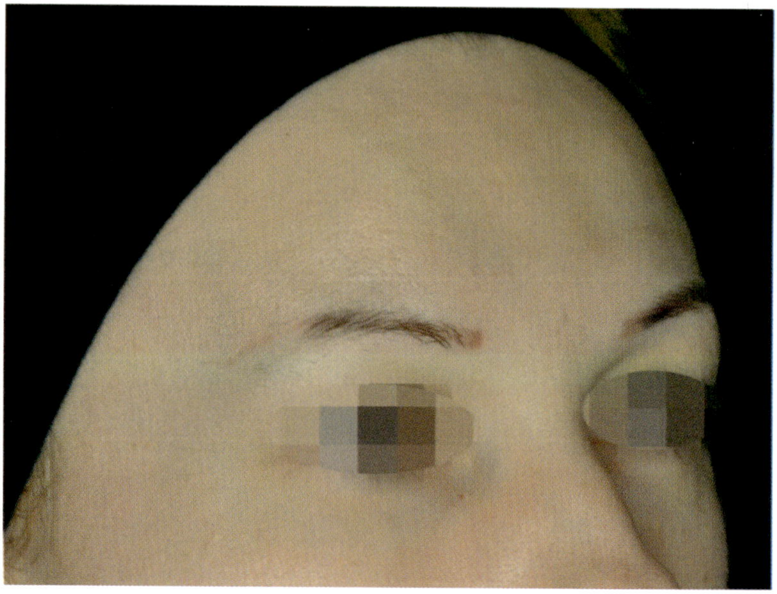

Figure 25 Same patient, static, before and thirty days after treatment of crow's feet with botulinum (right side)

CLINICAL CASES

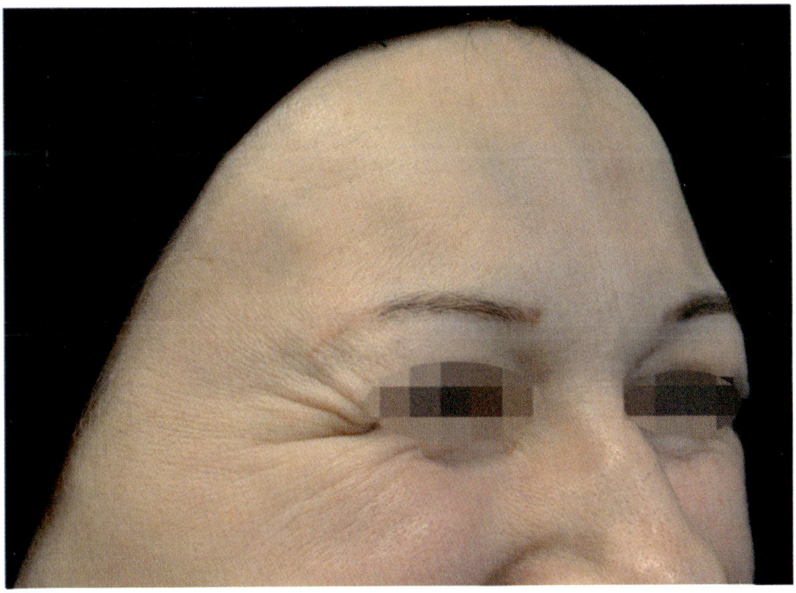

BEFORE <

AFTER >

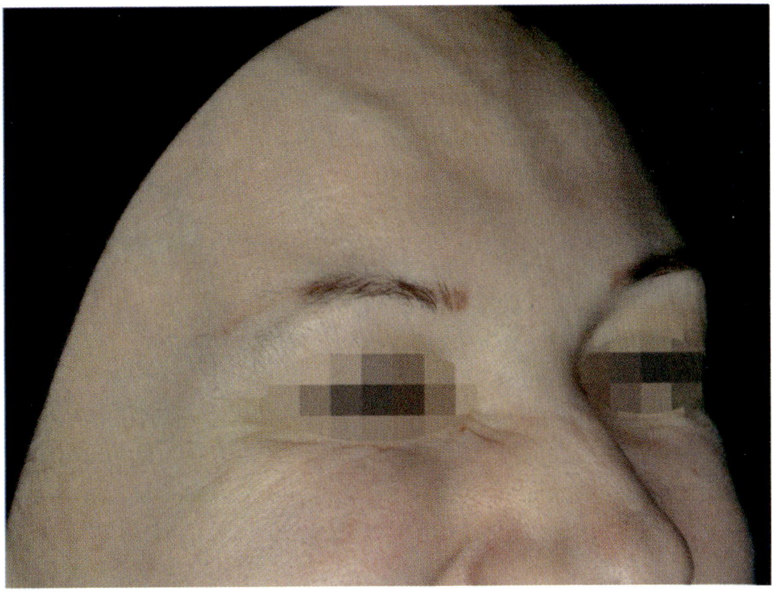

Figure 26 Same patient, dynamic, before and thirty days after treatment of crow's feet with botulinum (right side)

LIFTING THE LATERAL THIRD OF THE EYEBROW (GULL WING)

Patrizia Piersini

The position of the eyebrow varies according to gender, age and even ethnicity. An eyebrow that is considered too low in one patient may be normal in another.

In women, it is positioned over the upper orbital arch, curving upwards and outwards so that the apex of the eyebrow is at the lateral limbus of the cornea (junction line between cornea and sclera).

In men, it is located on or just above the upper orbital arch, and is straighter, almost horizontal in shape, arching only slightly to the side (fig. 27).

Ptosis of the eyebrow occurs slowly with advancing age, interfering with both eyebrow function and facial aesthetics, making the patient look tired and old.

The eyebrows are mobile and their ptosis is determined by muscular action, the force of gravity and skin elastosis. In addition, due to multiple factors, such as differences between the contraction of the right and left hemiface muscles, trauma, facial paralysis (e.g.: Bell's palsy) or simply the side on which the patient sleeps, ptosis is rarely symmetrical (fig. 28) [17].

Surgical correction, which for a long time was the only treatment option, was first proposed by the German surgeon Erich Lexer in 1910 in a brow lift. In 1957, Bames proposed an indirect brow lift by weakening the corrugator supercilii muscles [18]. The first endoscopic brow lifts were proposed in the early 1990s. Treatment with botulinum toxin as an alternative to surgery for eyebrow lifts was proposed in 1998 [19]. Non-surgical brow lift procedures are usually temporary but require less experience, and the management of an unsatisfactory result is easier [20].

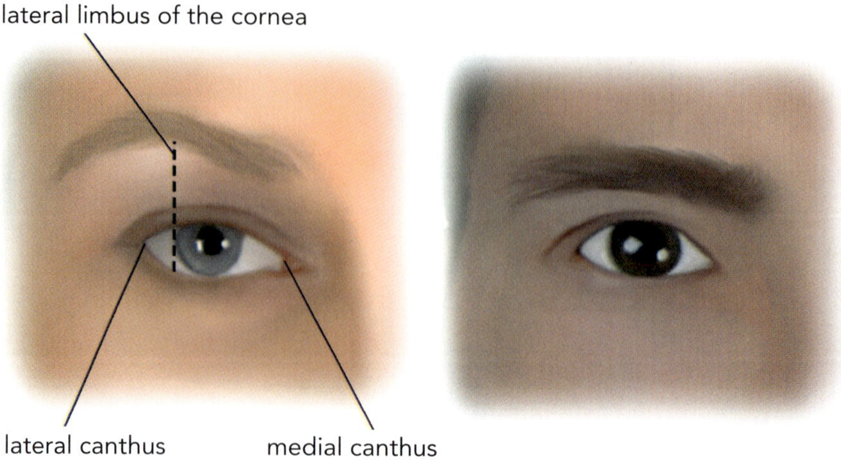

Figure 27 Difference between the female eyebrow and male eyebrow

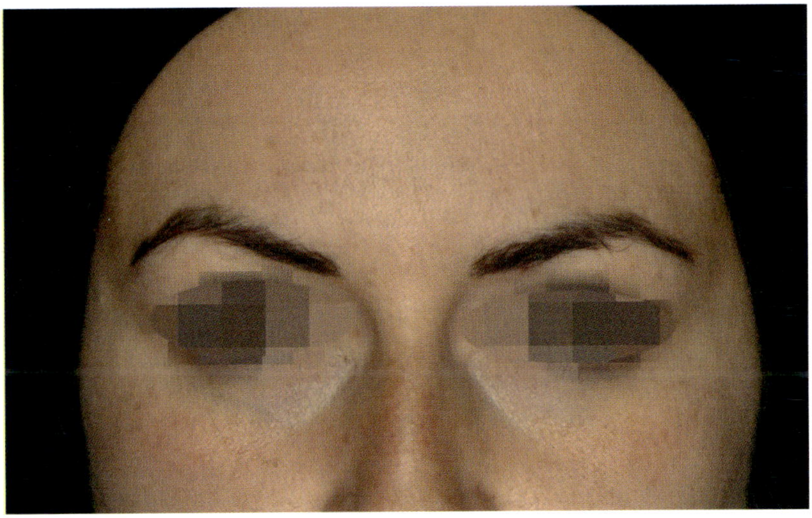

Figure 28 Static asymmetry of the eyebrow

Anatomy

The eyebrow (supercilium in Latin) is a mobile, arched, skin relief with a lower concavity, covered with small, coarse hairs, that separates the upper eyelid from the forehead. It has a more pronounced middle part, a head, a body and a thinner lateral end called the tail. It consists, from surface to depth, of skin, a slack subcutaneous layer with little fat, a muscular layer and a fat-rich periosteum adhering to the frontal bone.

The muscular layer is made up of the fibres of the orbicularis oculi, frontalis and corrugator supercilii muscles (see description of muscles in chapter 1). It is elevated by the frontal portion of the occipitofrontalis muscle.

The function of the eyebrow is mainly to protect the eye, preventing sweat and dust from entering the eye and disturbing vision, and preventing trauma thanks to the bony projection of the orbital arch. It also plays an important role in conveying emotions through facial expressions: a raised eyebrow indicates surprise, medially lowered is a sign of concentration or anger, and centrally lowered indicates fatigue.

Injection technique

The way botulinum toxin works is well known. It exploits the agonism and antagonism of muscle groups. Three points must be treated to raise the eyebrow: the first is in the glabella area, in the muscles that depress the eyebrow, and we use 7-10 U Botox (14-20 U Speywood).

Video 3.7 shows drawing of the treatment for mid brow lift in a patient with static asymmetry of the eyebrows.

Video 3.8 shows injection technique for mid brow lift using a 33 G/9 mm needle and botulinum diluted to 1.2 ml, with intramuscular injection.

The second and third points are injected with 1-2 U Botox to further raise the tail of the eyebrow if necessary, creating the so-called gull wing eyebrow. Video 3.9 shows drawing and

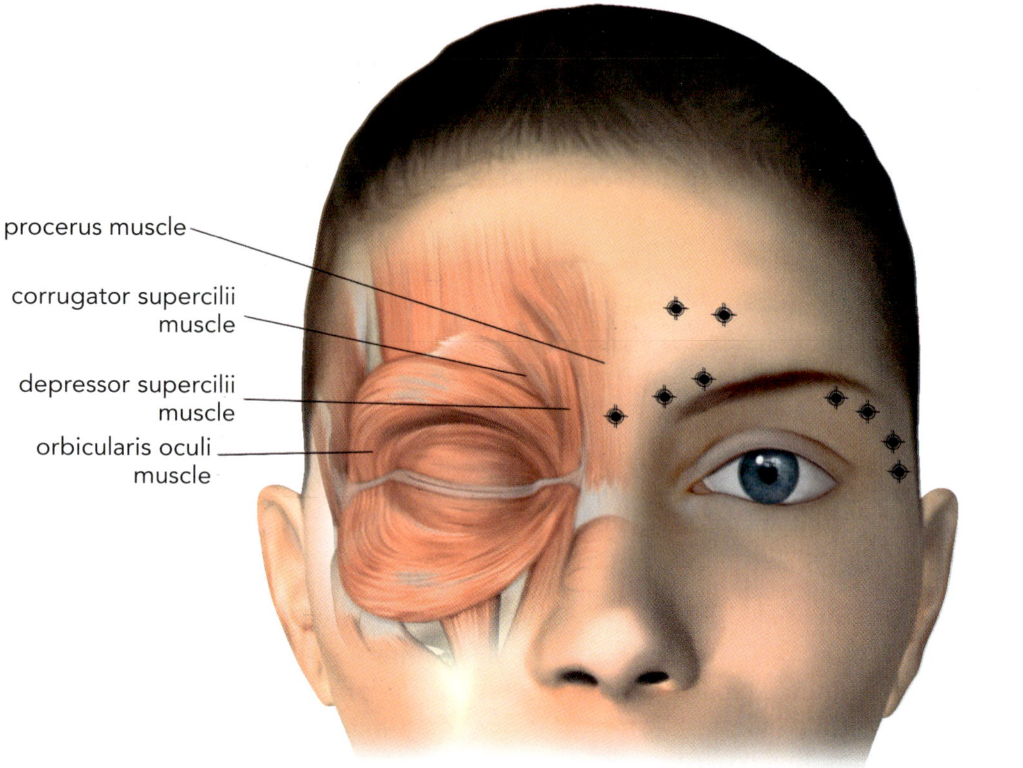

Figure 29 Anatomy of the eyebrow region

VIDEO 3.7

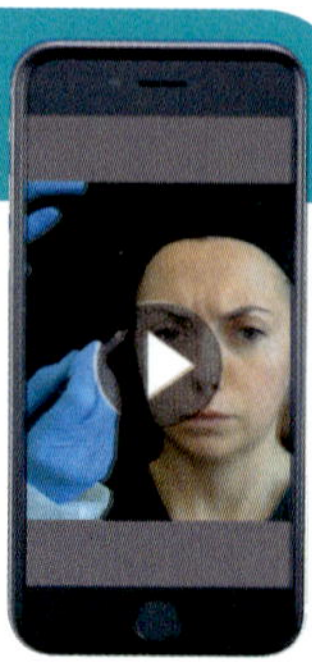

Drawing of the treatment for mid brow lift in a patient with static asymmetry of the eyebrows

VIDEO 3.8

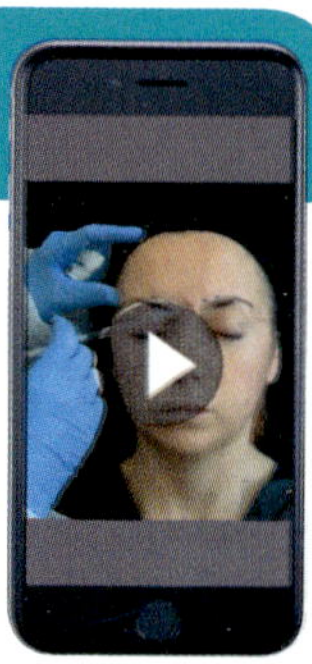

Injection technique for mid brow lift using a 33 G/9 mm needle

VIDEO 3.9

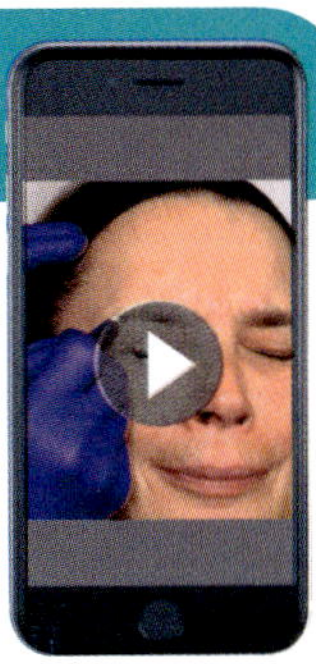

Drawing and injection technique for lateral brow lift using a 33 G/9 mm needle

injection technique for lateral brow lift (gull wing eyebrow) using a 33 G/9 mm needle and botulinum diluted to 1.2 ml, with intradermal injection.

Intradermal injection is performed at the point that often corresponds with the meeting of the temporal fusion line with the orbital arch, about 1 cm above the orbital arch, at the lateral canthus of the eye [21]. The effect is a brow lift of about 1-3 mm, which gives a more open and attractive appearance without detracting from the naturalness of the face. The elevation of the lateral part of the eyebrow can be further accentuated by lowering the head of the eyebrow and then injecting 2-3 U Botox (4-6 U Speywood) into the paramedial part of the frontalis muscle. A higher lift of the tail of the eyebrow is more indicated in female patients as it tends to make the eyes look more feminine.

When treating the depressor supercilia muscles, it is important to avoid paralysis of the frontalis muscle and prevent the opposite effect to that desired, i.e.: brow ptosis. Elderly patients may be more susceptible to lateral brow ptosis so it is important to select patients correctly.

The above can be summarised in two points (fig. 29):

- elevation of the medial part of the eyebrow, injections of botulinum toxin into the depressor supercilii muscles as used to treat glabella wrinkles. It is important to inject along the whole body of the corrugator supercilii muscle (fig. 30);
- elevation of the lateral part of the eyebrow, with very shallow intradermal injections of botulinum toxin at the point below the tail of the eyebrow (orbital rim with temporal crest), at the supero-lateral canthal points (as for eye wrinkles) and in the paramedial portion of the frontalis muscle if the head of the eyebrow is to be lowered to obtain an additional visual effect of tail elevation (figs. 31-32).

CLINICAL CASES

CLINICAL CASE 9

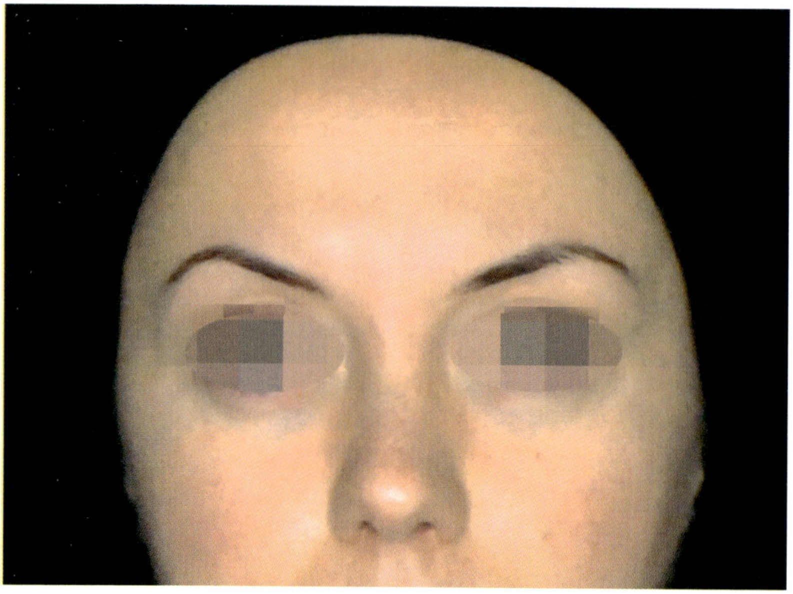

BEFORE

AFTER

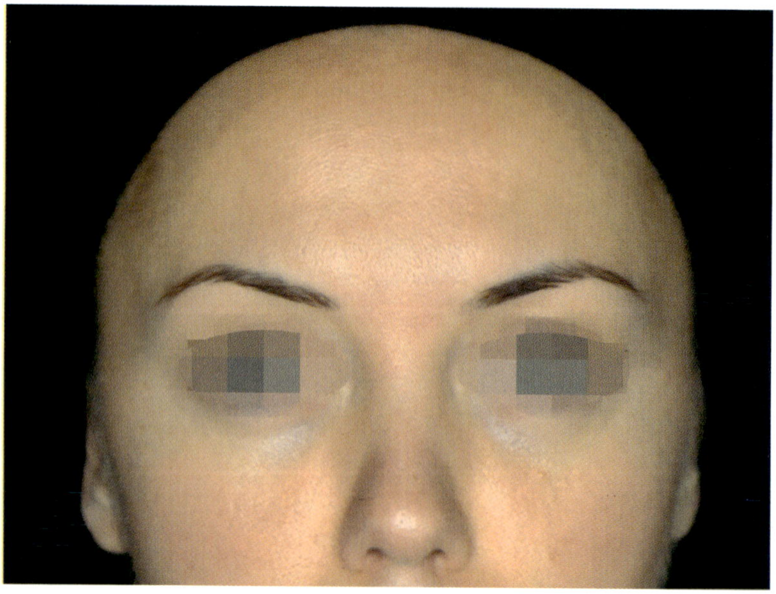

Figure 30 Before and thirty days after treatment with botulinum to lift the head of the eyebrow and make the eyebrows symmetrical

CLINICAL CASES

CLINICAL CASE 10

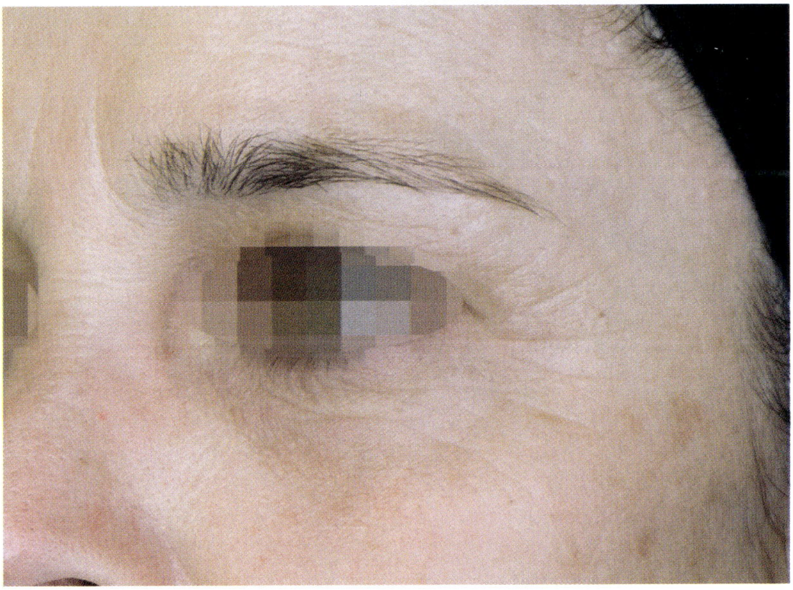

BEFORE
<

AFTER
>

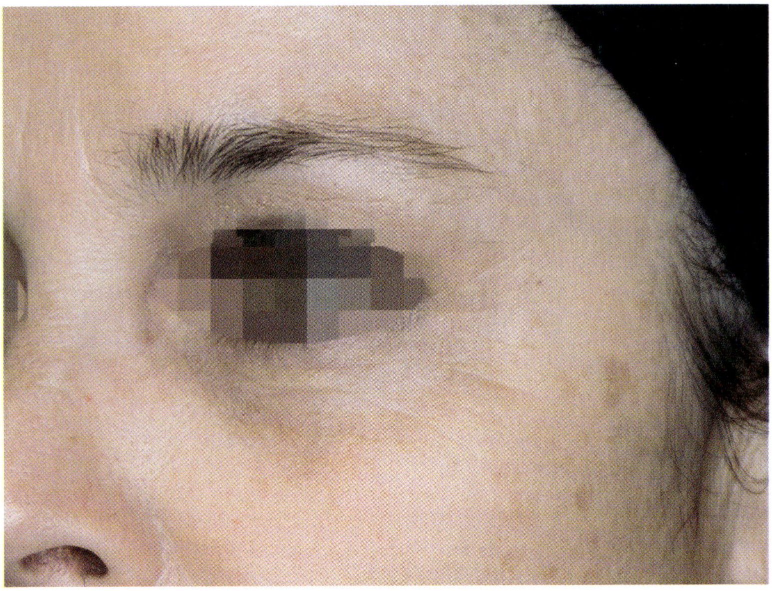

Figure 31 Before and thirty days after treatment with botulinum (side view) to lift the tail of the eyebrow (gull wing eyebrow)

CLINICAL CASES

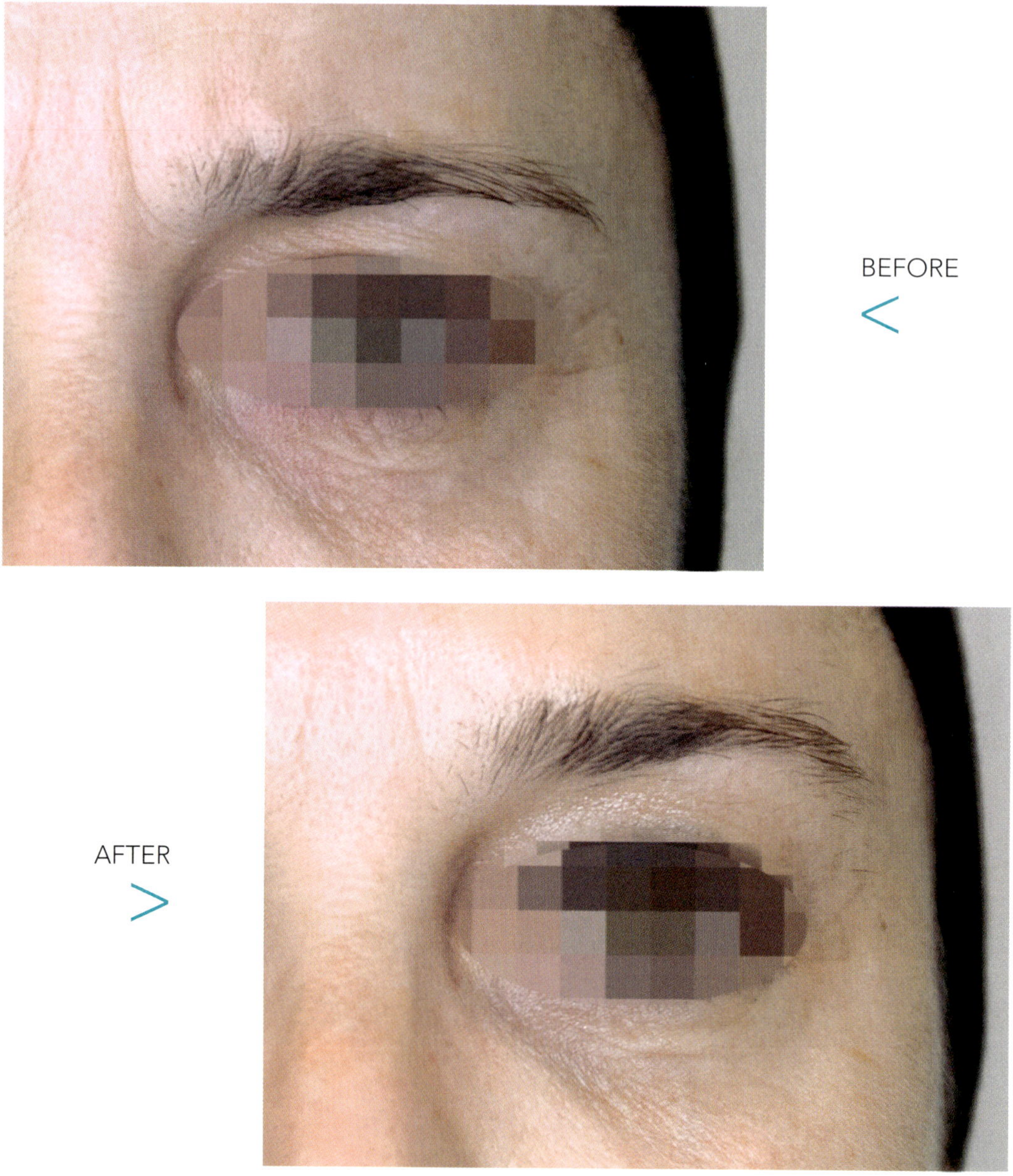

Figure 32 Before and thirty days after treatment with botulinum (front view) for mid and lateral brow lift, improving wrinkles around the eyes

MIDDLE THIRD

DEPRESSOR OF THE SEPTUM AND ELEVATION OF THE NASAL TIP

Alberto Diaspro

The nose is positioned in the centre of the face and is fundamental in determining its aesthetic balance. The projection and three-dimensional position of the tip of the nose are the result of complex surgical procedures, using grafts and sutures to shape the cartilaginous portion.

The use of botulinum to change the position of the tip, while having a temporary result, allows minor corrections in patients who prefer to avoid or are not eligible for surgery.

The injection of botulinum toxin can be used to treat moderate nasal tip ptosis, both static and dynamic [22], secondary to the excessive action of the nasal septum depressor muscle, which is hyperactive and hypertrophic in these cases.

Anatomy

It is advisable to consider the anthropometric points and angles of the nose as a clinical reference for correctly assessing the results of treatment:

- the subnasal point (Sn), is the midpoint on the nasolabial soft tissue contour between the crest of the columella and the upper lip;
- the subspinal point (Ss), is the most posterior midpoint of the philtrum;
- the labial superius point (Ls), is the midpoint of the line of the vermilion of the upper lip;
- naso-labial angle (SNA), is the angle between the base of the columella, the Sn point and the upper lip, Ls point, ideally between 90° and 100° in men and 95° and 110° in women (fig. 33).

The nasal septum depressor muscle is an extension of the orbicularis oris muscle which penetrates the base of the medial crura from the base of the columella and whose expressive contraction pulls the tip of the nose downwards; its action is most evident when we smile, due to the antagonistic effect of all the levator labii superioris muscles (figs. 34-35).

Its weakening determines the opening of the naso-labial angle by rotating and lifting the tip [23].

Injection technique

2 U Botox or 5 U Speywood, and up to 4 U Botox or 10 U Speywood are injected deeply into the point of origin of the muscle on the bone plane at the base of the columella.

In the case of a very mobile and drooping tip, at least another 2 U Botox or 5 U Speywood, up to 4 U Botox or 10 U Speywood, can be injected per side on the intra-nasal side of the tip, where the muscle penetrates the base of the alar cartilage in the crus (fig. 36).

The columellar artery, the terminal

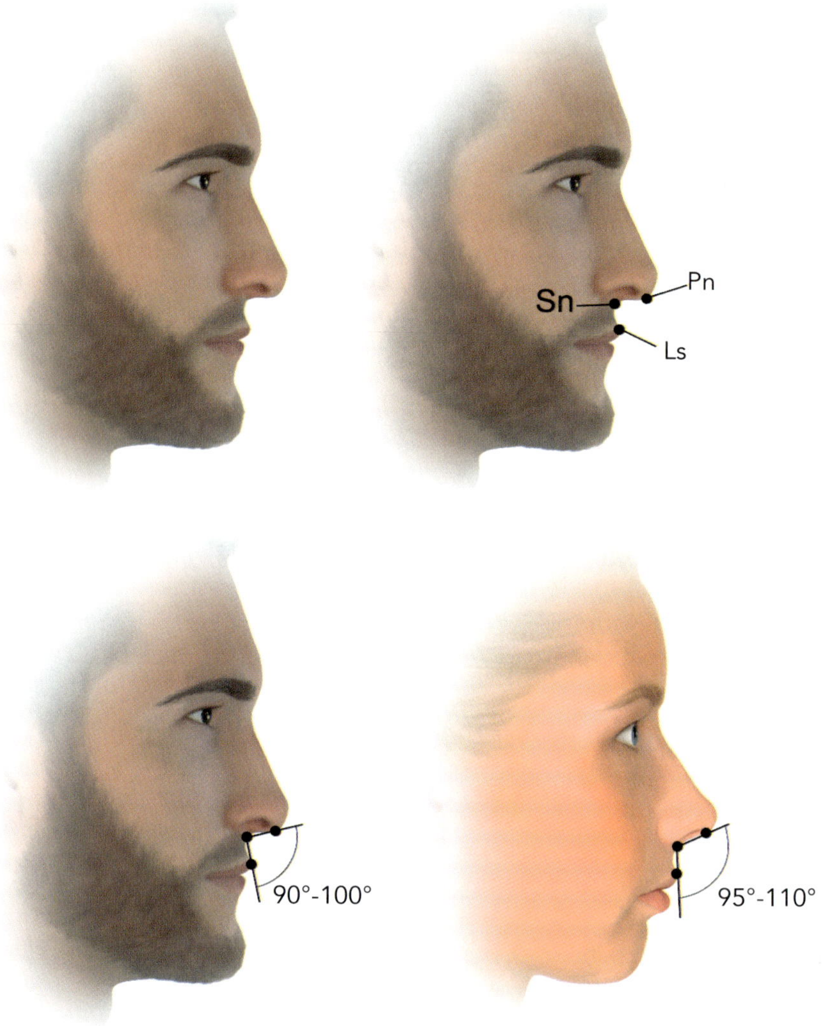

Figure 33 Anthropometric points of the naso-labial region and size of the naso-labial angle in women and men

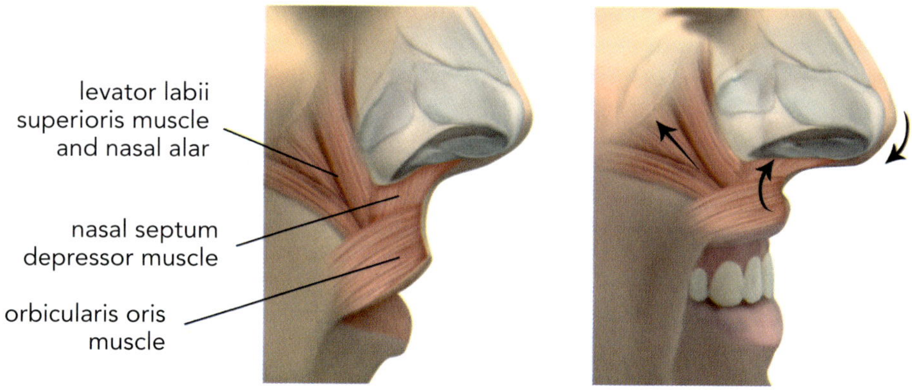

Figure 34 Functional diagram of the septum depressor muscle

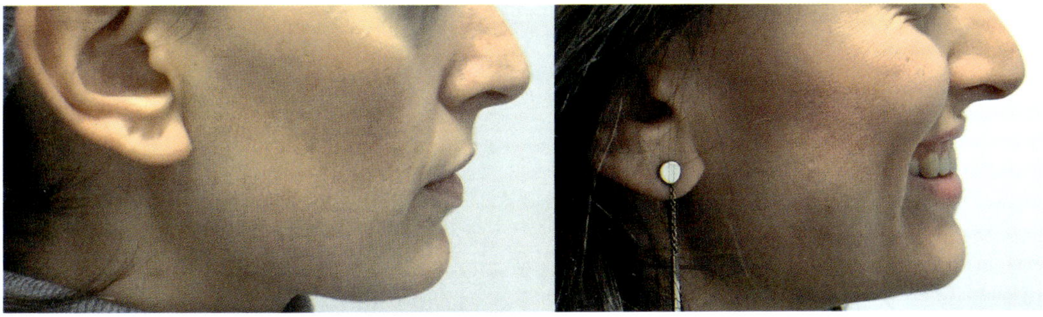

Figure 35 Synergistic activation of the levator labii and septum depressor muscles when smiling

branch of the superior labial artery, is the vessel that runs into the columella and whose accidental injection should be avoided so as not to release the botulinum into the bloodstream, losing its effect [24,25]. There is no risk of accidental ischaemia or necrosis.

Injecting into the base of the columella (origin of the muscle on the bone plane) either percutaneously at the Sn point (fig. 36, point A) or intra-nasally bilaterally, injecting the toxin into the same point (video 3.10, fig. 36, points B1 and B2).

If deemed appropriate, the tip can be injected intra-nasally (mucosal insertion, fig. 36, points C1 and C2), lifting the tip

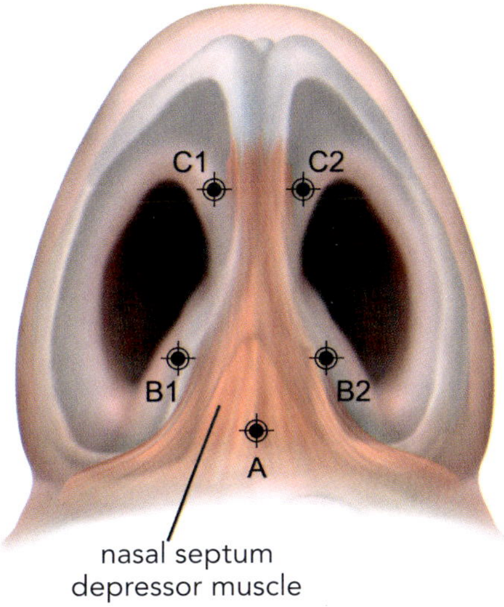

Figure 36 Injection point at the base of the columella, view from below

as it rotates upwards and opens the nasolabial angle.

This is a finishing technique and is not appropriate in the case of a very droopy tip with little mobility. The result is stable for up to three months and depends on the dose injected.

Excessive doses can lead to an increase in length up to ptosis of the upper lip due to migration of the botulinum effect to the orbicularis oris muscle. Consequently, this technique is contraindicated if the Sn-Ls prolabium is more than 19-22 mm long [26-28].

VIDEO 3.10

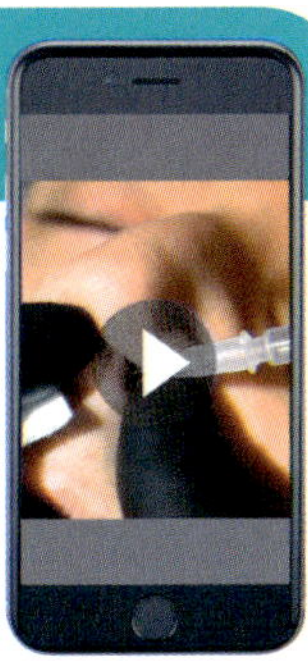

Septal depressor: injection technique

BUNNY LINES

Patrizia Piersini

Bunny lines, so named because they form when you wrinkle your nose bunny-style, are straight or slightly diagonal, dynamic fine lines that appear on both sides of the bridge of the nose when you laugh, smile broadly or sniff an unpleasant smell (fig. 37). Sometimes, however, they are caused by treatment with botulinum toxin: when the muscles of the glabella are blocked excessively, the nasal muscle can become overactive and accentuate or create these wrinkles (aka "botox signs") [29].

Anatomy

The nasal muscle is a mimetic muscle that covers the bridge of the nose and consists of an alar part (pars alaris or nostril dilator muscle, which is divided into an anterior part and a posterior part) and a transverse part (pars transversa or nostril constrictor muscle) (fig. 38).
The alar part originates from the maxilla, at the side of the lateral incisors, and penetrates the greater alar cartilage and the depressor septi nasi muscle. The transverse part also originates from the maxilla, above and to the side of the

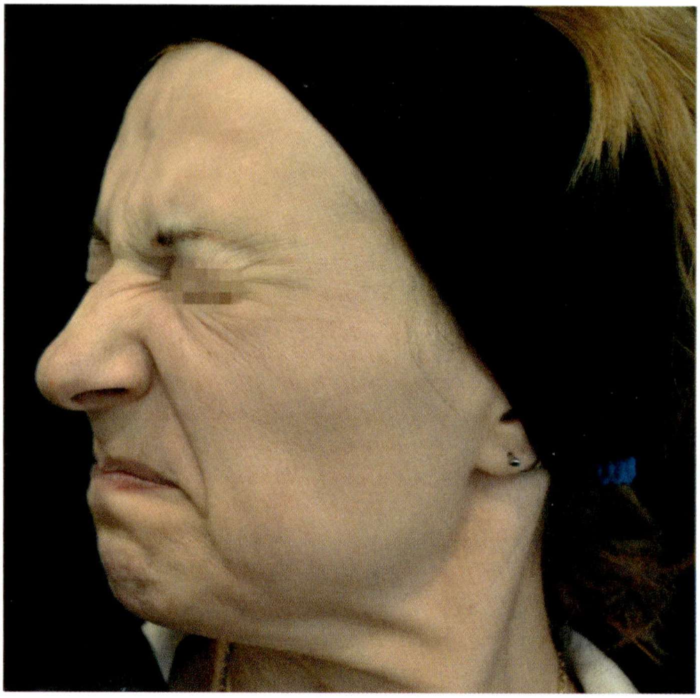

Figure 37 Bunny lines are fine, slightly diagonal lines that appear on both sides of the nose when the transverse portion of the nasal muscle is contracted

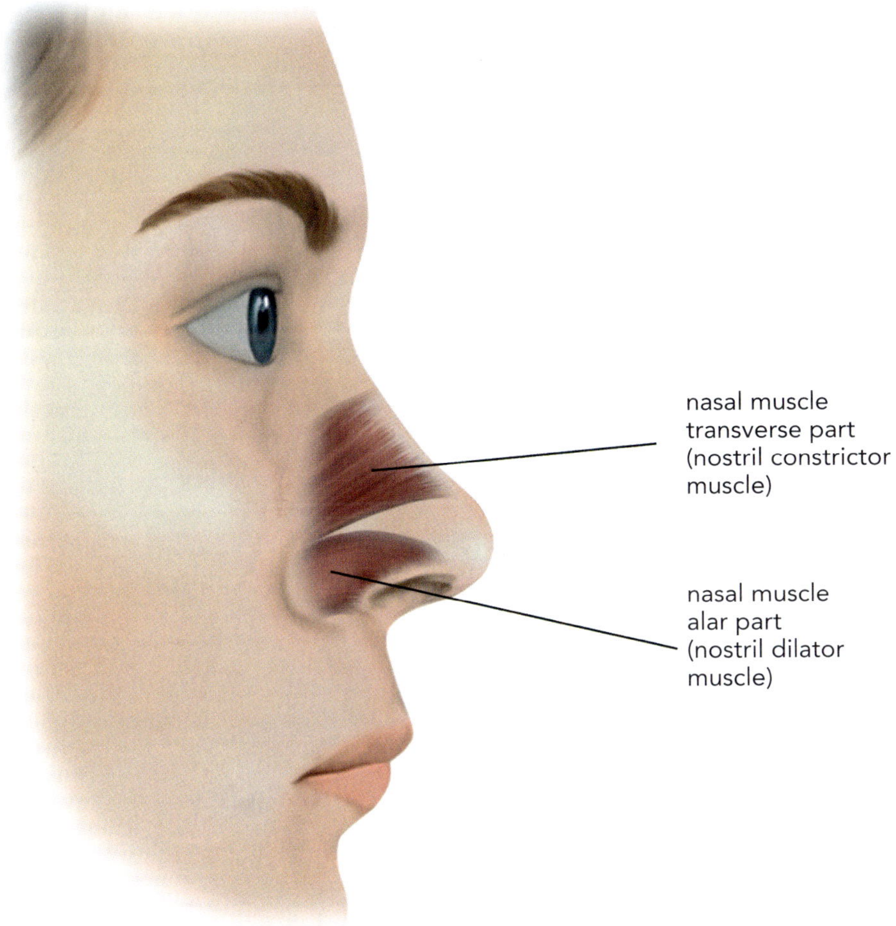

Figure 38 Anatomy and function of the nasal muscle

incisor fossa, and its fibres expand into a thin aponeurosis that joins with that of the nasal muscle on the opposite side of the nose and with the aponeurosis of the procerus muscle.

Its function is to mobilise the soft part of the nose and in particular to flare the nostrils (alar part), when inhaling deeply under stress or in certain emotional states, and to narrow (transverse part) the nostrils, like when some people use it to prevent water from entering the nose when diving. The contraction of the muscle fibres of the transverse portion of the nasal muscle causes the formation of a fan of wrinkles at the bridge of the nose, also known as bunny lines or scrunch lines [30].

The nasal muscle is innervated by the facial nerve (7th pair of cranial nerves).

Injection technique

Bunny lines can be corrected or, in the case of treatment of the glabella with

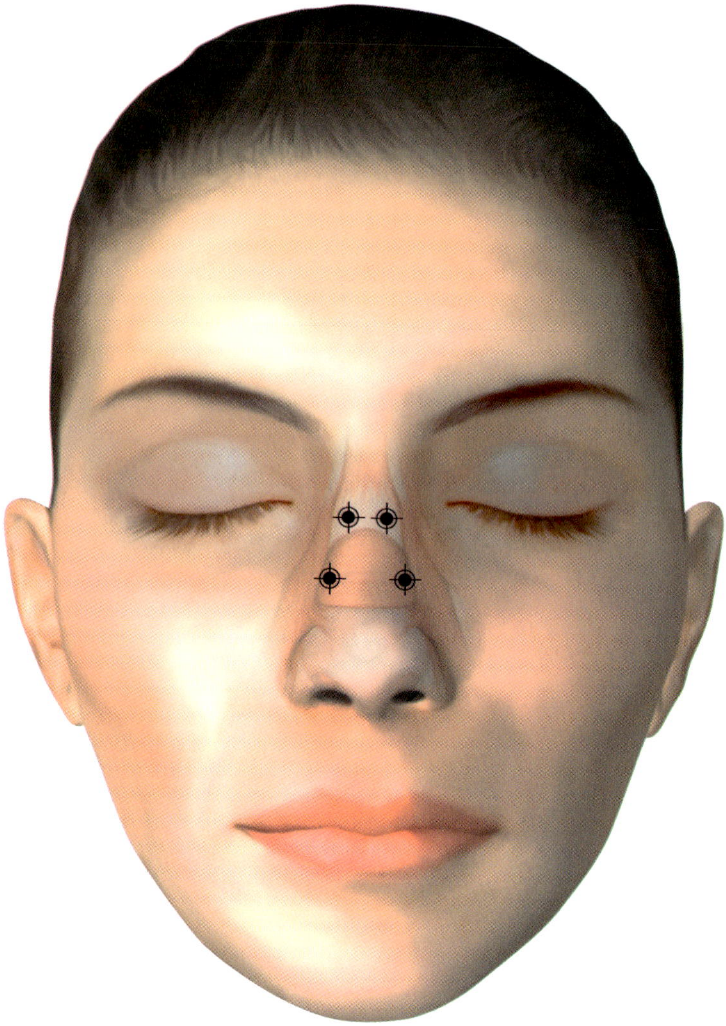

Figure 39 Injection points on the transversal part of the nasal muscle for the treatment of bunny lines with botulinum toxin

botulinum toxin, prevented by injecting a limited number of units of botulinum bilaterally into the nasal muscle or by performing a single central injection where the nasal muscle joins the procerus muscle (figs. 40-41). Three injection points can also be used, but the most recommended technique is two or four lateral injection points. The doses normally used vary from 2 to 5 U Botox per side (or 4-10 U Speywood) (fig. 39; videos 3.11 and 3.12).
Injection sites should be high on the nose and shallow to avoid excessive paralysis of the deeper, more caudal levator labii superioris muscle and the nasal alar. Excessive chemodenervation of this muscle can cause upper lip ptosis.

Injections should also be made above and medially to the angular vein, the uppermost segment of the facial vein, which runs deeply above and to the side of the nasal muscle; accidental puncture of its branches should be avoided due to the possibility of bruising [31].

VIDEO 3.11

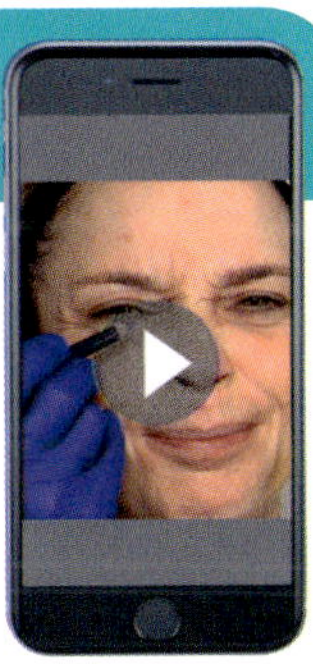

Bunny lines: contraction before treatment and drawing

VIDEO 3.12

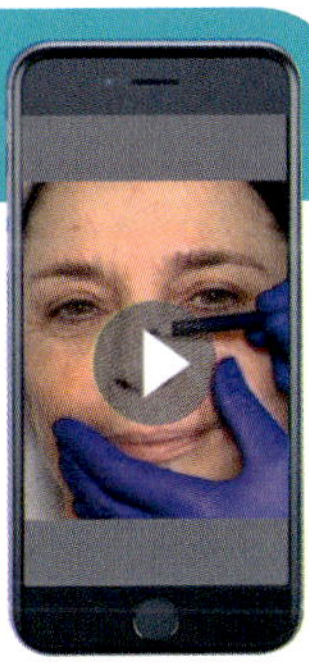

Bunny lines: injection technique with a dilution of 1.2 ml, a 33 G/9 mm needle, with intradermal injection

VIDEO 3.13

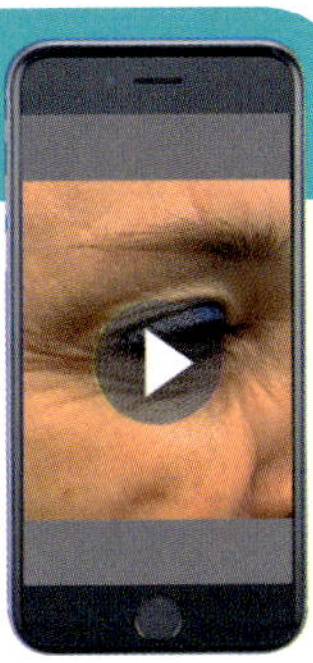

Bunny lines: contraction after treatment

CLINICAL CASES

CLINICAL CASE 11

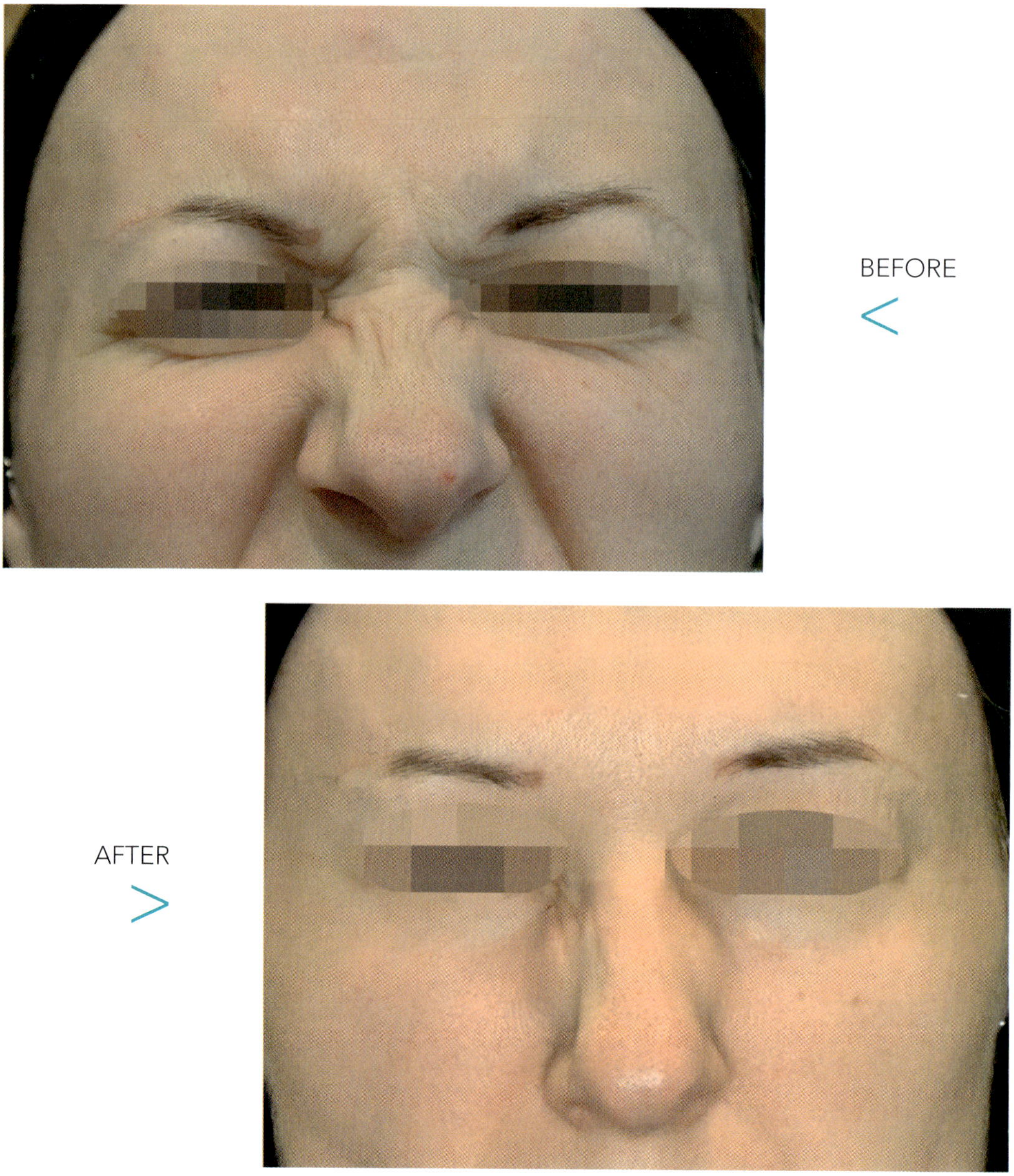

Figure 40 48 year-old patient before and after treatment of bunny lines with botulinum (frontal view, dynamic)

CLINICAL CASES

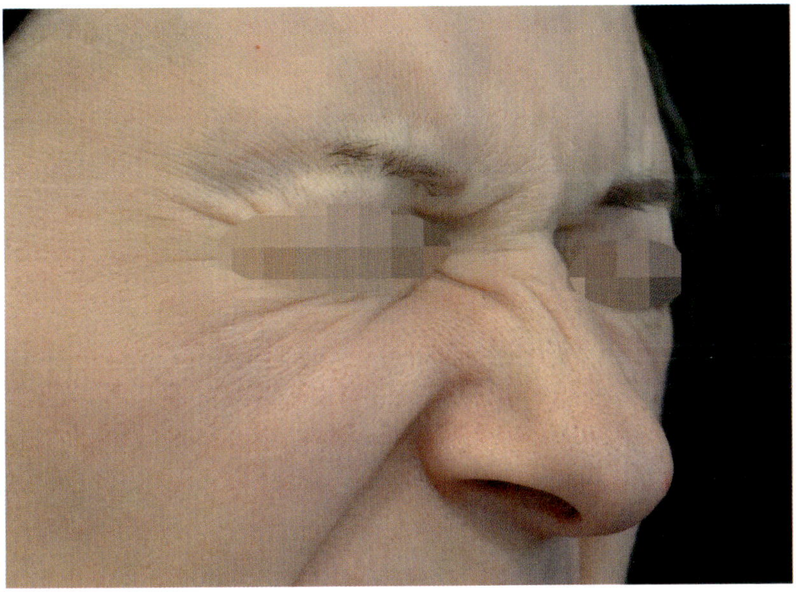

BEFORE

<

AFTER

>

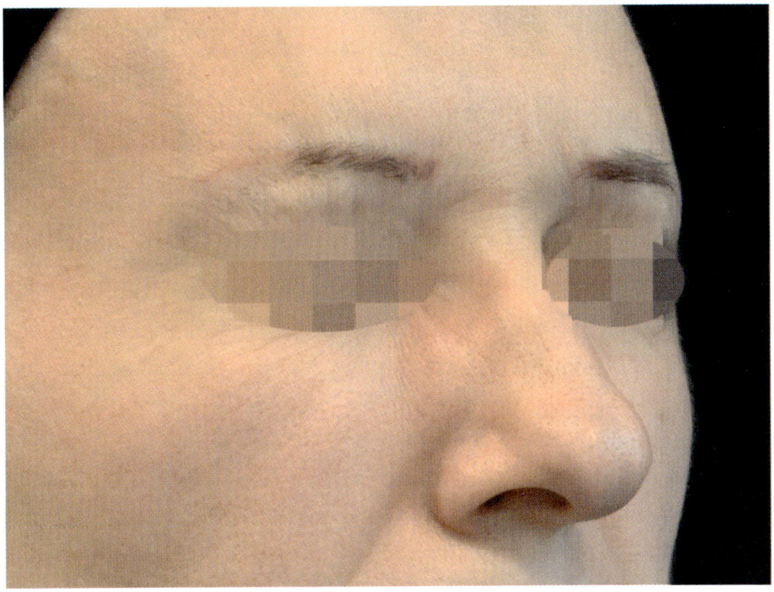

Figure 41 48 year-old patient before and after treatment of bunny lines with botulinum (right lateral view, static)

MASSETER HYPERTROPHY

Alberto Diaspro

Benign hypertrophy of the masseter muscle is characterised by the prominent profile of the angle of the mandible, which can be considered aesthetically unpleasant: it can be unilateral, resulting in facial asymmetry, or bilateral, resulting in the square appearance of the mandibular profile [32].

It is a phenomenon of uncertain aetiology attributable to a number of bio-psycho-social factors (emotional stress), neurogenic factors (primary or drug-induced bruxism) or altered facial development (facial hemiatrophy), so the aetiology is always multifactorial, in combination with a genetic predisposition.

The increase in muscle volume is not only secondary to excessive contraction, because the number of muscle fibres in the hypertrophic masseter is congenitally greater than in hyperactive muscles and normal masseter muscles (so-called functional hypertrophy).

The injection of botulinum is indicated for aesthetically defining the lower facial profile, leading to a reduction in muscle mass and therefore a less square appearance of the face, with an improvement especially in the female profile.

This treatment differs significantly depending on the geographic area: patients of Asian and Middle Eastern origin include this remodelling of the mandibular profile as one of the most popular treatments, due to the widespread presence of very prominent and hypertrophic masseter muscles compared to the Western population. In the European and American area, this correction is often concomitant with treatment of bruxism (see chapter 10) and more rarely required for aesthetic correction only [33].

Anatomy

The masseter muscle is one of the four fusiform masticatory muscles that elevate the mandible to allow the molar chewing of food. It is a strong quadrangular lamina in the outer part of the mandible, elevating it to open and close the mouth: it can be easily palpated from the corner of the mandible to the inferior and posterior edge and during contraction, when its anterior margin becomes easily perceptible. It originates from the lower edge of the middle and anterior third of the zygomatic arch, in front of the topographic projection of the temporomandibular joint and connects with the lateral surface of the angle of the mandible and the coronoid process of the mandible.

Injection technique

The most caudal portion of the muscle, topographically located below the trago-commissural line, is considered to be effective for treatment, to prevent the migration of botulinum to the zygomaticus major muscle, located more superficially and cranially in relation to the injection site, which results in a significant alteration of the smile (video 3.14).

It is also necessary to palpate the contracting muscle at its anterior edge,

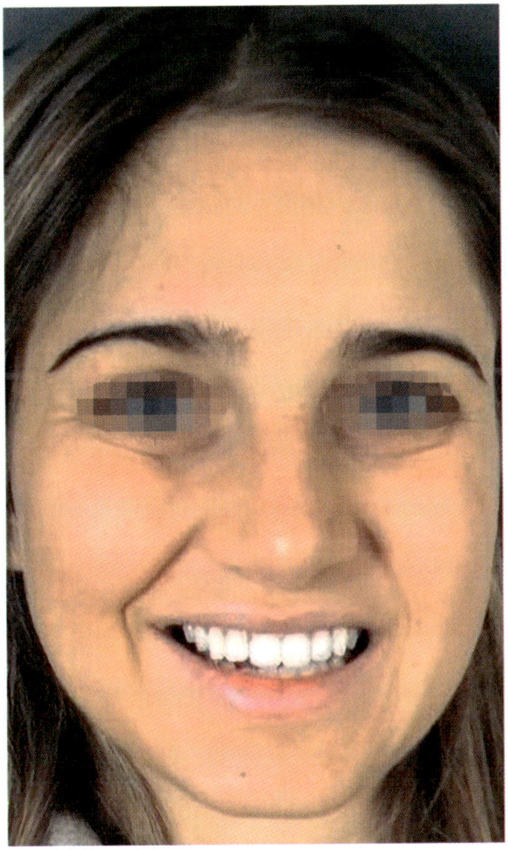

VIDEO 3.14

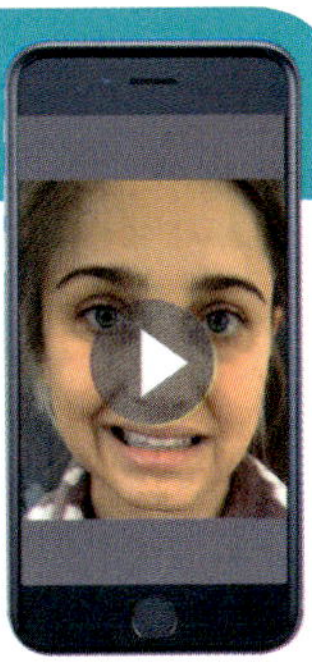

Masseter hypertrophy

Figure 42
Migration of the effect of the botulinum to the risorius muscle and the zygomaticus major and minor muscles on the left, due to excessively shallow injection: limitation of the exposure of the buccal corridors when smiling

and not to inject further forward into the cheek, or backward into the parotid gland. In the first case, the migration of botulinum can weaken the risorius muscle, with a limitation of the exposure of the buccal corridors when smiling (fig. 42, video 3.14), while in the second case, it can limit the secretion of saliva, which is not clinically significant but makes the treatment ineffective due to the incorrect injection site.
Once the injection area has been defined below the trago-commissural line, three injection points in topographical correspondence with the points of greatest hypertrophy during contraction are identified, all in the deep plane, after reaching the bone surface of the mandibular ramus with the tip of the needle, always asking the patient to keep the muscle relaxed during the injection (fig. 43).
As the injection is deep, a 30 G needle with a length of at least 13 mm is recommended, but the use of needles up to 25 mm is preferable as this muscle is very thick.
Up to 10 U Botox (20 U Speywood) per point are injected, depending on the volume of muscle treated, in a symmetrical injection pattern (video 10.1): the result, with reduction of the lower facial diameter (figs. 44-45), becomes clinically evident at between four and

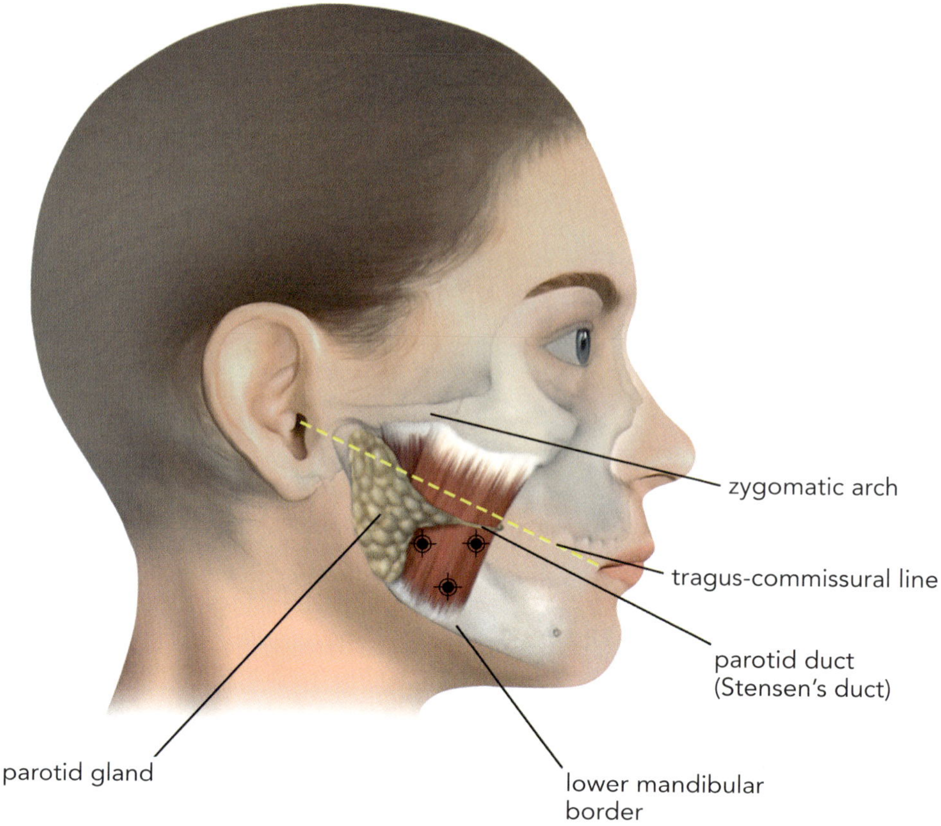

Figure 43 Masseter muscle injection sites

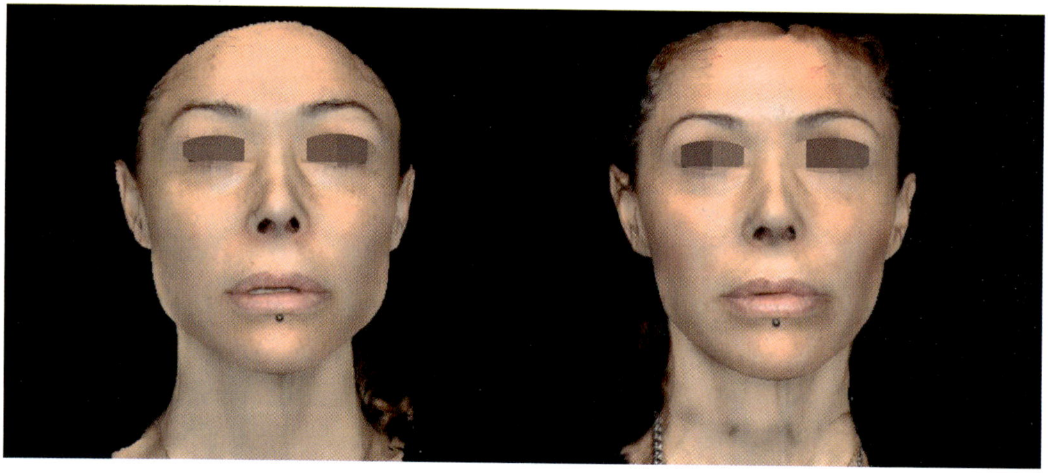

Figure 44 Frontal view before and thirty days after treatment with botulinum (computer-processed stereophotogrammetric images)

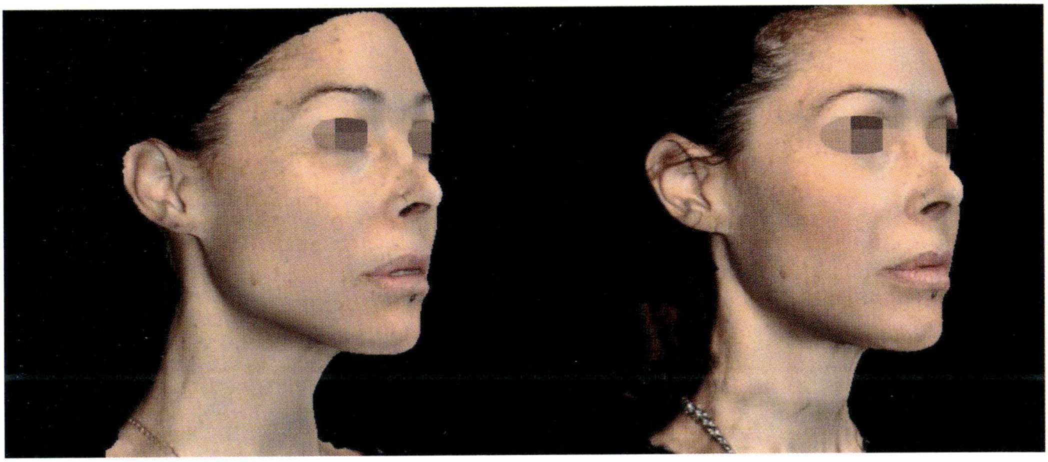

Figure 45 Lateral view before and thirty days after treatment with botulinum (computer-processed stereophotogrammetric images)

six weeks and is maintained for the following six months [34].

In the case of asymmetric hypertrophy, a different dose of botulinum per hemiface should be considered, but it is advisable to reserve this treatment for experienced injectors.

Overdose is rare and may result in perception of decreased mastication force, which is nevertheless guaranteed by the action of the temporalis muscle, with spontaneous resolution over time. It is important to bear in mind that overdosing can result in hypotrophy of the masseter muscle with excessive emptying of the cheek region, especially in individuals with a very thin face [35-36].

FLARING NOSTRILS

Alberto Diaspro

Flaring of the nostrils during breathing can be caused by certain pathological conditions (pneumonia, bronchiolitis, epiglottitis, asthma) or can occur after intense physical exercise, stimulated by the need to get more air into the lungs quickly. However, it can also be an expression of oromandibular dystonia, which is more common in women of African or Asian ethnicity.

The nostrils of a normally breathing person should not flare and a differential diagnosis of a primary respiratory disease, such as pneumonia or asthma, or cardiogenic dyspnoea, should always be made because of the risk of treating an epiphenomenon with botulinum.

However, it does occur in certain individuals following hyperactivity of the nostril dilator muscle, in which case it can be effectively treated with the injection of botulinum [37].

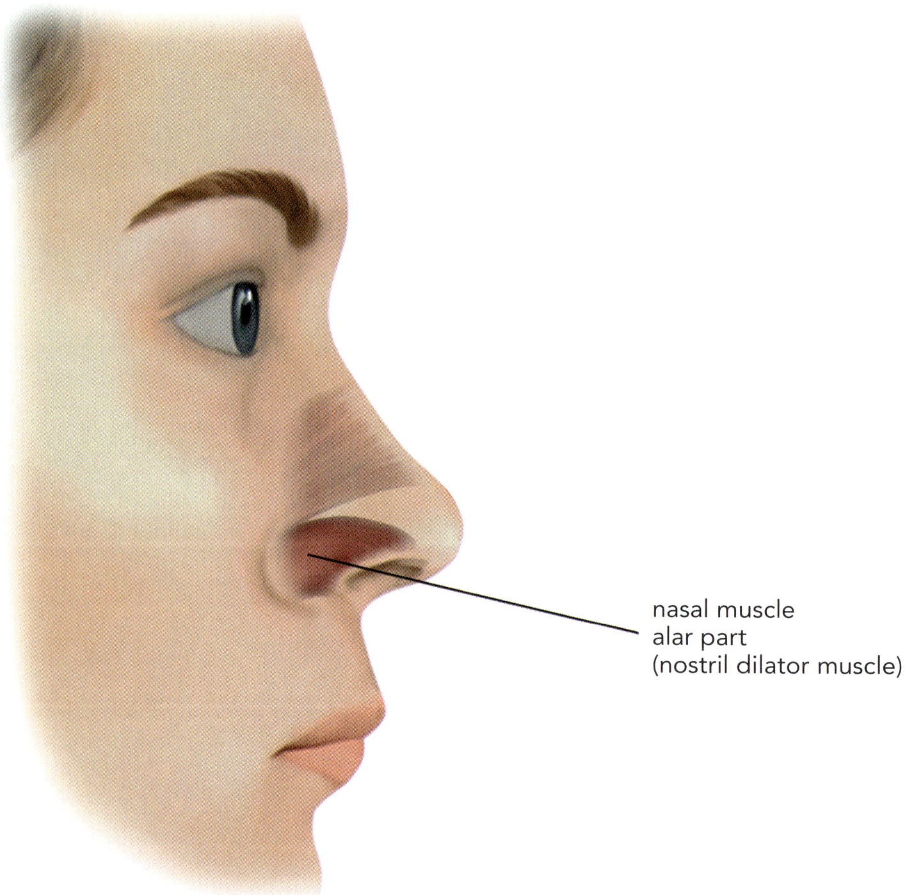

Figure 46 Anatomy of the nasal muscle, alar part

Anatomy

The nostril dilator muscle is located in the thickness of the lower edge of the nasal alar, made up of the caudal portion (pars alare) of the nasal muscle, extending to the lateral crus region of the alar cartilage (fig. 46). Its contraction causes the nostril to flare, displacing the nasal alar sideways (the transverse pars of the nasal muscle is responsible for lines caused by wrinkling the nose) [38].

Injection technique

An intramuscular injection is administered, then under the dermis and over the cartilage, 4 mm from the free edge between the tip of the nose and the naso-labial fold using 2 U Botox or 5 U Speywood [40]. Injection more posteriorly is to be avoided because of the risk of migration to the levator labii muscles.

Relaxation of the nostril dilator muscle leads to a reduction in the nostril opening, reducing the dilation of the nostrils and giving the nose a slimmer appearance when viewed from the front, with stable results for up to three months [40].

LOWER THIRD

PERIORAL LINES

Patrizia Piersini

As the lips age, there is involution of the skin and mucous membrane, attenuation or disappearance of the vermilion line and loss of firmness, with frequent vertical lines in the perioral region.

The lips are definitely an area of the face that is particularly affected by the ageing process. Remembering that the volume and, therefore, the vertical height of the upper and lower lips should be within the divine or golden ratio of 1:1.618 respectively [41], we can see that, as the years go by, the upper lip becomes longer, with a loss of projection and consequently less exposure of the vermillion (the red part of the lip) (fig. 47).

The flattening of the vermilion border, the dividing line between the mucous membrane and skin of the lip, leads to a loss of definition of the lips, and patients often complain of difficulty in applying lipstick due to the tendency for it to bleed into the peribuccal folds [42]. These fine, dynamic, vertical lines (which give this condition the name "barcode") are the result of the continuous movement of the orbicularis oris muscle (fig. 48) and the loss of elasticity in the skin, which makes them visible even at rest. They are not

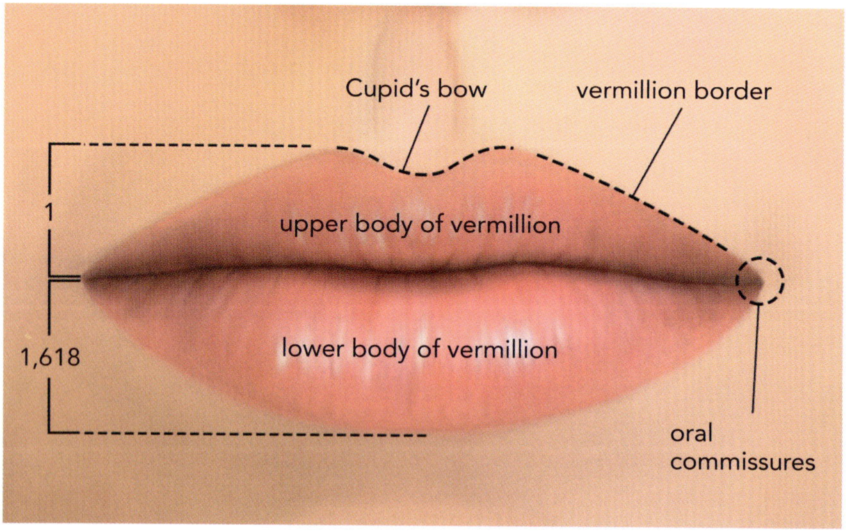

Figure 47 Anatomy of the lip surface

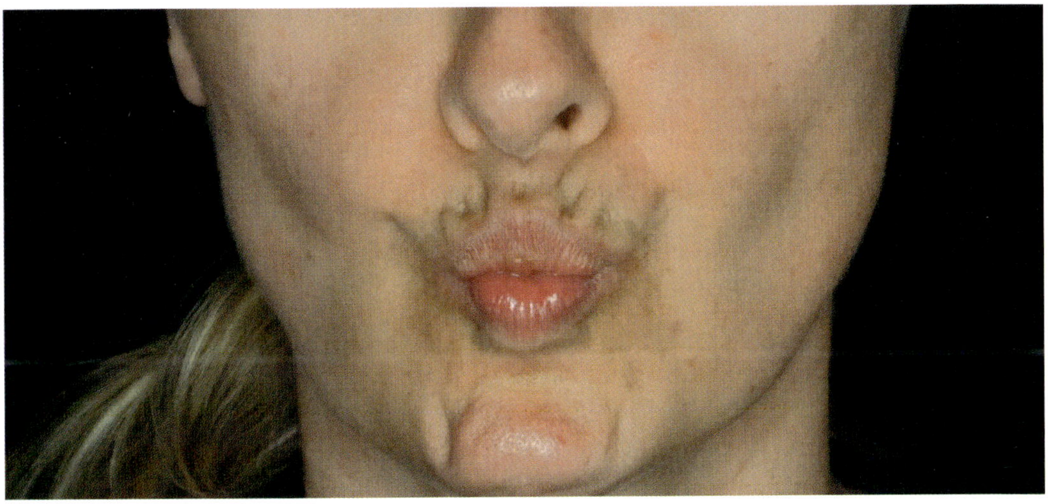

Figure 48 Repeated contraction of the orbicularis oris muscle leads to the formation of perioral lines

always age-related and occur earlier in female smokers, which is why they are also called "smoker's wrinkles", and in thin skin with actinic damage. Although they are very fine lines, they are hard to treat with fillers alone, because even the slightest overcorrection can lead to unsightly protrusion of the upper lip or the visibility of the implant as an unsightly ridge along the length of the wrinkle. The association of different techniques, such as chemical peeling, fractional laser, needling or botulinum, is recommended in order to obtain more satisfactory results in the treatment of this imperfection.

It is also essential to consider that the use of fillers in this region plays a more important role than the use of the neuromodulator, and fillers should always be used before considering the use of botulinum toxin, to restore the correct structure and provide support [43].

In this area, however, botulinum toxin achieves a further improvement, making the dynamic perioral lines less noticeable and creating a visual effect of increased fullness of the lip, thanks to a pleasant eversion of the upper lip [44].

Anatomy

The orbicularis oris muscle, from the Latin orbicularis meaning circular, is so called because it was previously thought to be a sphincter muscle, made up of a complete series of ellipses of striated muscles, surrounding the oral cavity. This theory is no longer considered current, as the fibres of this muscle do not branch out uniformly in a circular fashion but run in various directions [41]. The orbicularis oris is a complex muscle, attached to the dermis of the upper and lower lip by a thin, superficial muscular-aponeurotic system, and serves as an anchorage point for other muscles in the oral region. This muscle can be considered as a single muscle anatomically, but

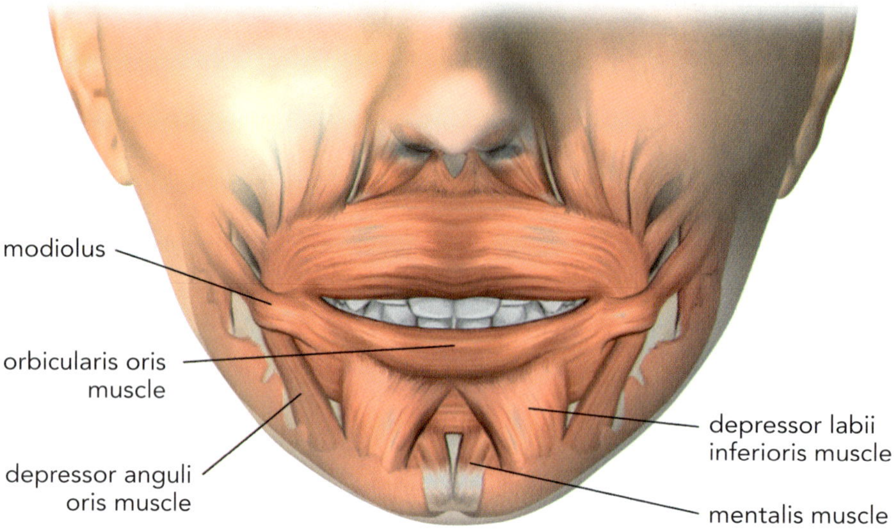

Figure 49 Anatomy of the muscles of the perioral region

functionally it appears to be made up of different parts acting both independently and together with other facial muscles [45]. It has no bone or tendon origin.

The orbicularis oris is made up of independent quadrants (superior, inferior, right and left), consisting of two well-defined parts, a more represented peripheral part and a marginal part found in all primate mammals but developed only in the human species, to be able to articulate sounds.

The peripheral part of each quadrant of the orbicularis oris muscle originates in the labial surface of the modiolus and it is thought that the muscle fibres are reinforced by fibres that, in the upper lip, originate from the buccinator, the levator anguli oris and the zygomaticus major, while in the lower lip they originate from the buccinator and the depressor anguli oris (fig. 49).

The orbicularis oris muscle has a dual function: the deep part performs a constricting action and is responsible for the sphincter action of the mouth; this is known as the "archaic" part of the muscle. The superficial part, on the other hand, is related to facial expressions and precise movements of the lips, necessary for the articulation of language.

The orbicularis oris also acts in association with the cheek muscles to maintain contact between the teeth and cheeks, which is necessary to prevent the stagnation of food during chewing. It helps with phonation and plays an important role in swallowing, chewing and sucking.

This muscle also allows the protrusion of the lips (when kissing or whistling, for example) and is used by musicians to play wind instruments. The muscle is innervated by the buccal and marginal mandibular ramifications of the facial nerve [46].

Injection technique

In order to relax the fibres of the orbicularis oris, without creating a real paresis that can seriously interfere with the important functions of this muscle, it is important to inject the muscle very superficially and with precise symmetry, with 1-2 U Botox (2 U Speywood) per injection point. The points are identified by asking the patient to pucker their lips, as if pronouncing the letter U. Two points per half-lip are drawn on the upper lip skin, about two mm above the edge of the vermilion and about five mm from both the philtrum ridge and the labial commissure. For the wrinkles of the lower lip, which are not always present, two or three points about five mm from the labial commissure, equidistant from each other and about two mm below the edge of the vermilion can be identified (fig. 50). Videos 3.15 and 3.16 show drawing and injection technique for perioral wrinkles (barcode) and vermilion eversion using a dilution of 1.2 ml, 33 G/9 mm needle, intradermal injection.
With this technique, the vertical lines will soften (figs. 51-52) and an eversion of the upper lip will also be achieved (figs. 53-54).
The injection should be performed slowly and with constant pressure to reduce the painful sensation of the injection and the possibility of bruising.

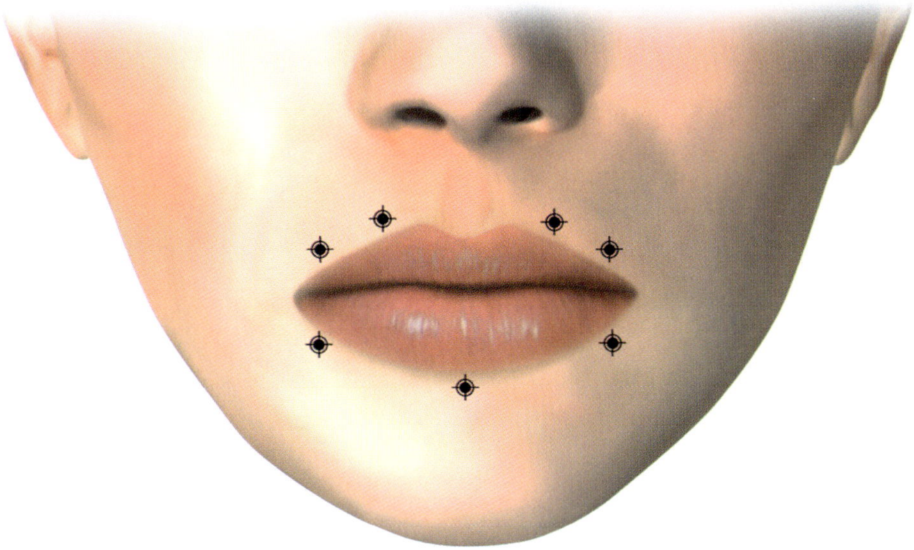

Figure 50 Injection points for the treatment of perioral lines of the upper and lower skin lip

VIDEO 3.15

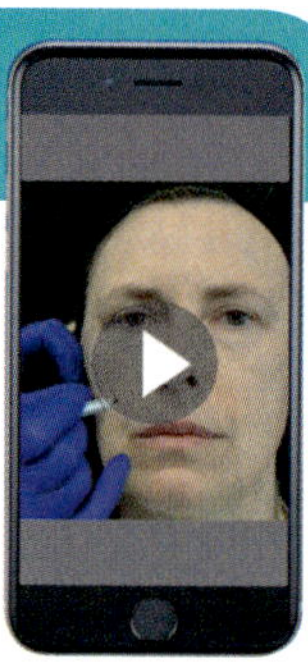

Perioral wrinkles (barcode) and vermilion eversion: injection point drawing

VIDEO 3.16

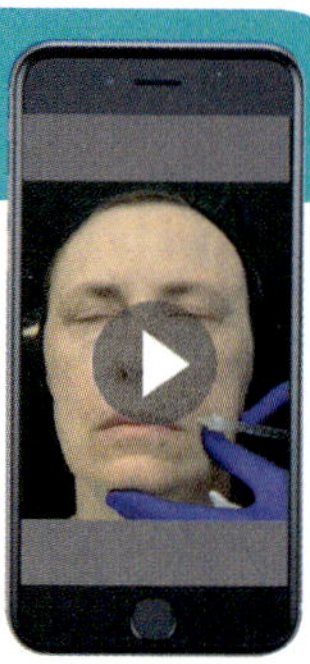

Perioral wrinkles (barcode) and vermilion eversion: injection technique using a 33 G/9 mm needle

The challenge in using botulinum toxin in this area is to be able to treat perioral lines while perfectly preserving the functionality of the orbicularis oris muscle, also considering that the duration is very limited in time due to the low doses injected. It is therefore clear that this is a technique for experienced injectors.

CLINICAL CASES

CLINICAL CASE 12

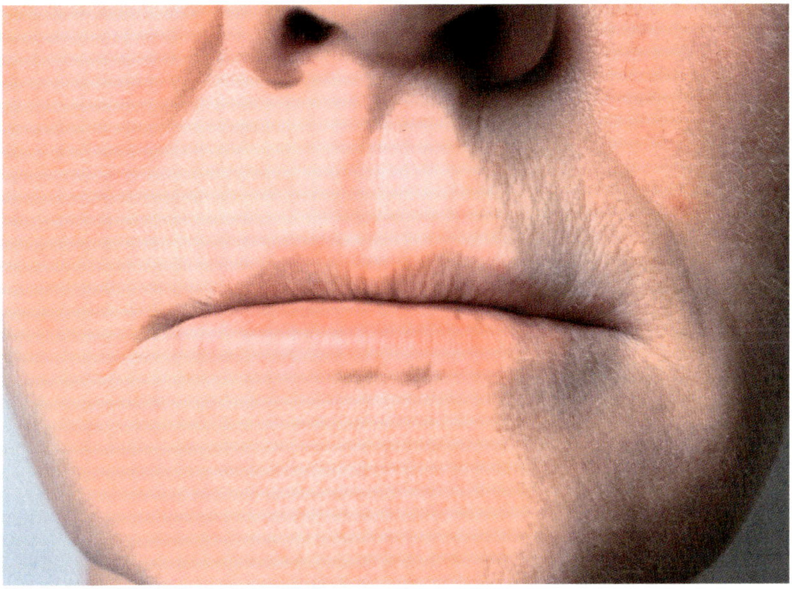

BEFORE

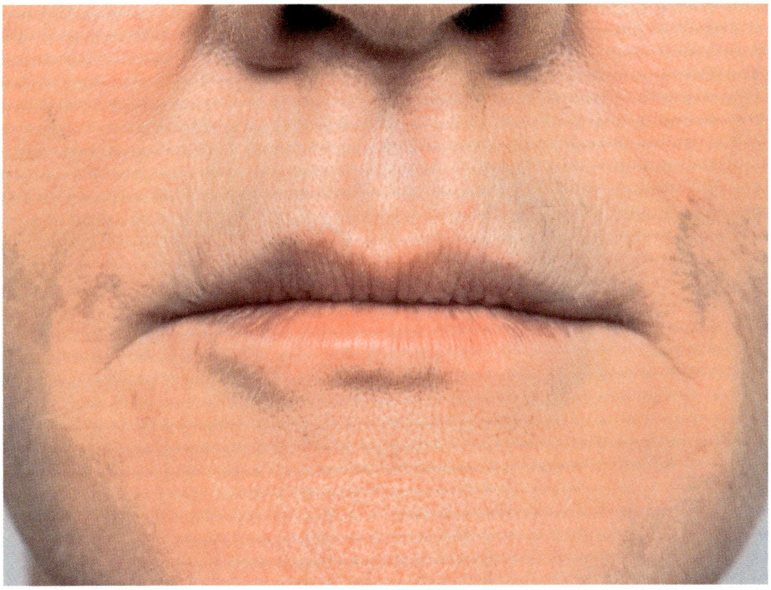

AFTER

Figure 51 61 year-old patient before and 30 days after treatment with botulinum for perioral lines and vermillion eversion (frontal view)

CLINICAL CASES

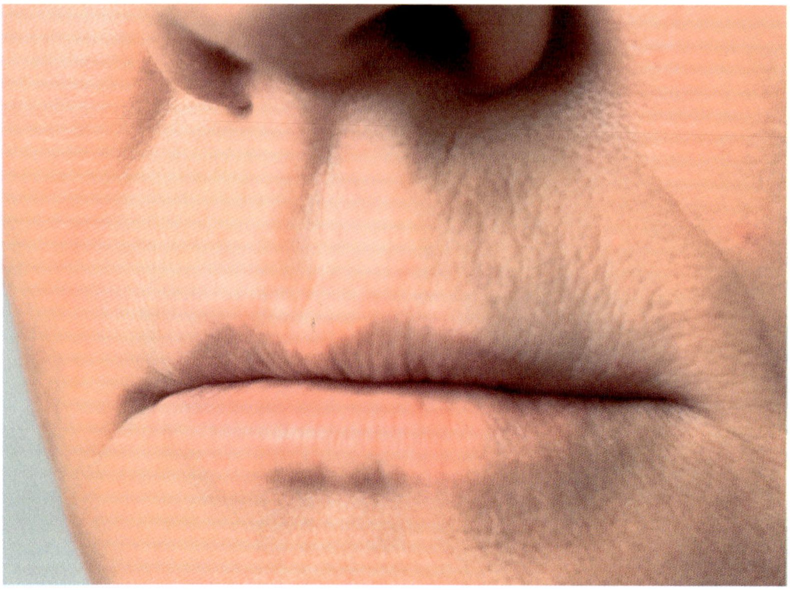

BEFORE

<

AFTER

>

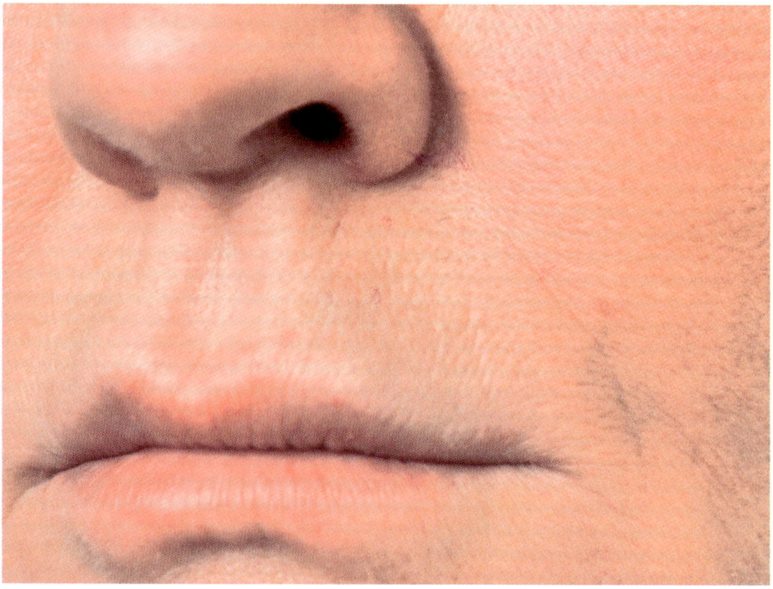

Figure 52 Same patient before and 30 days after treatment with botulinum for perioral lines and vermillion eversion (left side)

CLINICAL CASES

CLINICAL CASE 13

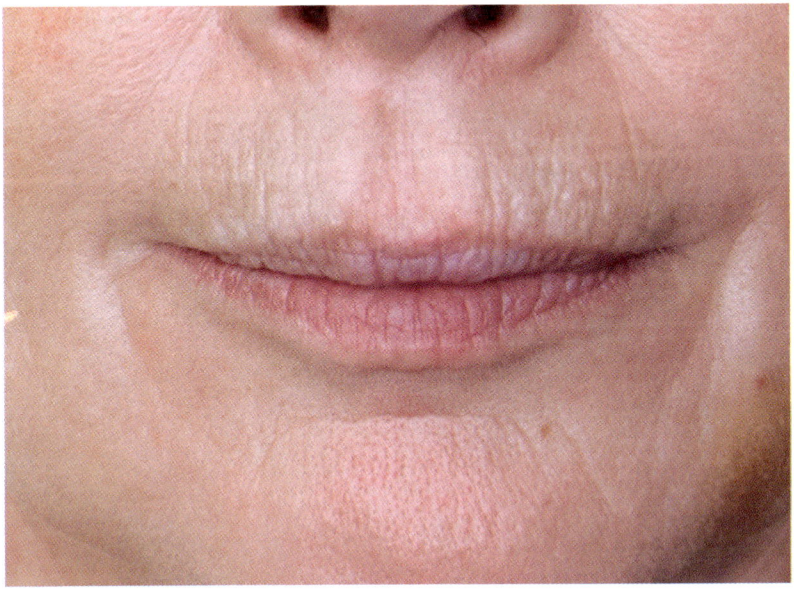

BEFORE

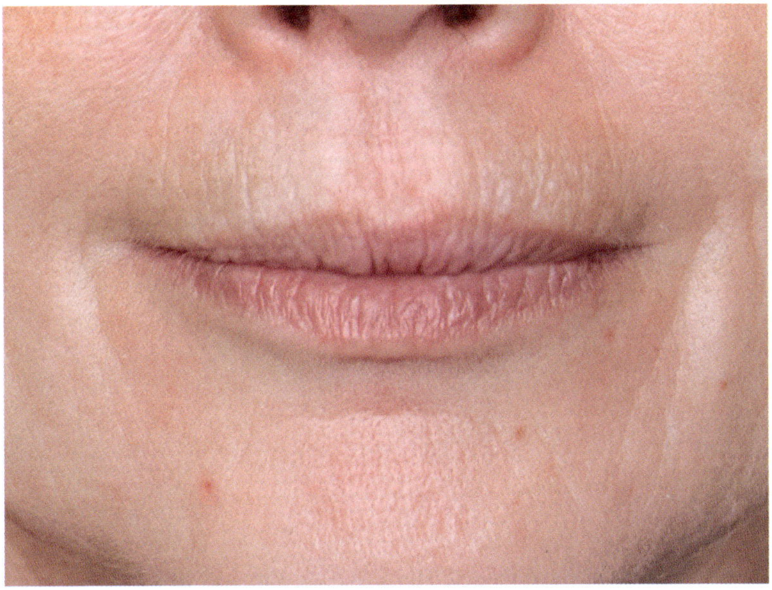

AFTER

Figure 53 53 year-old patient before and 30 days after treatment with botulinum for vermillion eversion (frontal view)

CLINICAL CASES

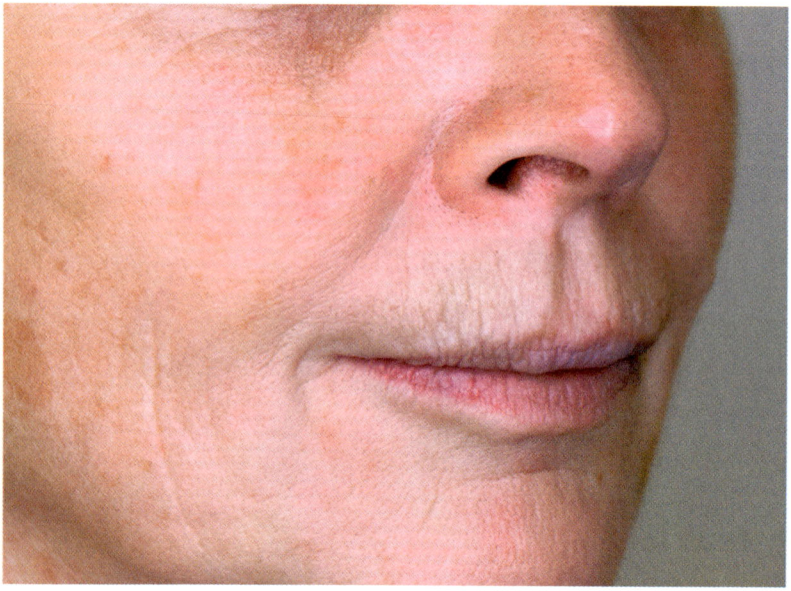

BEFORE

<

AFTER

>

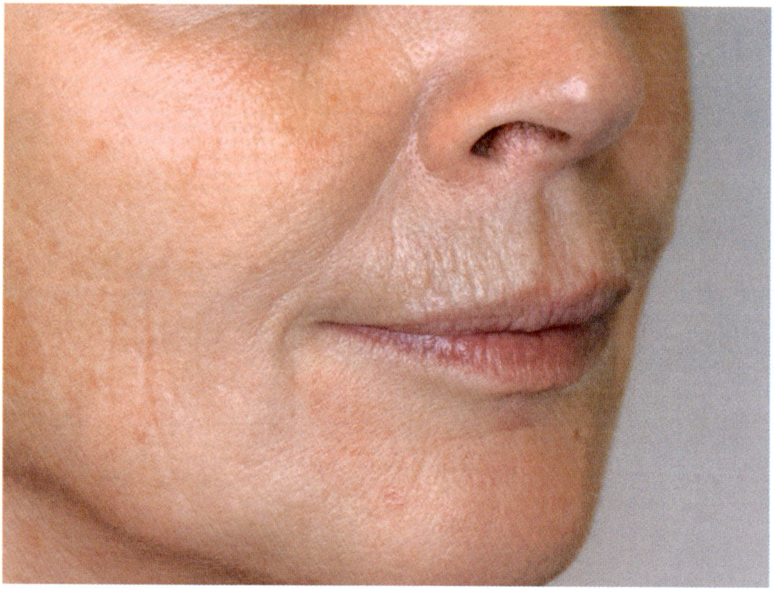

Figure 54 Same patient before and 30 days after treatment with botulinum for vermillion eversion (right side)

GUMMY SMILE

Alberto Diaspro

The smile is definitely an element of charm and powerful empathy: an upwardly curved upper lip exposes the incisors and gum line by 1-2 mm. An aesthetically pleasing smile, therefore, is the result of the visual balance between white (the teeth), pink (the gums) and the lips.

However, when it exposes the gums by more than 2 mm, it takes on an unsatisfactory aesthetic appearance, leading to increasing demand by patients for improvement (fig. 55).

Gummy smile affects about 7% of men and 14% of women [47].

This imperfection can be caused by various factors: excessive vertical growth of the maxilla, incomplete tooth eruption with reduced exposure of the crown of the upper incisors, an anatomically short upper lip or muscular overactivity of the upper lip, either individually or combined, can lead to its appearance.

Excessive gum exposure, secondary to excessive vertical maxillary growth or excessive extrusion of the dento-alveolar complex, can be treated by dento-alveolar or orthognathic surgery in combination with orthodontic treatment, which may be sufficient on its own in some cases.

Excessive gum exposure due to delayed tooth eruption, on the other hand,

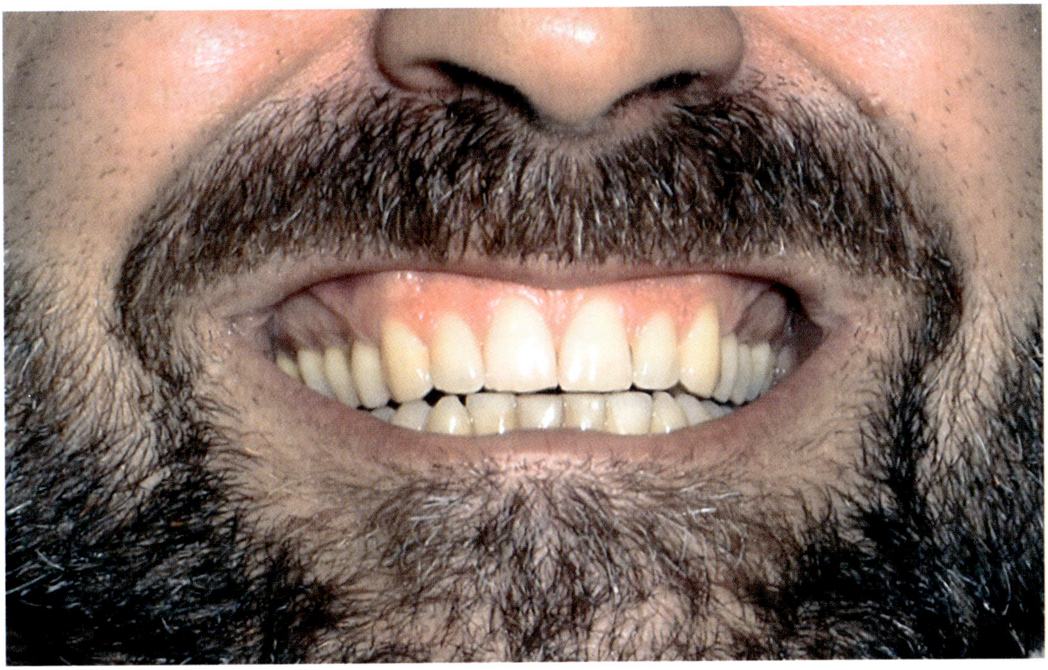

Figure 55 Exposure of more than 2 mm of gum while smiling, indication for correction

can be treated with surgical, periodontal and pre-prosthetic dental procedures, changing the shape of the tooth to define a more apical (cranial) gum margin.

The presence of an incompetent or short upper lip, another cause of gummy smile but, unlike the previous ones, not of skeletal origin, can be effectively treated by surgical repositioning, limiting the action of the elevator muscles consisting of the zygomaticus major muscle and zygomaticus minor muscle (ZMJ and ZMI), the orbicularis oris (OO), the levator labii superioris (LLS) and the levator labii superioris alaeque nasi (LLSAN) [48].

Lastly, if the gummy smile is caused by hyperactivity of the upper lip, it can be treated on an outpatient basis, to the patient's satisfaction, using minimally invasive treatments such as hyaluronic acid fillers [47] or botulinum toxin.

Anatomy

Lip movement is the result of synergistic activity between the levator labii superioris, the levator labii superioris alaeque nasi, the zygomaticus minor and the zygomaticus major muscles.

The levator labii superioris alaeque nasi lifts the lip upwards while the other mimetic muscles, the levator labii superiori, the zygomaticus minor and the zygomaticus major, lift the lip and the corner of the mouth superolaterally.

The insertion of the levator labii superioris muscle is covered by that of the levator labii superioris alaeque nasi and of the zygomaticus minor, and these three muscles converge in the lateral area of the alar cartilage, precisely at the ideal injection point for the action of botulinum toxin A.

The levator labii superioris alaeque nasi muscle is, therefore, the only muscle that lifts the lip supero-medially, in particular with its deep portion (fig. 56), while the more superficial part determines the synergistic movements of the nasal alar, with the nasal muscle receiving some fibres from the levator labii superioris and the alaeque nasi (fig. 57).

Injection technique

Gummy smile due to overactivity of the upper lip is treated by injecting botulinum toxin laterally to the alar cartilage of the nose, where the naso-labial fold begins, at the insertion site of the levator labii superioris, levator labii superioris alaeque nasi and zygomaticus minor (fig. 58).

The action of the toxin leads to a reduction in the action of the levator labii superioris muscles, with reduced lifting of the lip when we smile.

A total of 5 U Botox or 2-3 U Speywood are injected into the muscle bilaterally (2-3 on each side) where the three muscles converge: this causes the smile line to lower at maximum contraction, with results appearing within 7-14 days and generally lasting about four months (fig. 58) [49].

The effective dose must be assessed by the doctor in relation to the patient's facial activity, bearing in mind that the dosage may vary between women and men, with men generally requiring a higher dosage due to their greater muscle volume.

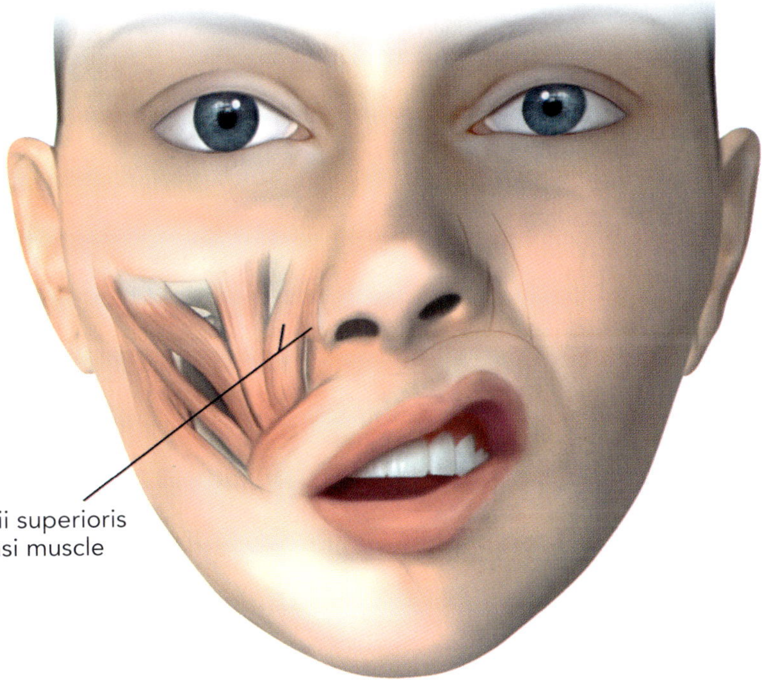

Figure 56 The levator labii superioris alaeque nasi (LLSAN) muscle is the only muscle that lifts the lip supero-medially, with its deep portion, while the more superficial part determines the synergistic movements of the nasal alar

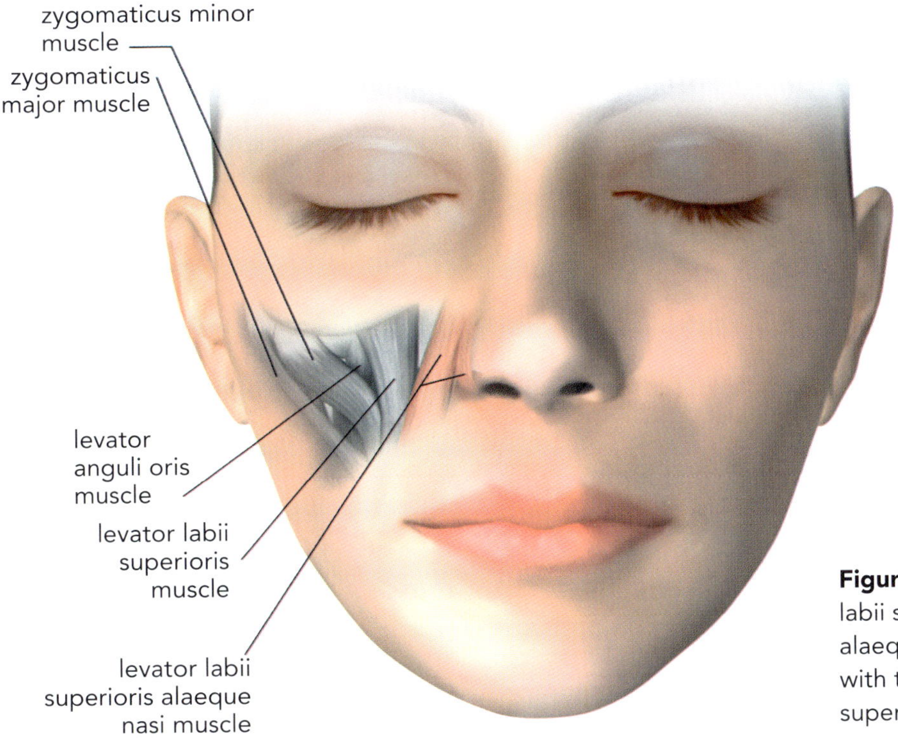

Figure 57 Levator labii superioris alaeque nasi (LLSAN) with the deep and superficial portions

It is also important to bear in mind that excessive doses can lead to ptosis and elongation of the lip, with consequent non-exposure of the teeth while smiling. This is especially true in patients where this is already present for age-related reasons [50]. In addition, unexpected muscle synkinesis or lip asymmetry may appear while smiling [51]. This treatment is usually requested by young patients or young adults, who benefit most from the result obtained, not only from an aesthetic point of view but also psychologically, because gummy smile often lowers the patient's self-esteem and leads them to hide or control their smile.

CLINICAL CASES

CLINICAL CASE 14

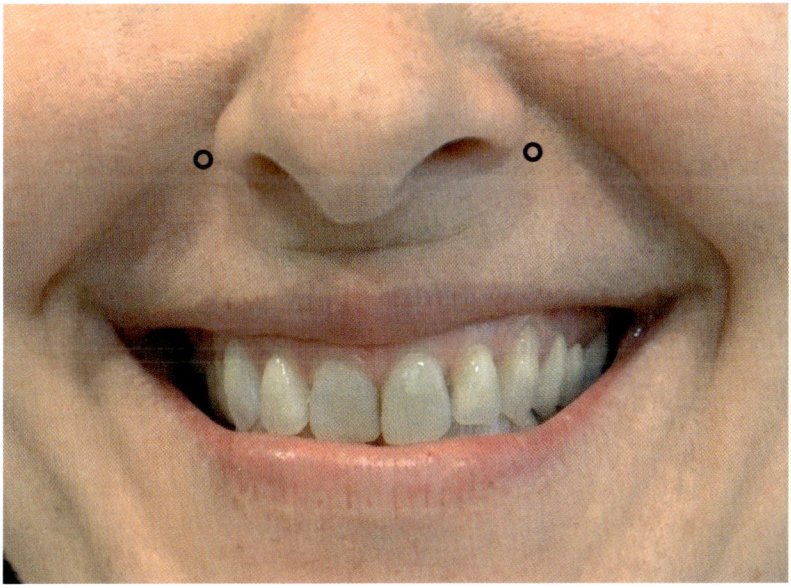

BEFORE

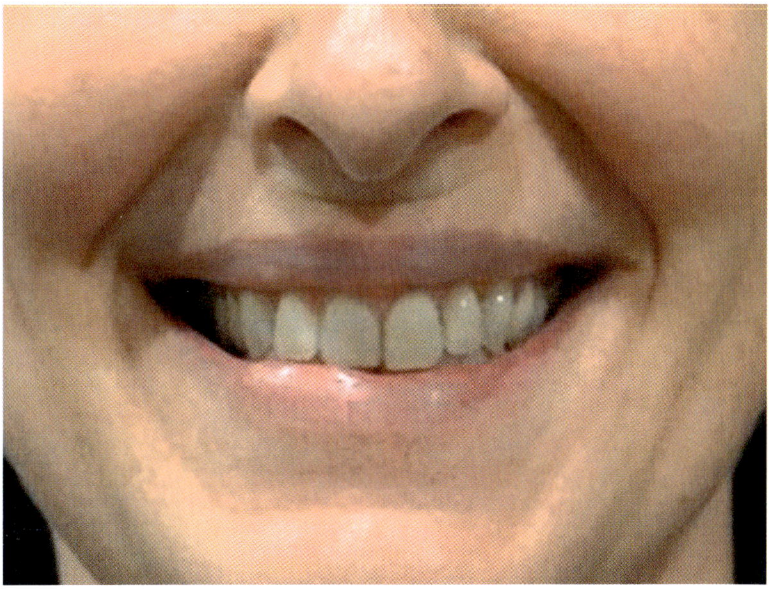

AFTER

Figure 58 Botulinum injection points. Before treatment and 15 days after injection with botulinum (photo courtesy of Patrizia Piersini)

MARIONETTE LINES

Gabriele Muti

Marionette lines are wrinkles that evoke a rather clear image. A puppet on a string has a split jaw, so that the puppeteer can open and close its mouth, so that it looks as though the puppet is talking. Humans develop folds in exactly the same area over time. These lines run from the outer corners of the lips to the outer corners of the chin. Because of their droopy appearance, marionette lines can make a face look perpetually sullen. As always, treatment is not simple and can be complicated.

Apart from hereditary factors, gravity is the main factor responsible when it comes to marionette lines. Over many years, the force of gravity exerts its control over our faces, causing the initially firm and taut skin to sag downwards and medially. The skin tissue collects on the chin, often forming lines on both sides.

This process is aggravated by a general loss of volume that occurs with age (the breakdown of soft tissue, fat and structural proteins such as collagen and elastin), resulting in a sagging effect. As with any other sign of skin ageing, lifestyle factors such as suntanning and smoking can also have a negative impact.

Anatomically, the marionette line extends from the lateral modiole of the lip to the medial insurgence of the muscle that turns down the corner of the mouth, better known as the DAO (depressor anguli oris) (fig. 59). The same muscle develops at the side of the marionette line as a triangle, where the upper point is represented by the modiole, while the two lower points are located medially on the marionette line and about one cm to the side of it. Originating from the periosteum of the mandibular margin, its contraction tends to lateralise and lower the corner of the mouth. The DAO partially covers the DLI (depressor labii inferioris) with its most medial portion and cooperates with it in lip movement. This is a key point to consider when treating the DAO with botulinum toxin.

The buccal ramus of the facial nerve enters the muscle through the middle third of the lateral margin of the DAO and then spreads out. At the same time, the mandibular marginal ramus of the facial nerve enters the muscle through the lower third of the lateral margin of the DAO [52,53].

As we know, the best results can be obtained when the toxin is used in the upper third, while the lower middle third should be more the preserve of very experienced doctors. The DAO is treated in patients with pronounced hypertrophy or in support of treatment with hyaluronic acid. The filler acts by filling the gap that forms between the chin and the cheek, lending continuity to the skin. Treatment of the DAO, which is usually carried out 15 days before treatment with filler, occurs when its movement directly affects the visibility of the marionette line.

There are two different techniques for treating the DAO, each of which have different pros and cons [54-56].

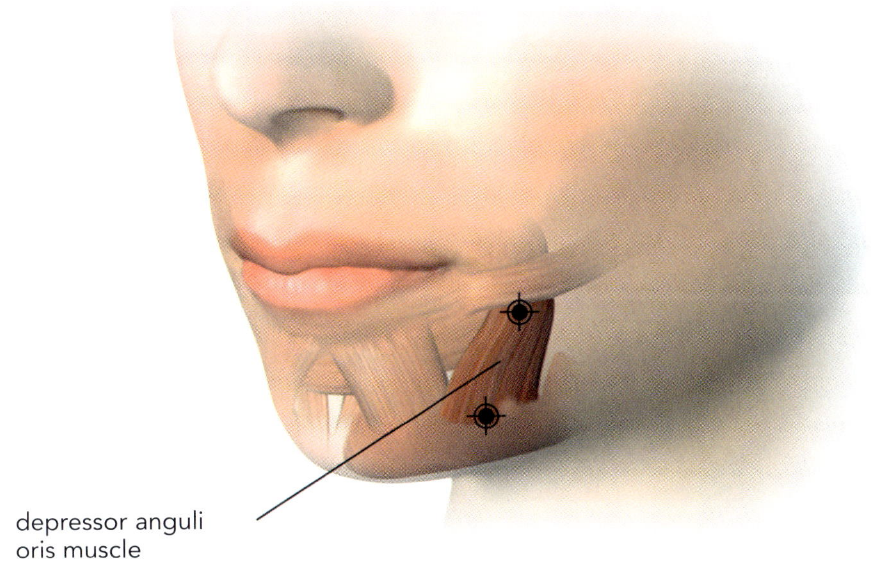

Figure 59 The anatomy of the marionette line is also determined by the position of the depressor anguli oris (DAO) muscle and its action upon contraction. The injection points, as indicated, are also chosen to avoid impairment of the depressor labii inferioris (DLI) muscle

In the first technique, action is taken directly on the main portion of the muscle belly. The injection point is one cm above the mandibular margin and 1 cm to the side of the prolongation of the line joining the nasal alar to the corner of the oral commissure (fig. 59). The cephalic portion of the DAO does not overlap with the DLI and this ensures that, in the event of an injection error or excessive diffusion of the toxin, it cannot interact with a different muscle and thereby induce a distortion of the lower lip. In this case, 2-4 U of onabotulinum or incobotulinum and 5-10 U of abobotulinum are injected.

The other technique involves injecting 0.5 cm to the side of the cheilion (modiolus) and 0.5 cm below the line joining the two corners of the oral commissure. This prevents distortion of the lip due to the involvement of the DLI, but it is harder to act directly on the DAO. Again, 2-4 U of onabotulinum or incobotulinum and 5-10 U of abobotulinum are injected.

In both techniques, the 12 mm needle penetrates one third of its length and is inserted perpendicularly to the skin. As already mentioned, the clinical effect can be improved by injecting hyaluronic acid a fortnight later.

CLINICAL CASES

CLINICAL CASE 15

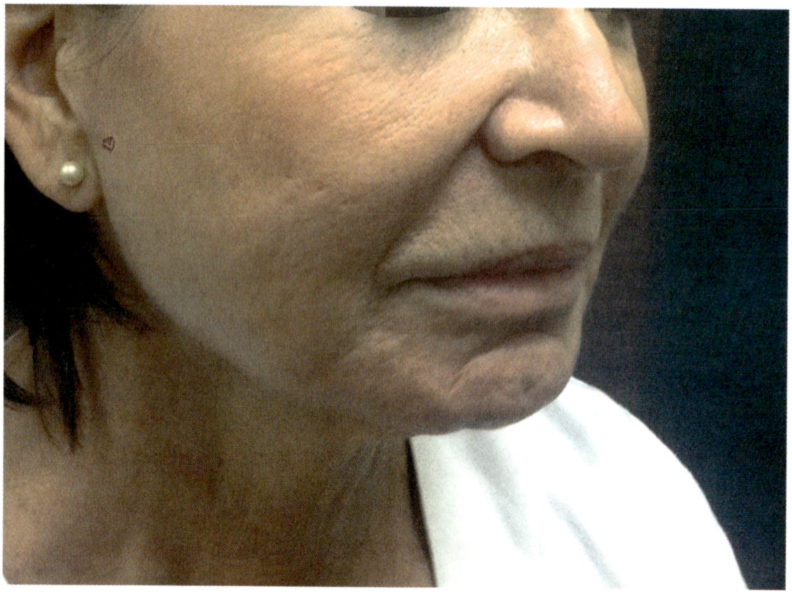

BEFORE
<

AFTER
>

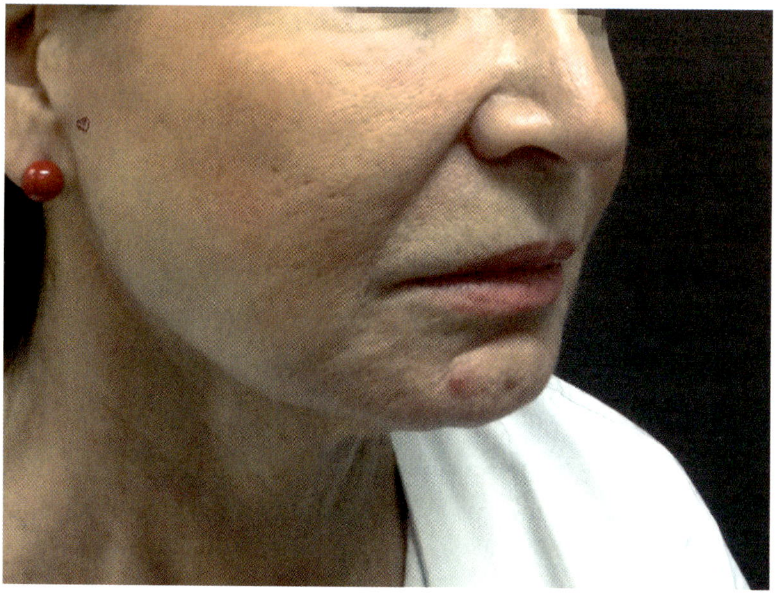

Figure 60 Patient treated with injection of botulinum toxin into the depressor anguli oris (DAO) muscle. Pictures taken before and after treatment. The reduction of muscle tone favours the improvement of the marionette line even in a situation of facial relaxation

CHIN PROFILE AND POPPY CHIN

Patrizia Piersini

In men, a square, more prominent chin accentuates the virility of the face and gives a more powerful appearance, while in women, a smaller, softer chin with rounded contours lends femininity and grace to the face (fig. 61).

Thanks to the use of fillers and botulinum toxin, the shape of the chin can be redefined and the skin surface can be adjusted. It can also be given an enhanced three-dimensional projection, making the face look more interesting and the proportions more correct.

Botulinum toxin can help improve the appearance of the chin in patients in which it tends to recede due to excessive contraction of the mentalis muscle. The pogonion (the central cephalometric point of the chin) is repositioned, creating a more harmonious profile [57]; this is achieved by limiting the contraction of the mentalis muscle, which leads to the shortening and thickening of the muscle, and results in the forward projection of the pogonion on the sagittal plane. Thanks to the action of botulinum, it is possible to reposition the pogonion further back on the sagittal plane, limiting the contraction of the chin muscle

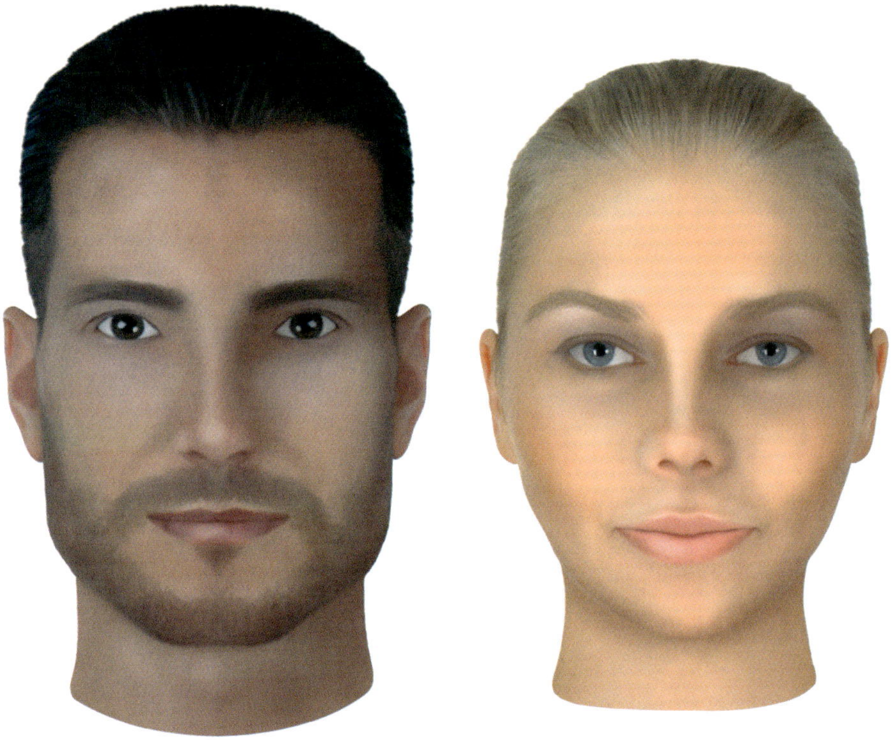

Figure 61 Differences between the male and female chin: in men the chin is square and prominent, while in women it is smaller and rounded

and consequently shortening it.
There is also another imperfection that we can improve with the help of type A botulinum toxin: so-called "poppy chin" (fig. 62). This condition is also known as orange-peel chin, cobblestone chin, pebble chin and dimpled chin [58] and is caused by hyperkinesis of the mentalis muscle. It consists in the formation of hollows on the surface of the chin with accentuation of the chin furrow where the muscle enters the soft tissues. Hypertone often, but not always, becomes evident with age, due to the loss of skin structure and subcutaneous fat; moreover, due to the atrophy of the mandibular bone, the mentalis muscle tends to be more voluminous and hypertonic because it is shorter.

Anatomy

The mentalis muscle is a conical and centrally-positioned mimetic muscle located deep in the tip of the chin. Its fibres originate from the incisive canal of the alveolar process of the mandible, in the lateral incisor region, spreading out and penetrating the skin and soft tissues of the chin, running vertically from the deep to the superficial plane [60]. The two ends of the muscle are usually separate, with fatty tissue between their origins. To the side of the mentalis muscle is the depressor labii inferioris (DLI), which overlaps the middle portion of the mentalis muscle, and even further to the side is the depressor anguli oris (DAO) (fig. 63).
The functions of the mentalis muscle are to raise the central portion of the lower lip and the soft tissues of the chin, to give stability to the lower lip and also, in conjunction with the action of the orbicularis oris muscle, to allow the lip to protrude, during a kiss for example. Those who want to emphasise an expression of sorrow or sadness also use this muscle [59].
The mentalis muscle is innervated by the mandibular ramus of the facial nerve (7th pair of cranial nerves).

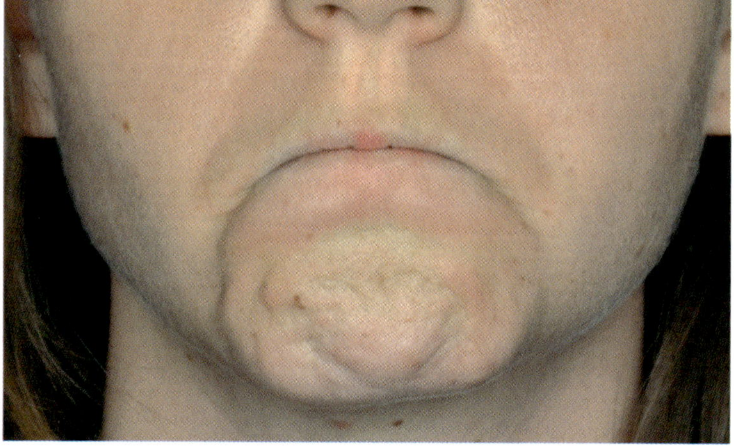

Figure 62 Voluntary contraction of the mentalis muscle, with formation of the so-called "popply" chin, and of the tiny depressor anguli oris muscle (DAO)

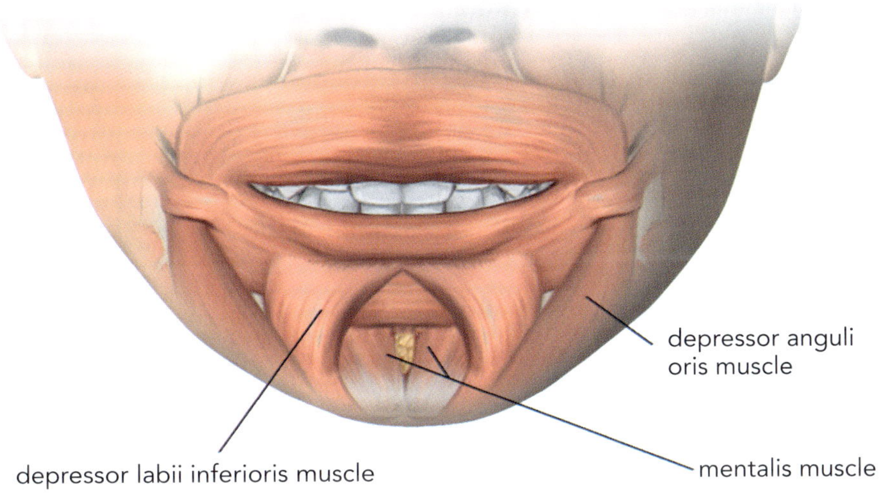

Figure 63 Anatomy of the chin region

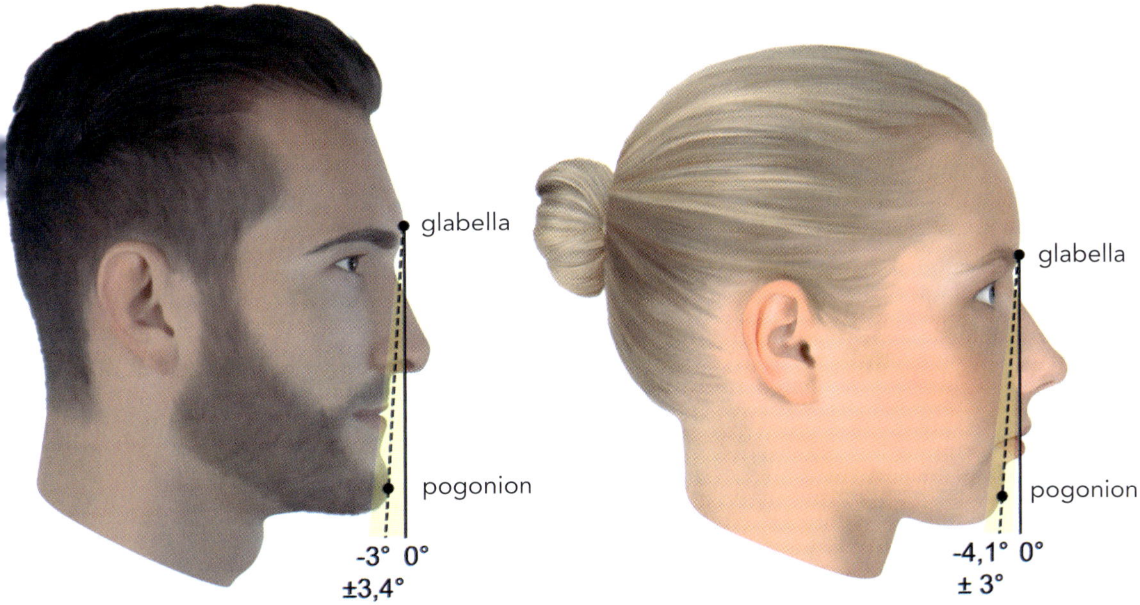

Figure 64 The inclination of the facial profile is defined by a line drawn from the glabella to the pogonion. In men, the chin projects further forward (-3 ± 3.4 degrees) than in women (-4.1 ± 3.0). Source: based on Farkas et al.

An important aspect to consider in the evaluation of the chin is undoubtedly its projection on the sagittal plane, when viewed in profile. According to the anthropometric studies of Farkas et al. [60], the average inclination of the facial profile is defined by a line that runs from the glabella to the pogonion. The anterior projection of the chin is greater in men (-3±3.4 degrees) than in women (-4,1±3,0) (fig. 64).

Injection technique

The mentalis muscle is considered a key structure in aesthetic medical procedures for the rejuvenation of the lower third of the face.

Botulinum toxin injections into the mentalis muscle should include the entire thickness of the muscle to prevent asymmetrical blockage and paradoxical protrusion of the chin, bearing in mind that the muscle below the skin is set at a depth of approximately 6.7-10.7 mm.

In order to avoid complications, the injection should be performed approximately 0.5 cm from the lower edge of the chin and at least 2 cm from the lower lip, bearing in mind that the mentalis muscle is approximately 5-10 mm from the midline and 20-30 mm from a horizontal line connecting the corners of the mouth. For both the repositioning of the pogonion and the correction of the poppy chin (figs. 66-67), it is possible to perform a single central injection or, even better, two to four symmetrical injections at a distance of no more than 5-7 mm from the midline of the chin (fig. 65, video 3.17). Video 3.17 shows drawing and injection technique for repositioning the pogonion and for poppy (or dimpled) chin using a dilution of 1.2 ml, a 33 G/12 mm needle, and injection into the intramuscular plane.

The more lateral the injections, the less superficial they have to be, while the central portion of the muscle can be injected from deep down to the surface without risk of migration, because the other mimetic muscles of the lower lip are far enough away from it.

The units of botulinum toxin used for this correction can vary depending on the force of contraction of the muscle from 3 to 10 U Botox per side or 6-20 U Speywood per side.

It is important to remember, as we have already seen in the anatomical description, that the mentalis muscle overlaps at the top with the orbicularis oris muscle and at the side of the top with the depressor labii inferioris (DLI) muscle. If the injections are performed too close to the lower lip or too far to the side of the centre of the chin, the action of these muscles may

VIDEO 3.17

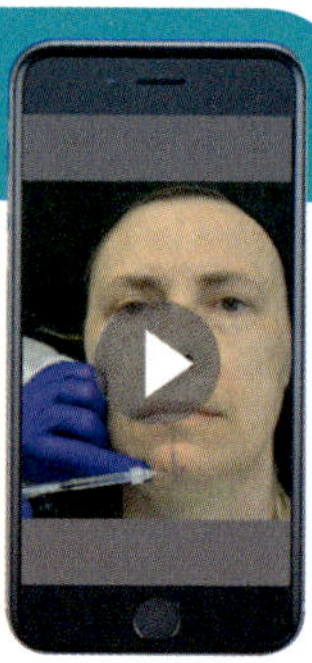

Drawing and injection technique for repositioning the pogonion and for poppy (or dimpled) chin

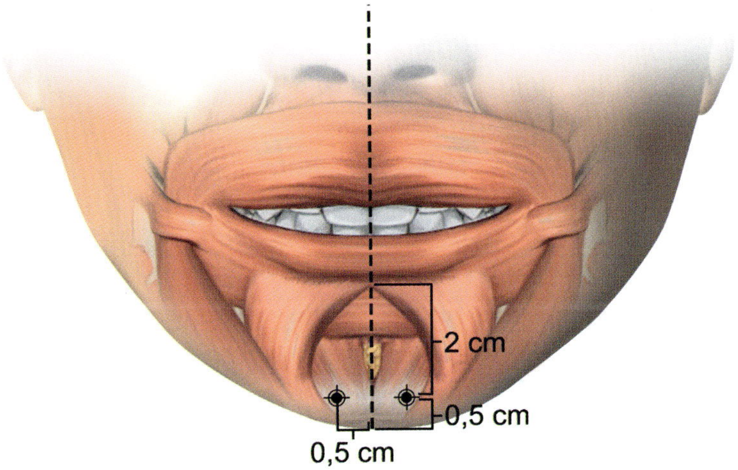

Figure 65 Injection points for treatment of a poppy chin with botulinum

be weakened or movement asymmetries may occur. For example, injections that accidentally weaken the depressor labii inferioris may result in speech difficulties, while accidental injection of the orbicularis oris may result in an incompetent lower lip or facial asymmetry [62,63].

CLINICAL CASES

CLINICAL CASE 16

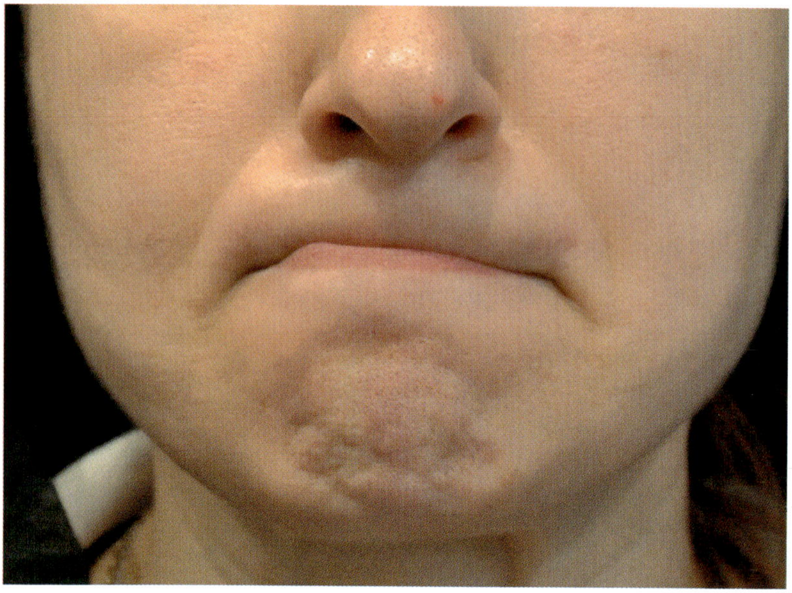

BEFORE

<

AFTER

>

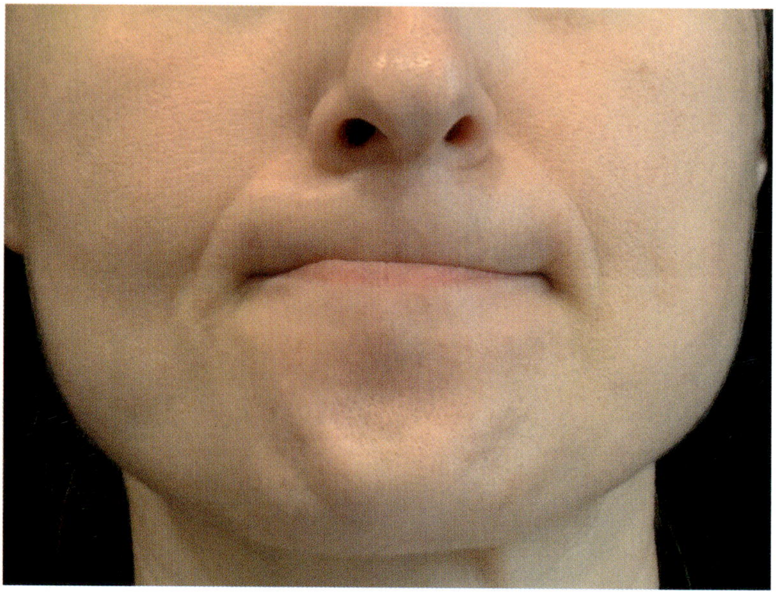

Figure 66 48-year-old patient before and 30 days after botulinum treatment for a poppy chin

CLINICAL CASES

CLINICAL CASE 17

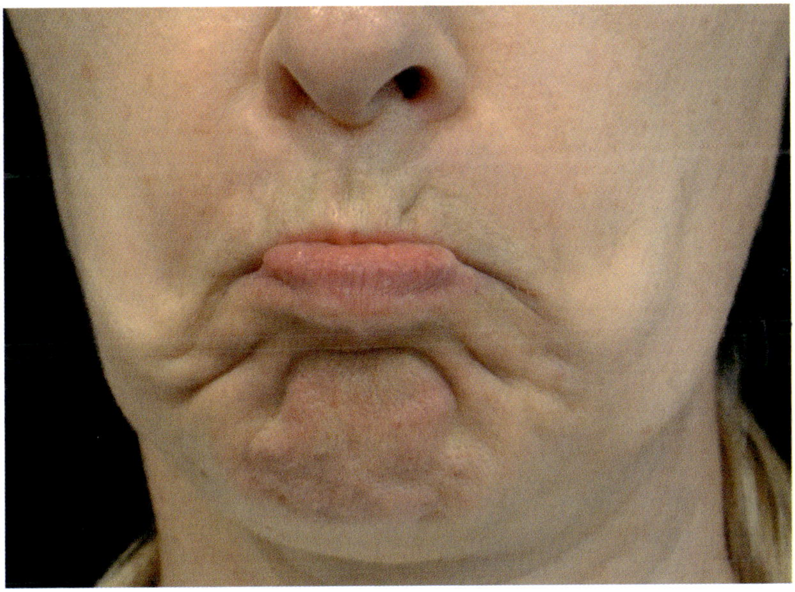

BEFORE

AFTER

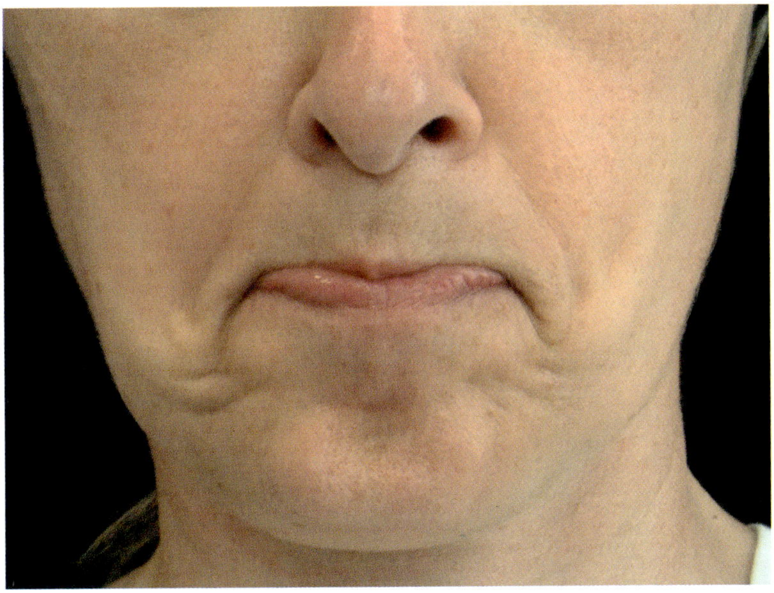

Figure 67 52-year-old patient before and 30 days after botulinum treatment for a poppy chin

NEFERTITI LIFT

Giovanni Brunelli

The Nefertiti Lift is a rejuvenation technique for the lower third of the face and neck described by Phillip Levy in 2007 [67]. It is named after the beautiful Egyptian queen Nefertiti, who was famous for the beautiful definition of her jawline and neck.

The technique is aimed in particular at treating the platysma, a flat, even and symmetrical skin muscle, which extends inferiorly from the deltoid and pectoral fascia and partially inserts into the mandible (its only connection to bone), while the rest of the fibres join and mix with those of the other muscles leading to the modiolus and the depressor anguli oris, and the depressor labii inferioris, ending in the SMAS and the skin of the cheeks (fig. 68).

These insertions allow the platysma to pull down the skin of the cheeks and lower the corners of the mouth. The anterior and posterior platysmal bands are evident during the contraction of this muscle, which is innervated by the cervical ramifications of the facial nerve.

To understand whether our treatment will be successful, it is necessary to ask our patients to contract the platysma; often, to achieve this, it is necessary for the doctor to contract the muscle first because, surprisingly, many people are unable to do this when asked.

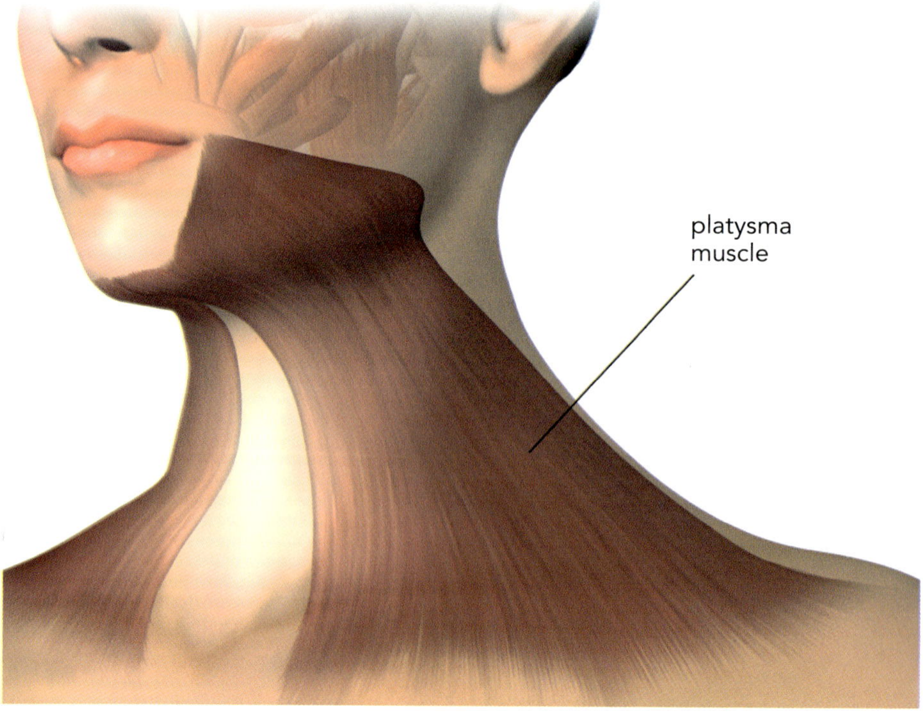

Figure 68 Schematic drawing: anatomy of the platysma muscle

The disappearance of the definition of the mandibular border and the appearance of a strong posterior platysmal band upon contraction are good indications for the Nefertiti lift (fig. 69).
As with the eyebrow, the height of the jaw line depends on the balance between the elevator muscles and the platysma, which is a depressor. As we age, and partly due to the force of gravity, the jawline tends to become less defined and to slide downwards. Botulinum decreases the caudal traction force and lifts the affected area.
The posterior platysmal band should be pinched between the thumb and forefinger of the non-dominant hand to isolate it. Four or five equidistant injection points are then marked on it. Immediately afterwards, we mark the mandibular angle on the mandibular line and the intersection with a line that continues the nasolabial fold. We mark four equidistant points within this area, below the mandible, where we inject the botulinum (video 3.18).
The treatment can be carried out with all three types of toxin currently available; 50 units of onabotulinum and incobotulinum, or 125 of abobotulinum, are usually not exceeded.
Patients should, as always, be checked after 15 days to assess the need for any adjustments.
In video 3.19 we can appreciate the results of this treatment after two weeks.
The effect of the treatment lasts between four and six months.
Of course, the anterior platysmal bands can also be treated in the same session, taking care not to inject too many units.
Side effects are rare and minimal and consist mainly of dysphagia; this can be avoided by reducing the dilution and dose of botulinum and using a good injection technique.
To improve the quality of the result of the Nefertiti Lift it can be beneficial, in many cases, to complete the treatment with hyaluronic acid to further define the jawline. Of course, the filler must not be injected into the jowls as this could make them heavier, but should be injected in front of and behind them.

CLINICAL CASES

CLINICAL CASE 18

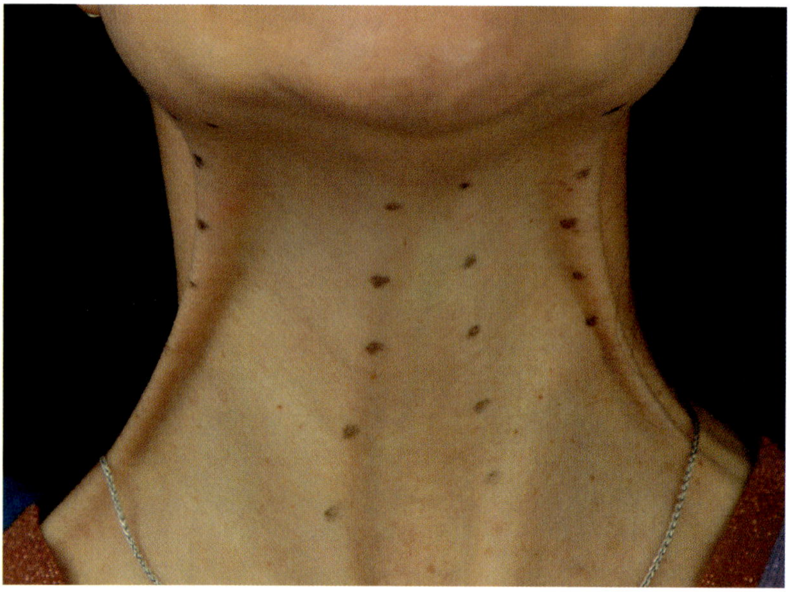

BEFORE

<

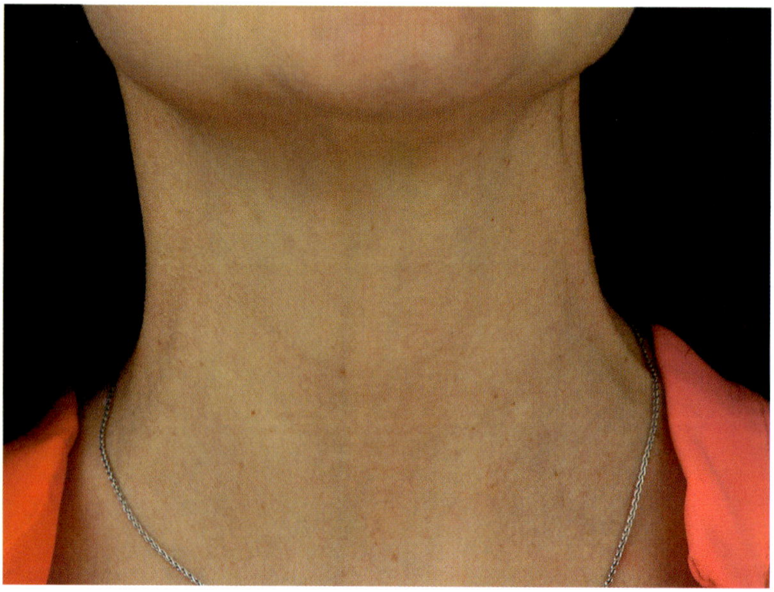

AFTER

>

Figure 69 Maximum platysma contraction: pre-treatment image and result at 15 days (frontal)

CLINICAL CASES

BEFORE

AFTER

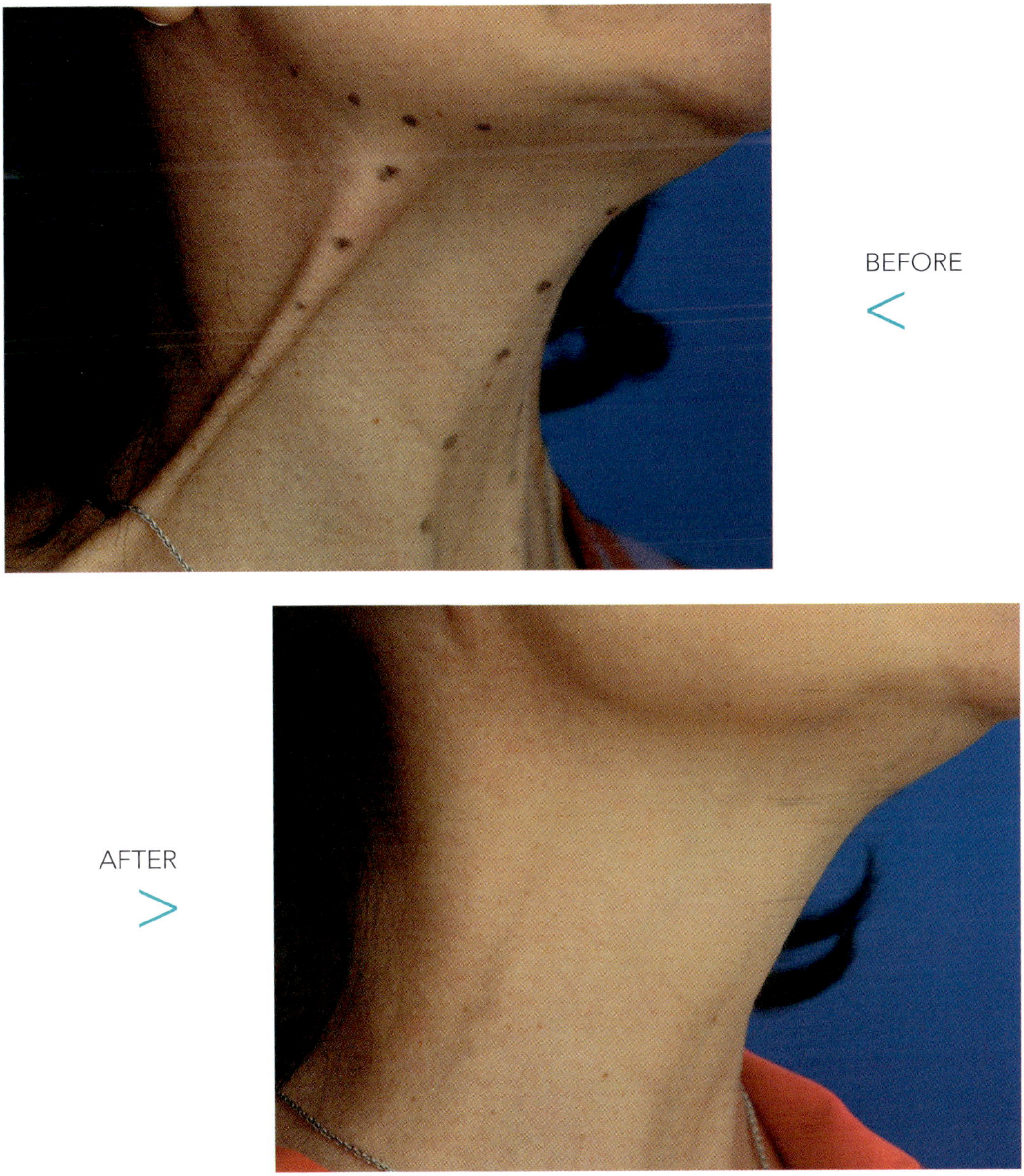

Figure 70 Maximum platysma contraction: pre-treatment image and result at 15 days (right side)

CLINICAL CASES

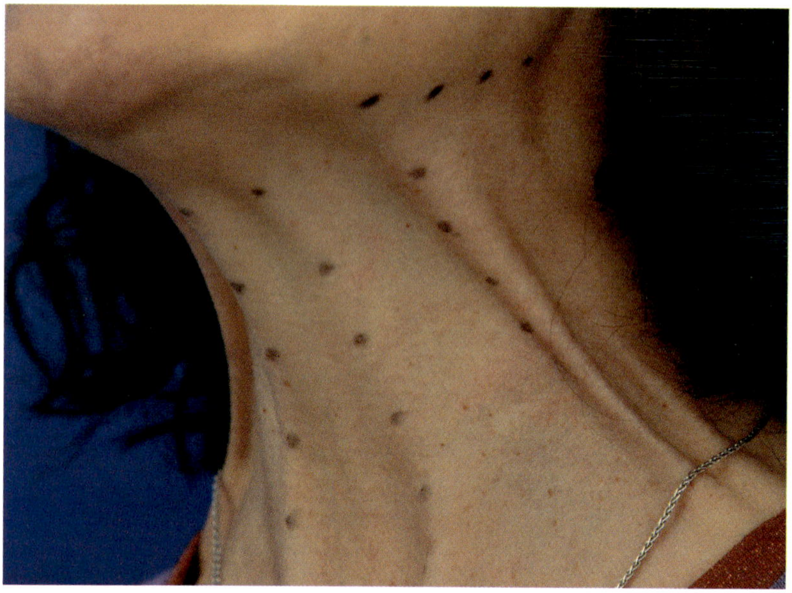

BEFORE

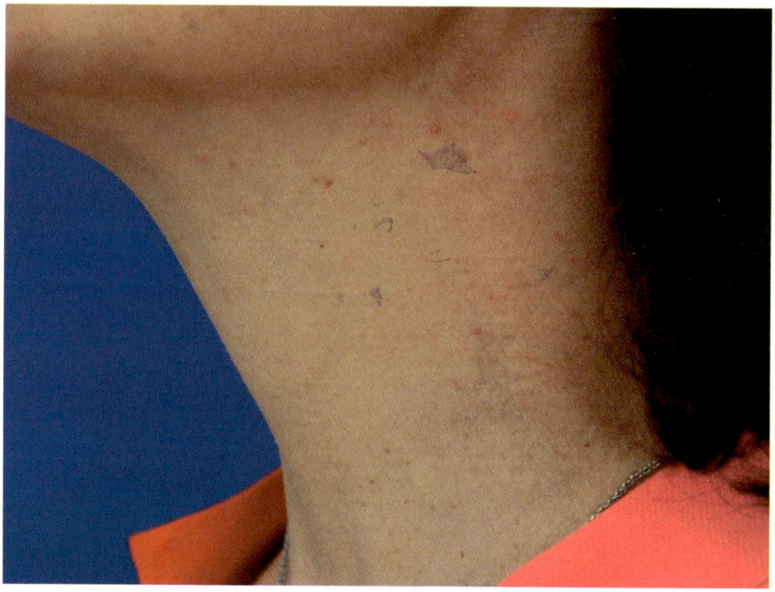

AFTER

Figure 71 Maximum platysma contraction: pre-treatment image and result at 15 days (left side)

CLINICAL CASES

VIDEO 3.18

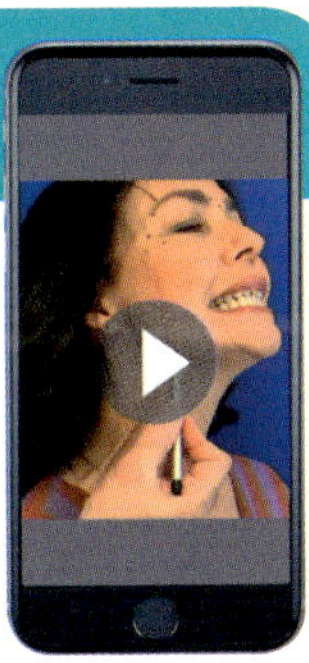

Nefertiti lift: drawing and injection technique

VIDEO 3.19

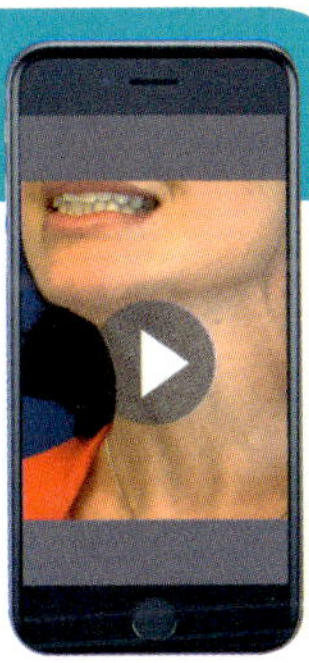

Nefertiti lift: results after two weeks

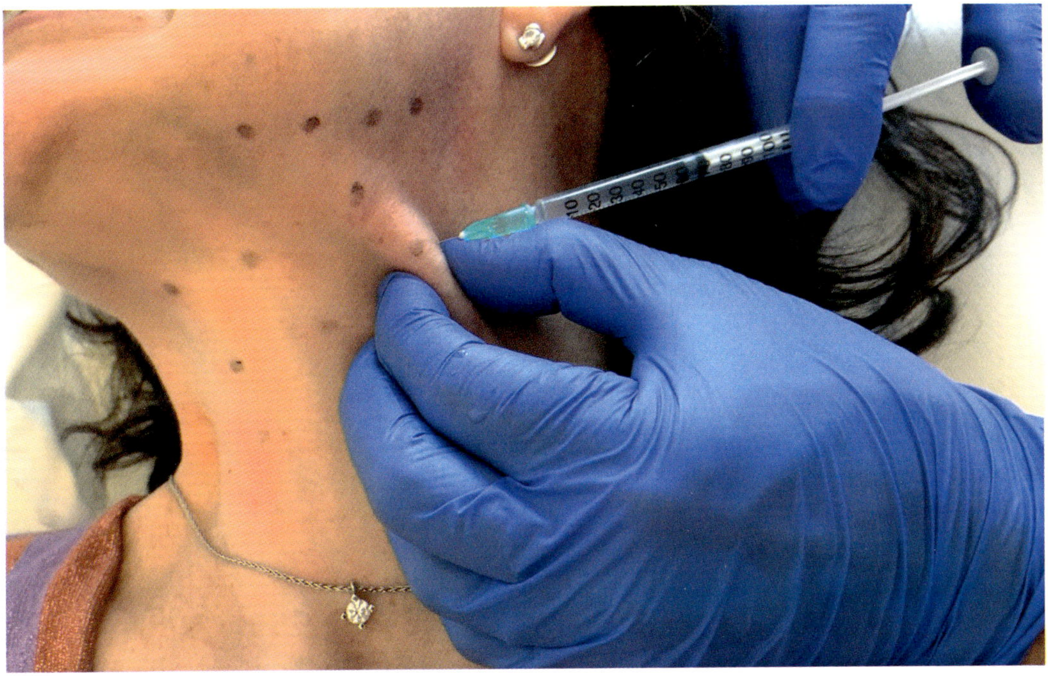

NECK

PLATYSMA BANDS, HORIZONTAL NECK LINES AND CLEAVAGE

Giovanni Brunelli

The neck and cleavage regions have always been a challenge for plastic surgeons and aesthetic doctors and continue to be so today.

The neck and hands are the areas of the body that reveal the true age of our patients, even when the face is very well cared for, plumped up and rejuvenated by all the treatments we carry out.

Treatment of the neck was strictly surgical for many years. However, this approach is not suitable for all patients, who may be too young or not ready for surgery, or unsuitable candidates for various reasons.

The treatments on offer are often valid, but the results in these areas are not always particularly satisfactory, despite the presence of numerous medical and energy-based devices (EBD).

The doctor is often obliged to propose different types of treatment, all of which complement each other. These include fillers, biostimulation, PDO biostimulation threads, and laser or pulsed light, all of which improve the appearance of these areas but undoubtedly have their limitations. Patients need to be informed of these limitations as they often expect miraculous results that cannot be achieved.

Even surgery, which definitely offers the best solution despite being more invasive, encounters its weak point in the neck. Countless surgical techniques have been described for treating a sagging neck. Some of them are very effective, others less so, demonstrating that there is no single surgical procedure that is universally recognised as the best.

The neck is a disadvantaged area for several reasons:

- due to the effect of gravity, which causes the skin on the neck to droop downwards;
- due to the accumulation of fat under the chin, both preplatysmal and retroplatysmal;
- due to the contraction of the platysma muscle (for details of the anatomy of this muscle see the chapter on the "Nefertiti lift")
- due to the lack of skin appendages, which greatly limits the possibility of using EBD because of the poor regenerative capacity:
- due to the elastosic damage caused by very frequent exposure to the sun, especially in patients who are currently aged 50-60 years and over and who have been exposed to the sun in the past without paying much attention to the use of creams with high sun filters, or even using mirrors or oils that caused the skin to really burn, as was common years ago.

In aesthetic medicine, botulinum definitely plays an important role in these areas of the body, where it has become a viable alternative, as it is a minimally invasive treatment with very few side effects.
Let's take a closer look at the various fields of application.

Platysma bands

The platysma is a flat, even muscle, and is the largest mimic muscle in the human body. Enveloped by its own fascia, it covers the cervical fascia and is firmly attached to the skin.
Platysma bands are caused by the contraction of the platysma, the anterior and posterior margins of which tend to contract over time and become hypertonic, forming cords covered by the overlying skin, which follows their movement. It has been noted that patients with facial nerve palsy do not have platysma bands on the affected side.
To properly treat platysma bands, patients should be asked to clench their teeth tightly while lowering the corners of their mouth; this movement will highlight the muscular cords.
Using the non-dominant hand, take each band of the platysma between the thumb and forefinger and use a pencil to mark dots approximately 1.5-2 cm apart; the usual number of dots per band is 4-5 (fig. 76).
The botulinum toxin is then infiltrated using the technique described in video 3.20.
2-3 units of botulinum (onabotulinum or incobotulinum) or the corresponding number of abobotulinum units are injected into each injection site.
The treatment is safe, but care must be taken to avoid overdosing or the undesirable migration of the product, which may cause dysphagia, dysphonia or weakness of the neck muscles, although this happens very rarely.
Side effects, mainly related to injection, include oedema, erythema and ecchymosis, but these are all temporary.
Results are visible from day 5-7, but can improve up to day 14, bearing in mind that a significant amount of excess skin may make them less noticeable (fig. 76).

VIDEO 3.20

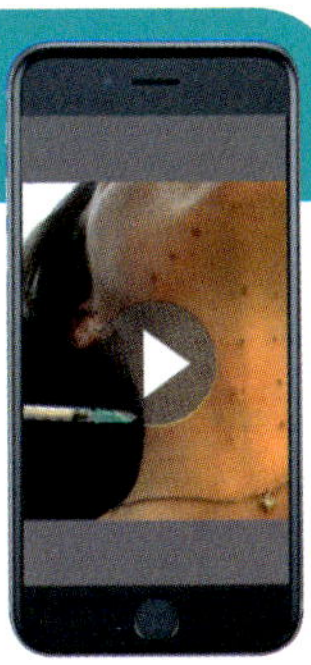

Platysma bands: infiltration technique

Horizontal neck lines

Horizontal neck lines usually form around the neck in numbers of two to four, and can occur when relatively young. They are caused by the basal tone of the platysma muscle fibres and run transversally to these fibres. They extend between the two sternocleidomastoid muscles, from the submandibular region to the collarbones (fig. 72).
Their depth is also favoured by the

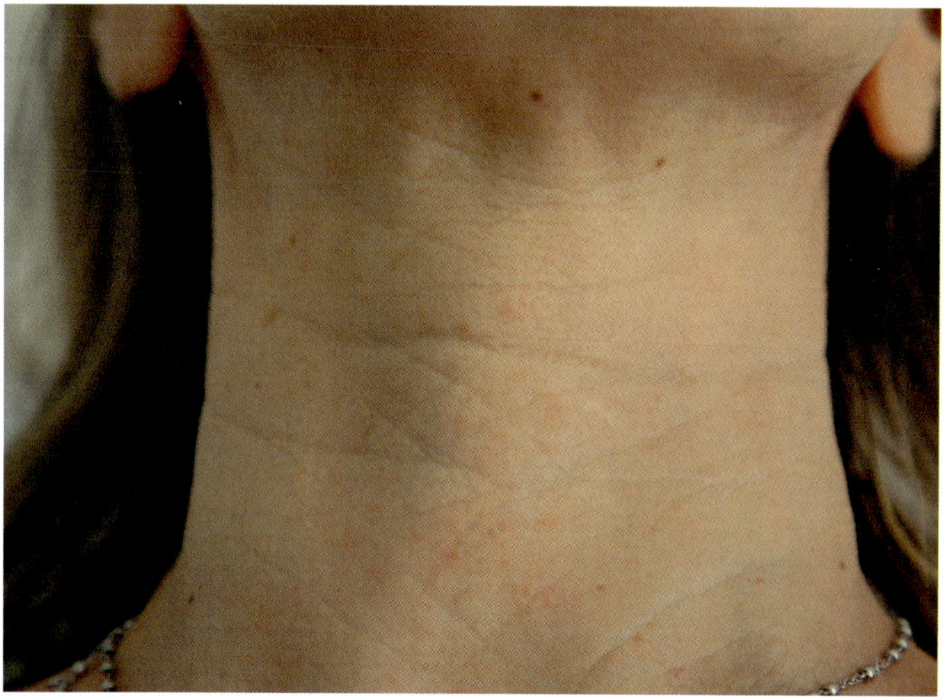

Figure 72 Example of horizontal neck lines in older patients

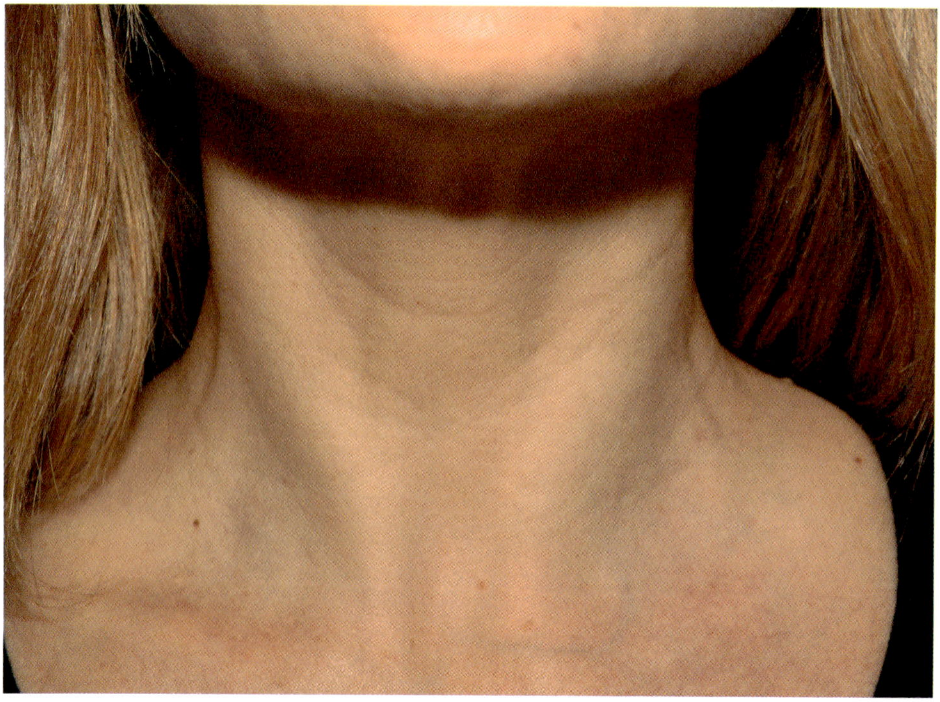

Figure 73 Example of horizontal neck lines in younger patients

scarce thickness of the dermis in this region; in the case shown in figure 73, in a younger patient, they are less evident.
The treatment of horizontal neck lines involves the infiltration of two units of botulinum, at a standard dilution, at points approximately 2 cm apart (fig. 77), taking care to inject very superficially, intradermally if possible, causing the formation of the characteristic bump. Some resistance should be felt when pressing on the plunger, confirming that the needle is positioned intradermally. Infiltration without resistance would mean that the needle has gone too deep. To facilitate intradermal infiltration it is best to use very small needles, such as 33 G/4 mm. About 10-15 U of botulinum are usually injected for each horizontal line.

The side effects are similar to those described for the treatment of the platysma and are temporary.
Horizontal neck lines can be further improved with the infiltration of a "soft" filler when patients come in for a check-up, typically after about two weeks.
The results of this treatment usually last no longer than four months, although repeated applications may prolong its effect (fig. 77).

Cleavage

The cleavage is another area of the body prone to premature ageing. It has a considerably reduced dermo-epidermal thickness and a lack of skin appendages, especially in women.
This region is very often exposed to sunlight from a very young age and therefore suffers frequent and constant

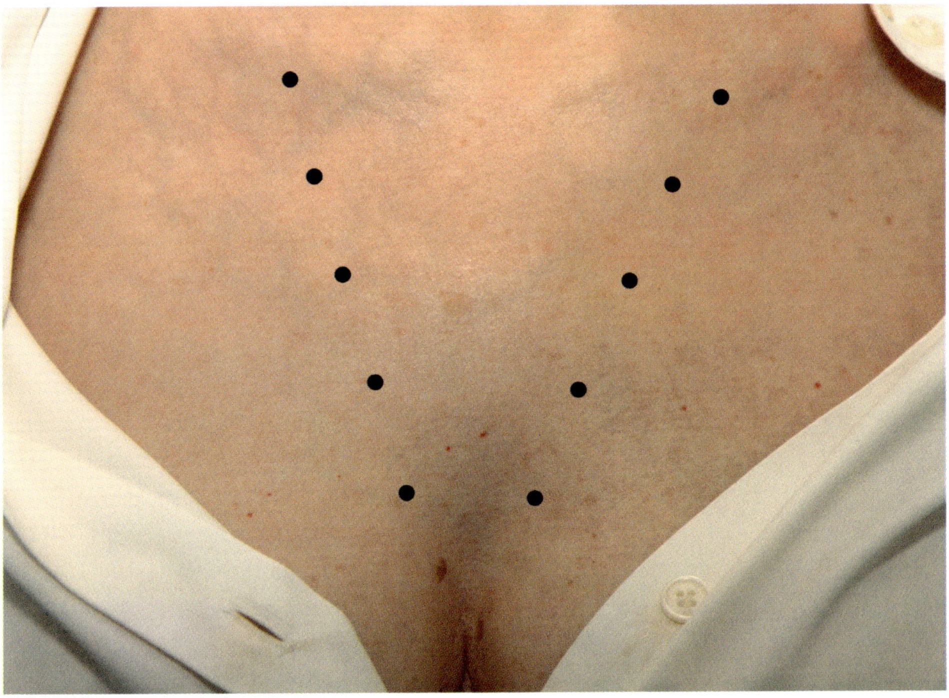

Figure 74 Narrow V pattern for cleavage treatment

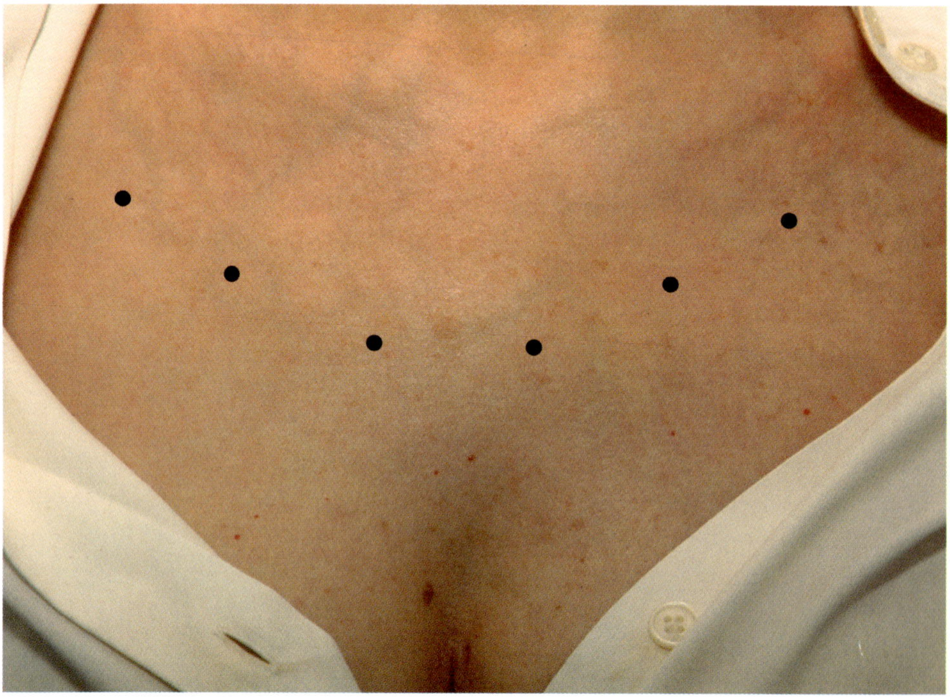

Figure 75 Wide V pattern for cleavage treatment

actinic damage, the effects of which add up over time, leading to elastosis with impoverished, wrinkled and blotchy skin.

Treatment of the cleavage is not restricted to botulinum toxin, which can only partially improve the appearance of the skin in this area. This region benefits particularly from treatments involving hyaluronic acid and biostimulation, as well as PDO threads and laser and pulsed light treatments, bearing in mind that the absence of skin appendages limits the power of devices.

Botulinum injections in this area are very safe and free from complications, apart from the possibility of bruising, which will last a few days.

It is necessary to remain as close to the surface as possible, so it is better to use small needles (33 G/4 mm) with an insulin syringe with a luer-lock connector; after injection, we should see a series of bumps intradermally or just below the dermis.

A V-shaped pattern is usually followed, starting from the presternal intermammary region and rising up to the collarbones (fig. 74), but it can be a little wider, as in the case shown in figure 75, depending on the type of flaw to be corrected. For each point, 3-5 U up to a total of 50 U can be injected. Of course, it is also possible to treat this entire region with the microbotulinum technique, details of which can be found in the specific chapter.

CLINICAL CASES

CLINICAL CASE 19

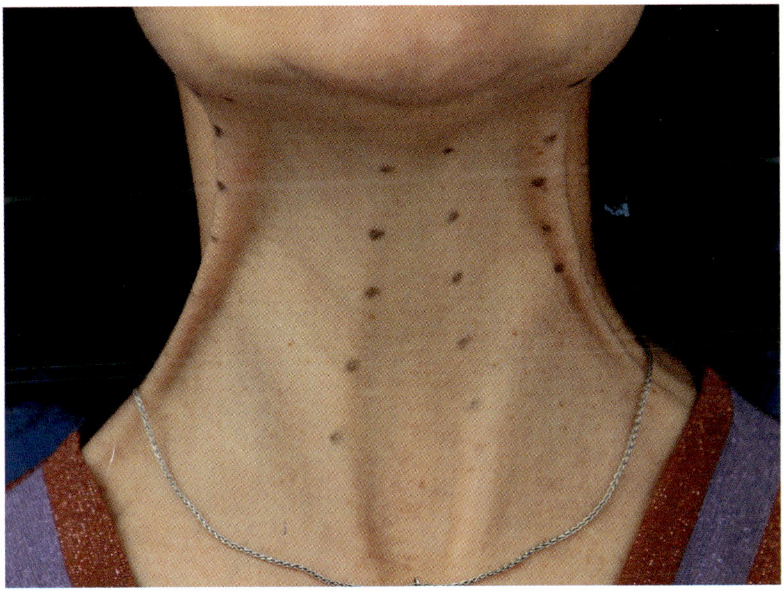

BEFORE

AFTER

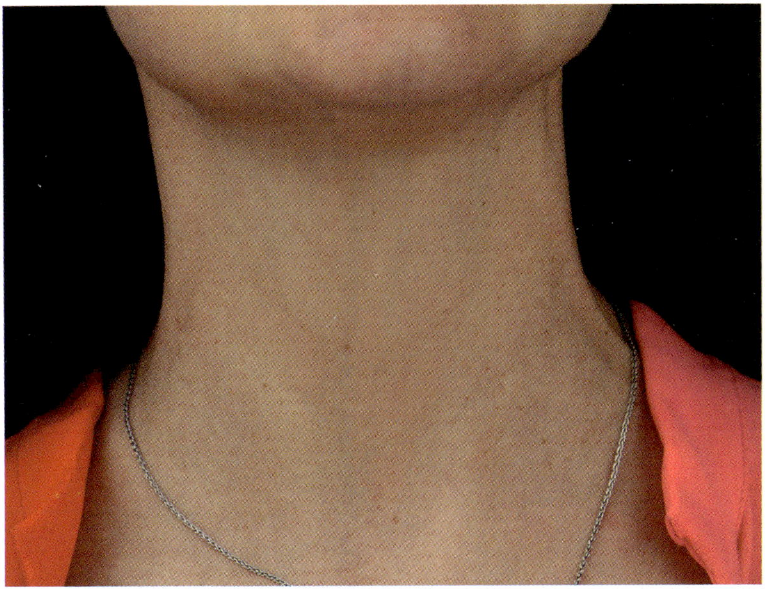

Figure 76 Contraction of the platysma and drawing of the injection points on the anterior and posterior bands. Result of infiltration of platysma bands after 15 days

CLINICAL CASES

CLINICAL CASE 20

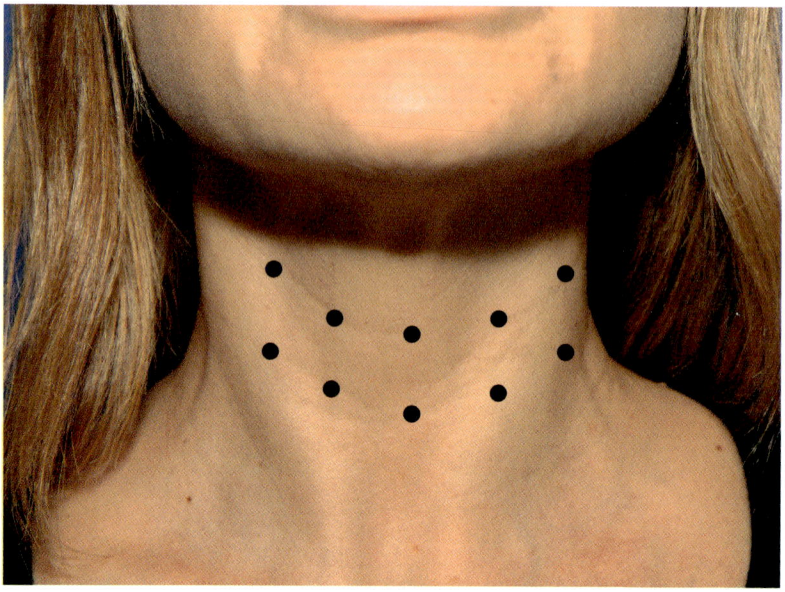

BEFORE

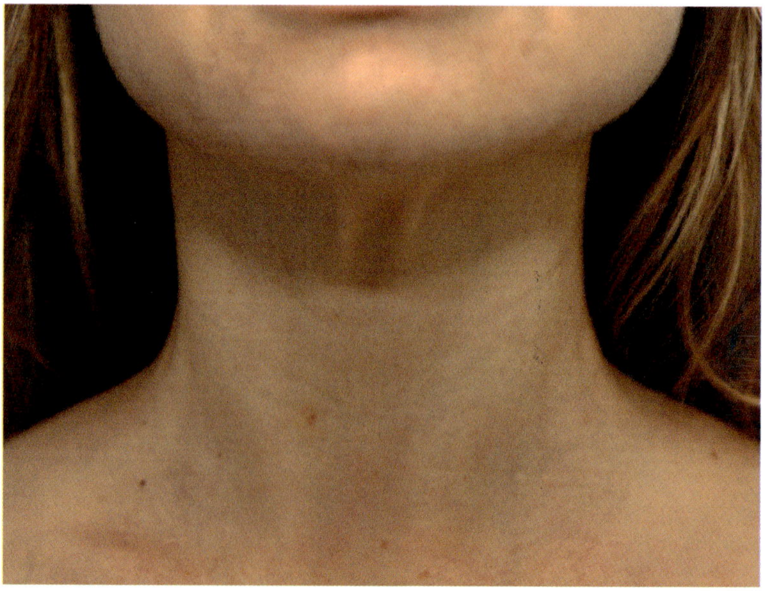

AFTER

Figure 77 Drawing of botulinum injection points into horizontal neck lines and result one month after infiltration of botulinum

SALIVARY GLANDS

Gabriele Muti

The idea of treating the salivary glands and parotid glands in aesthetic medicine originated in clinical practice for the treatment of sialorrhea.

K. O. Bushara first proposed parotid botulinum toxin infiltration for the treatment of sialorrhea in patients with amyotrophic lateral sclerosis in 1997 [75].

The salivary glands are controlled by the autonomic nervous system and are mainly regulated by cholinergic tone. The secretory activity of the submandibular and sublingual glands is maintained at a constant level (mainly adrenergic tone). Salivary secretion is stimulated by sensitive responses to olfactory and gustatory stimuli (mainly cholinergic tone). Hence the predominance of parotid secretory activity in the presence of heightened salivary flows. The rationale for the use of botulinum toxin in salivary pathology is based on selective chemical denervation by cleavage of proteins of the neuroexocytosis apparatus (SNARE complex) and on the consequent presynaptic inhibition of acetylcholine release in the glands. In this way, the parasympathetic dependent salivary secretory capacity is depressed, while no effect is exerted on the adrenergic system, so that basal secretory activity is maintained, reducing the risk of xerostomia.

Following treatment of sialorrhea, a reduction was assessed not only in salivary production but also in the volume of the salivary and parotid glands, as demonstrated on rat salivary glands in the work of Teymoortash [76]. It was then re-assessed in humans by Bae, using computed tomography [77].

Enlarged parotid glands can contribute to a square-shaped lower face, especially in Asian patients. As acetylcholine acts as a neurotransmitter, it can be blocked by botulinum toxin in both the salivary glands and in the neuromuscular junction as we have already seen (fig. 78).

The injection of an enlarged or protruding parotid gland can reduce the width of the face, as a complement to treatment of the masseter muscles. Injection of the parotid gland rarely results in a dry mouth, as most salivary production (71%) comes from the submandibular gland. The most prominent part of the parotid gland around the mandibular angle is the preferred injection site. Based on clinical experience, 4-6 injection sites are typically used for the parotid gland, with a dose of 4-6 U of inco-onabotulin, 10-15 U of abobotulin, per injection site. The injection of botulinum toxin in very thin patients with a submandibular salivary gland can improve lines on the neck (fig. 79). It is preferable to perform an initial ultrasound check, to assess the position and be sure of the diagnosis [78]. The treatment is administered by direct injection into the submandibular gland, palpating it with the fingers and using a 12 mm needle. 10 to 20 units of inco-onabotulinum, 25 to 50 units of abobotulinum, are usually injected,

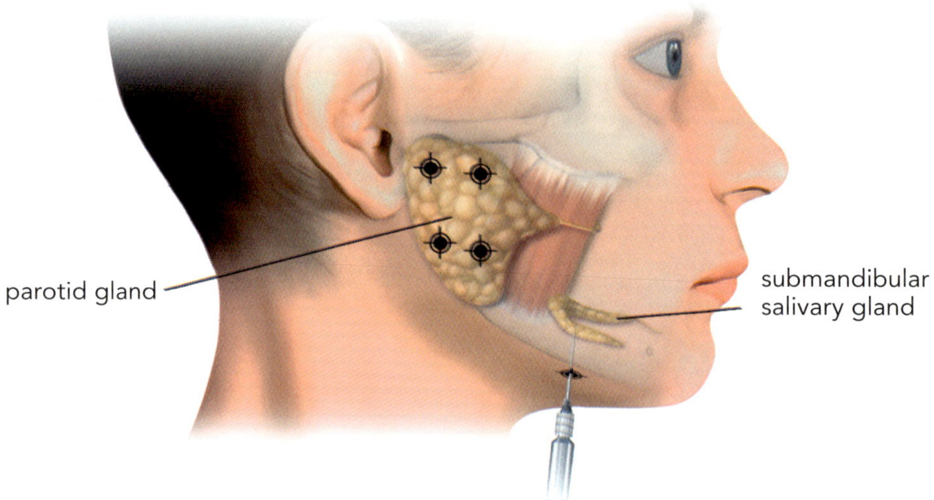

Figure 78 The position of the parotid and salivary glands can alter the shape of the face. The parotid gland is treated with injection of botulinum toxin into the marked points using a 12 mm needle which enters the skin perpendicularly, penetrating it by 2/3 of the length of the needle. The submandibular salivary glands assessed with ultrasound are injected, after drawing on the skin, with a 12 mm needle, which completely enters the tissue below the jawline

possibly divided into two doses at a distance of about one month.
Side effects are temporary and may consist of pain, bruising, haematomas, hyperaemia, infection and sometimes initially xerostomia with increased susceptibility to stone formation, caries and local infections. Dysphagia and difficulty in chewing may occur in the oral cavity in the event of an injection error.

CLINICAL CASES

CLINICAL CASE 21

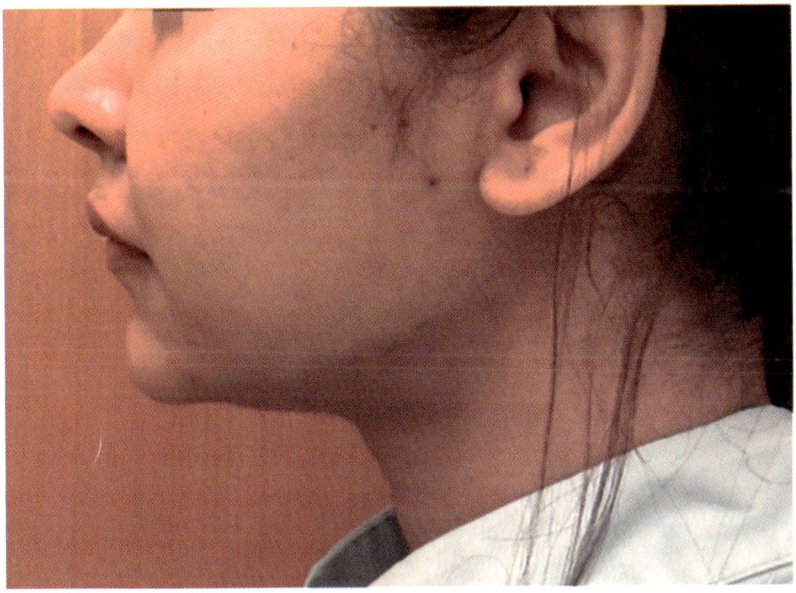

BEFORE

<

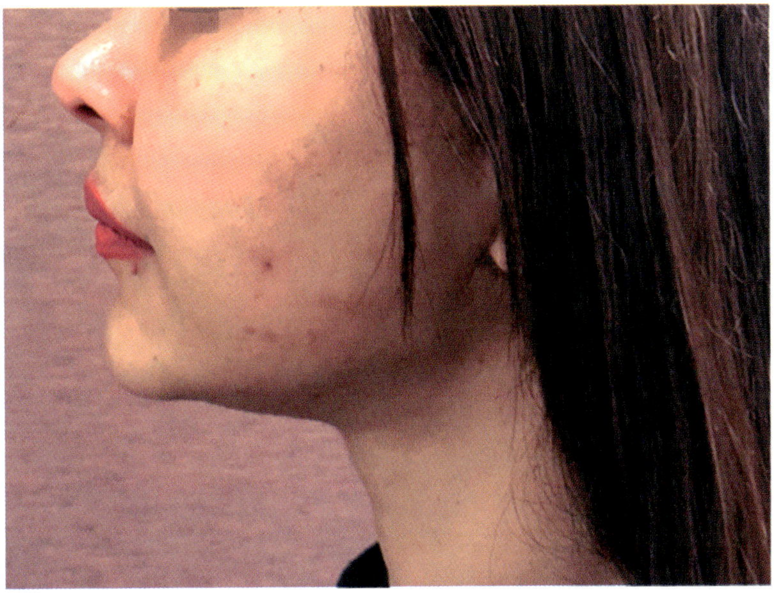

AFTER

>

Figure 79 Example of treatment of the submandibular salivary glands, pictures before and after treatment. Note the change in cervical conformation below the jawline one month after treatment

Bibliography

Forehead

1. Sarit Cohen, MD, Ofir Artzi, MD, Lior Heller, MD, Forehead Lift Using Botulinum Toxin, Aesthetic Surgery Journal, Volume 38, Issue 3, March 2018, Pages 312–320.
2. Williams, Bannister, Berry, Collins, Dyson, Dussek, Ferguson. Anatomia del Gray. Zanichelli IV ed./ XXXVIII English ed. 2001.
3. Cotofana S, Freytag DL, Frank K, Sattler S, Landau M, Pavicic T, Fabi S, Lachman N, Hernandez CA, Green JB. The Bidirectional Movement of the Frontalis Muscle: Introducing the Line of Convergence and Its Potential Clinical Relevance. Plast Reconstr Surg. 2020 May;145(5):1155-1162.
4. Moqadam M, Frank K, Handayan C, Hakami M, Benslimane F, Gotkin RH, Sadick NS, Cotofana S. Understanding the Shape of Forehead Lines. J Drugs Dermatol. 2017 May 1;16(5):471-477.
5. Carruthers J, Carruthers A. Using Botulinum Toxins Cosmetically. A practical Guide. Martin Dunitz. Taylor & Francis Group. 2003.

Glabella

6. Lewis MB, Bowler PJ. Botulinum toxin cosmetic therapy correlates with a more positive mood. J Cosmet Dermatol 2009;8(1):24-6.
7. Cook BE Jr, Lucarelli MJ, Lemke BN. Depressor supercilii muscle: anatomy, histology, and cosmetic implications. Ophthalmic Plast Reconstr Surg. 2001;17(6):404-411.
8. Lorenc ZP, Smith S, Nestor M, Nelson D, Moradi A. Understanding the functional anatomy of the frontalis and glabellar complex for optimal aesthetic botulinum toxin type A therapy. Aesthetic Plast Surg. 2013 Oct;37(5):975-83.
9. Williams, Bannister, Berry, Collins, Dyson, Dussek, Ferguson. Anatomia del Gray. Zanichelli IV ed./ XXXVIII English ed. 2001.
10. De Almeida AR, da Costa Marques ER, Banegas R, Kadunc BV. Glabellar contraction patterns: a tool to optimize botulinum toxin treatment. Dermatol Surg. 2012 Sep;38(9):1506-15.

Crow's feet

11. Tsukahara K, Tamatsu Y, Sugawara Y, Shimada K. The Relationship Between Wrinkle Depth and Dermal Thickness in the Forehead and Lateral Canthal Region. Arch Dermatol. 2011;147(7):822-828.
12. Contet-Audonneau JL, Jeanmaire C, Pauly G. A histological study of human wrinkle structures: comparison between sun-exposed areas of the face, with or without wrinkles, and sun-protected areas. Br J Dermatol. 1999;140(6).
13. Tong J, Lopez MJ, Patel BC. Anatomy, Head and Neck, Eye Orbicularis Oculi Muscle. [Updated 2020 Jul 27]. In: StatPearls [Internet]. Treasure Island (FL): StatPearls Publishing; 2021 Jan.
14. Cao Y, Yang JP, Zhu XG, Zhu J, Chang HQ, Guo SH, Luo D, Zhou BR. A Comparative In Vivo Study on

Three Treatment Approaches to Applying Topical Botulinum Toxin A for Crow's Feet. Biomed Res Int. 2018 Jul 3.
15. Gart MS, Gutowski KA. Overview of Botulinum Toxins for Aesthetic Uses. Clin Plast Surg. 2016 Jul;43(3):459-71.
16. Carruthers J, Carruthers A. Using Botulinum Toxins Cosmetically. A practical Guide. Martin Dunitz. Taylor & Francis Group. 2003

Lifting the lateral third of the eyebrow (gull wing)

17. Patel BC, Malhotra R. Mid Forehead Brow Lift. In: StatPearls. Treasure Island (FL): StatPearls Publishing; September 14, 2021.
18. Bames HO. Frown disfigurement and ptosis of eyebrows. Plast Reconstr Surg (1946). 1957;19(4):337-340.
19. Frankel AS, Kamer FM. Chemical browlift. Arch Otolaryngol Head Neck Surg. 1998;124(3):321-323.
20. Karimi N, Kashkouli MB, Sianati H, Khademi B. Techniques of Eyebrow Lifting: A Narrative Review. J Ophthalmic Vis Res. 2020;15(2):218-235.
21. Huilgol SC, Carruthers A, Carruthers JD. Raising eyebrows with botulinum toxin. Dermatol Surg. 1999;25(5):373-376.

Depressor of the septum and elevation of the nasal tip

22. Redaelli A, Limardo P. Minimally invasive procedures for nasal aesthetics. J Cutan Aesthet Surg. 2012 Apr;5(2):115-20.
23. Redaelli A. Medical rhinoplasty with hyaluronic acid and botulinum toxin A: a very simple and quite effective technique. J Cosmet Dermatol. 2008 Sep;7(3):210-20.
24. Dayan SH, Kempiners JJ. Treatment of the lower third of the nose and dynamic nasal tip ptosis with Botox. Plast Reconstr Surg. 2005 May;115(6):1784-5.
25. Ghavami A, Janis JE, Guyuron B. Regarding the treatment of dynamic nasal tip ptosis with botulinum toxin A. Plast Reconstr Surg. 2006 Jul;118(1):263-4.
26. Cohn JE, Greco TM. Advanced Techniques for the Use of Neurotoxins in Non-Surgical Facial Rejuvenation. Aesthetic Plast Surg. 2020 Oct;44(5):1788-1799.
27. Cigna E, Sorvillo V, Stefanizzi G, Fino P, Tarallo M. The use of botulinum toxin in the treatment of plunging nose: cosmetic results and a functional serendipity. Clin Ter. 2013;164(2):e107-13.
28. Pascali M, Marchese G, Diaspro A. The Rhino-Lip-Lifting: A Novel Proposal for Midface Profileplasty Performed as a Single Surgical Procedure. Facial Plast Surg. 2021 Jun;37(3):340-347.

Bunny lines

29. de Maio M, DeBoulle K, Braz A, Rohrich RJ; Alliance for the Future of Aesthetics Consensus Committee. Facial Assessment and Injection Guide for Botulinum Toxin and Injectable Hyaluronic Acid Fillers: Focus on the Midface. Plast Reconstr Surg. 2017 Oct;140(4):540e-550e.
30. Carruthers J, Carruthers A. Using Botulinum Toxins Cosmetically. A practical Guide. Martin Dunitz. Tay-

lor & Francis Group. 2003.
31. Gart MS, Gutowski KA. Overview of Botulinum Toxins for Aesthetic Uses. Clin Plast Surg. 2016 Jul;43(3):459-71.

Masseter hypertrophy

32. Fedorowicz Z, van Zuuren EJ, Schoones J. Botulinum toxin for masseter hypertrophy. Cochrane Database Syst Rev. 2013 Sep 9;2013(9):CD007510.
33. Almukhtar RM, Fabi SG. The Masseter Muscle and Its Role in Facial Contouring, Aging, and Quality of Life: A Literature Review. Plast Reconstr Surg. 2019 Jan;143(1):39e-48e.
34. Chang CS, Lin S, Wallace CG, Hsiao YC, Lin CM, Kang GC, Chen ZC, Chen PK, Lo LJ, Chen YR, Chen JP. Masseter Muscle Volume Changes Evaluated by 3-Dimensional Computed Tomography After Repeated Botulinum Toxin A Injections in Patients With Square Facial Morphology. Ann Plast Surg. 2019 Jan;82(1S Suppl 1):S29-S32.
35. Yeh YT, Peng JH, Peng HP. Literature review of the adverse events associated with botulinum toxin injection for the masseter muscle hypertrophy. J Cosmet Dermatol. 2018 Oct;17(5):675-687.
36. Peng HP, Peng JH. Complications of botulinum toxin injection for masseter hypertrophy: Incidence rate from 2036 treatments and summary of causes and preventions. J Cosmet Dermatol. 2018 Feb;17(1):33-38.

Flaring nostrils

37. Dayan SH, Kempiners JJ. Treatment of the lower third of the nose and dynamic nasal tip ptosis with Botox. Plast Reconstr Surg. 2005 May;115(6):1784-5.
38. Sundaram H, Signorini M, Liew S, Trindade de Almeida AR, Wu Y, Vieira Braz A, Fagien S, Goodman GJ, Monheit G, Raspaldo H; Global Aesthetics Consensus Group. Global Aesthetics Consensus: Botulinum Toxin Type A--Evidence-Based Review, Emerging Concepts, and Consensus Recommendations for Aesthetic Use, Including Updates on Complications. Plast Reconstr Surg. 2016 Mar;137(3):518e-529e.
39. Gassia V, Raspaldo H, Niforos FR, Michaud T. Global 3-dimensional approach to natural rejuvenation: recommendations for perioral, nose, and ear rejuvenation. J Cosmet Dermatol. 2013 Jun;12(2):123-36.
40. Gassia V, Beylot C, Béchaux S, Michaud T. Les techniques d'injection de la toxine botulique dans le tiers inférieur et moyen du visage, le cou et le décolleté. Le "Néfertiti lift" [Botulinum toxin injection techniques in the lower third and middle of the face, the neck and the décolleté: the "Nefertiti lift"]. Ann Dermatol Venereol. 2009 May;136 Suppl 4:S111-8. French.

Perioral lines

41. Jain P, Rathee M. Anatomy, Head and Neck, Orbicularis Oris Muscle. In: StatPearls. Treasure Island (FL): StatPearls Publishing; August 11, 2021.
42. Coleman WP III. Cosmetic Surgery of the Skin. Principles and Techniques. Mosby 1997.
43. de Maio M, Wu WTL, Goodman GJ,

Monheit G; Alliance for the Future of Aesthetics Consensus Committee. Facial Assessment and Injection Guide for Botulinum Toxin and Injectable Hyaluronic Acid Fillers: Focus on the Lower Face. Plast Reconstr Surg. 2017;140(3):393e-404e.
44. Semchyshyn N, Sengelmann RD. Botulinum toxin A treatment of perioral rhytides. Dermatol Surg. 2003 May;29(5):490-495.
45. Williams L, Bannister L, Berry MM, Collins P, Dyson M, Dussek JE, Ferguson M. Anatomia del Gray. Zanichelli, IV ed., 2001.
46. Vinkka-Puhakka H, Kean MR, Heap SW. Ultrasonic investigation of the circumoral musculature. J Anat. 1989 Oct; 166:121-33.

Gummy smile

47. Diaspro A, Cavallini M, Piersini P, Sito G. Gummy Smile Treatment: Proposal for a Novel Corrective Technique and a Review of the Literature. Aesthet Surg J. 2018 Nov 12;38(12):1330-1338.
48. Gong X, Huang H, Gu C, Li F, Zou L, An Y, Han X, Tang Z. Individual Factors of Botulinum Type A in Treatment of Gummy Smile: A Prospective Study. Aesthet Surg J. 2020 Dec 15:sjaa366.
49. Vergara-Buenaventura A, Mayta-Tovalino F, Correa A, Breen E, Mendoza-Azpur G. Predictability in Lip Repositioning with Botulinum Toxin for Gummy Smile Treatment: A 3-Year Follow-up Case Series. Int J Periodontics Restorative Dent. 2020 Sep/Oct;40(5):703-709.
50. Rajagopal A, Goyal M, Shukla S, Mittal N. To evaluate the effect and longevity of Botulinum toxin type A (Botox®) in the management of gummy smile - A longitudinal study up to 4 years follow-up. J Oral Biol Craniofac Res. 2021 Apr-Jun;11(2):219-224.
51. Chen G, Oranges CM, Giordano S, Huang R, Wang W. Horizontal animation deformity as unusual complication of neurotoxin modulation of the gummy smile. Dermatol Online J. 2019 Aug 15;25(8):13030/qt49s9h9zh.

Marionette lines

52. Hur MS, Hu KS, Cho JY, Kwak HH, Song WC, Koh KS, Lorente M, Kim HJ. Topography and location of the depressor anguli oris muscle with a reference to the mental foramen. Surg Radiol Anat. 2008 Jul;30(5):403-7.
53. Choi YJ, We YJ, Lee HJ, Lee KW, Gil YC, Hu KS, Tansatit T, Kim HJ. Three-Dimensional Evaluation of the Depressor Anguli Oris and Depressor Labii Inferioris for Botulinum Toxin Injections. Aesthet Surg J. 2021 May 18;41(6):NP456-NP461.
54. de Maio M, Swift A, Signorini M, Fagien S; Aesthetic Leaders in Facial Aesthetics Consensus Committee. Facial Assessment and Injection Guide for Botulinum Toxin and Injectable Hyaluronic Acid Fillers: Focus on the Upper Face. Plast Reconstr Surg. 2017 Aug;140(2):265e-276e.
55. Sundaram H, Signorini M, Liew S, Trindade de Almeida AR, Wu Y, Vieira Braz A, Fagien S, Goodman GJ, Monheit G, Raspaldo H; Global Aesthetics Consensus Group. Glo-

bal Aesthetics Consensus: Botulinum Toxin Type A--Evidence-Based Review, Emerging Concepts, and Consensus Recommendations for Aesthetic Use, Including Updates on Complications. Plast Reconstr Surg. 2016 Mar;137(3):518e-529e.

56. Sundaram H, Liew S, Signorini M, Vieira Braz A, Fagien S, Swift A, De Boulle KL, Raspaldo H, Trindade de Almeida AR, Monheit G; Global Aesthetics Consensus Group. Global Aesthetics Consensus: Hyaluronic Acid Fillers and Botulinum Toxin Type A-Recommendations for Combined Treatment and Optimizing Outcomes in Diverse Patient Populations. Plast Reconstr Surg. 2016 May;137(5):1410-1423.

Chin profile and poppy chin

57. Hsu AK, Frankel AS. Modification of Chin Projection and Aesthetics with OnabotulinumtoxinA Injection. JAMA Facial Plast Surg. 2017 Dec 1;19(6):522-527.

58. Yu N, Liu Y, Chen C, Dong R, Yang E, Wang X. Paradoxical bulging of mentalis after botulinum toxin type A injection. J Cosmet Dermatol. 2020 Jun;19(6):1290-1293.

59. Zarins U. Anatomy of Facial Expression. Anatomy Next, Inc. Third Edition 2019.

60. Farkas LG, Katic MJ, Forrest CR, Alt KW, Bagic I, Baltadjiev G, Cunha E, Cvicelová M, Davies S, Erasmus I, Gillett-Netting R, Hajnis K, Kemkes-Grottenthaler A, Khomyakova I, Kumi A, Kgamphe JS, Kayo-daigo N, Le T, Malinowski A, Negasheva M, Manolis S, Ogetürk M, Parvizrad R, Rösing F, Sahu P, Sforza C, Sivkov S, Sultanova N, Tomazo-Ravnik T, Tóth G, Uzun A, Yahia E. International anthropometric study of facial morphology in various ethnic groups/races. J Craniofac Surg. 2005 Jul;16(4):615-46.

61. D'Souza A, Ng CL. (2020). Applied Anatomy for Botulinum Toxin Injection in Cosmetic Interventions. Current Otorhinolaryngology Reports. 8. 10.1007.

62. Yu N, Liu Y, Chen C, Dong R, Yang E, Wang X. Paradoxical bulging of mentalis after botulinum toxin type A injection. J Cosmet Dermatol. 2020 Jun;19(6):1290-1293.

63. Choi DY, Bae H, Bae JH, Kim HJ, Hu KS. Effective Locations for Injecting Botulinum Toxin into the Mentalis Muscle; Cadaveric and Ultrasonographic Study. Toxins (Basel). 2021 Jan 27;13(2):96.

Nefertiti lift

64. Levy PM. The 'Nefertiti lift': a new technique for specific re-contouring of the jawline. J Cosmet Laser Ther. 2007;9(4):249-252.

65. Levy PM. Neurotoxins: Current Concepts in Cosmetic Use on the Face and Neck--Jawline Contouring/Platysma Bands/Necklace Lines. Plast Reconstr Surg. 2015;136(5 Suppl):80S-83S.

66. Cohn JE, Greco TM. Advanced Techniques for the Use of Neurotoxins in Non-Surgical Facial Rejuvenation. Aesthetic Plast Surg. 2020;44(5):1788-1799.

67. Jabbour SF, Kechichian EG, Awaida CJ, Tomb RR, Nasr MW. Botulinum

Toxin for Neck Rejuvenation: Assessing Efficacy and Redefining Patient Selection. Plast Reconstr Surg. 2017;140(1):9e-17e.
68. Awaida CJ, Jabbour SF, Rayess YA, El Khoury JS, Kechichian EG, Nasr MW. Evaluation of the Microbotox Technique: An Algorithmic Approach for Lower Face and Neck Rejuvenation and a Crossover Clinical Trial. Plast Reconstr Surg. 2018;142(3):640-649.

Platysma bands, horizontal neck lines and cleavage

69. Trévidic P, Sykes J, Criollo-Lamilla G. Anatomy of the Lower Face and Botulinum Toxin Injections. Plast Reconstr Surg. 2015;136(5 Suppl):84S-91S.
70. Awaida CJ, Jabbour SF, Rayess YA, El Khoury JS, Kechichian EG, Nasr MW. Evaluation of the Microbotox Technique: An Algorithmic Approach for Lower Face and Neck Rejuvenation and a Crossover Clinical Trial. Plast Reconstr Surg. 2018;142(3):640-649.
71. Cohn JE, Greco TM. Advanced Techniques for the Use of Neurotoxins in Non-Surgical Facial Rejuvenation. Aesthetic Plast Surg. 2020;44(5):1788-1799.
72. Trévidic P, Criollo-Lamilla G. Platysma Bands: Is a Change Needed in the Surgical Paradigm?. Plast Reconstr Surg. 2017;139(1):41-47.
73. Pelle-Ceravolo M, Angelini M, Silvi E. Complete Platysma Transection in Neck Rejuvenation: A Critical Appraisal. Plast Reconstr Surg. 2016;138(4):781-791.
74. Lee JH, Park YG, Park ES. A Prospective Observational Study of the Effectiveness and Safety of Botulinum Toxin in the Horizontal Neck Lines. Aesthetic Plast Surg. 2018;42(5):1370-1378.

Salivary glands

75. Bushara KO. Sialorrhea in amyotrophic lateral sclerosis: a hypothesis of a new treatment--botulinum toxin A injections of the parotid glands. Med Hypotheses. 1997 Apr;48(4):337-9.
76. Teymoortash A, Sommer F, Mandic R, Schulz S, Bette M, Aumüller G, Werner JA. Intraglandular application of botulinum toxin leads to structural and functional changes in rat acinar cells. Br J Pharmacol. 2007 Sep;152(1):161-7.
77. Bae GY, Yune YM, Seo K, Hwang SI. Botulinum toxin injection for salivary gland enlargement evaluated using computed tomographic volumetry. Dermatol Surg. 2013 Sep;39(9):1404-7.
78. Sundaram H, Huang PH, Hsu NJ, Huh CH, Wu WT, Wu Y, Cassuto D, Kerscher MJ, Seo KK; Pan-Asian Aesthetics Toxin Consensus Group. Aesthetic Applications of Botulinum Toxin A in Asians: An International, Multidisciplinary, Pan-Asian Consensus. Plast Reconstr Surg Glob Open. 2016 Dec 7;4(12):e872.

4

MICROBOTULINUM

Alberto Diaspro, Lucia Calvisi

The use of botulinum to reduce facial wrinkles is one of the leading treatments in aesthetic medicine and surgery.
The desire to avoid a rigid and artificial looking appearance has led patients to demand more natural treatment results. Consequently, doctors have started to vary the dose of the drug and the dilution in order to achieve optimal reduction of wrinkles, preserving facial expression as much as possible. While those learning the injection technique are taught to inject fixed doses in traditional sites, this has evolved, developing off-label indications to customise the dosage and injection sites on an individual basis.
In order to achieve the non-artificial result desired by both the doctor and the patient, more detailed technical aspects, such as the anatomy of the muscles in relation to the points of penetration into the dermis, where expression lines appear, and the attenuation of muscle strength rather than its suppression, were taken into consideration, with the aim of ensuring a natural expression following treatment [1].

Indications

The main indication of the microbotulinum technique are:
- treatment of the forehead and eye area (fig. 5);
- rejuvenation of the jawline and neck (fig. 1);
- improvement of skin quality (fig. 2).

For the treatment of the forehead and eye area, this technique has a lower incidence of brow ptosis and preserves a more natural facial expression than intramuscular injection, especially in older people, as the frontalis muscles become progressively thinner as we age. This different effect is presumably due to the reduced thickness of the skin and subcutaneous layer of the forehead, which facilitates propagation to the portion of muscle responsible for the formation of the wrinkle and better results despite the use of a reduced dose [2,3].
The improvement in skin quality is due to a reduction in surface microwrinkles, secondary to the effect of the drug on the dermal attachment of the mimic muscles [4]. It also acts on the cholinergic fibres of the sebaceous glands, limiting seborrhoea, and of the capillaries, controlling redness (see chapter on botulinum in dermatology).
Facial rejuvenation is achieved with injection into the mandibular edge, the pre-parotid and temporal regions and the eye area, enhancing the action of the elevator muscles with respect to the depressor antagonists. This attenuates the gravitational ptosis of the tissues, decreasing the depth of nasolabial folds and marionette lines, and improves the definition of the jawline [5,6]. Facial ageing is also characterised by an imbalance between the action of the depressor muscles which, together with the effect of gravity, prevails over that of the elevator muscles, leading to superficial sagging of the facial tissues [7].

Injection techinque

The microbotulinum injection technique involves the repeated injection of hyperdiluted botulinum toxin micro injections into the dermis, following a repetitive pattern over the entire treatment area (fig. 5).

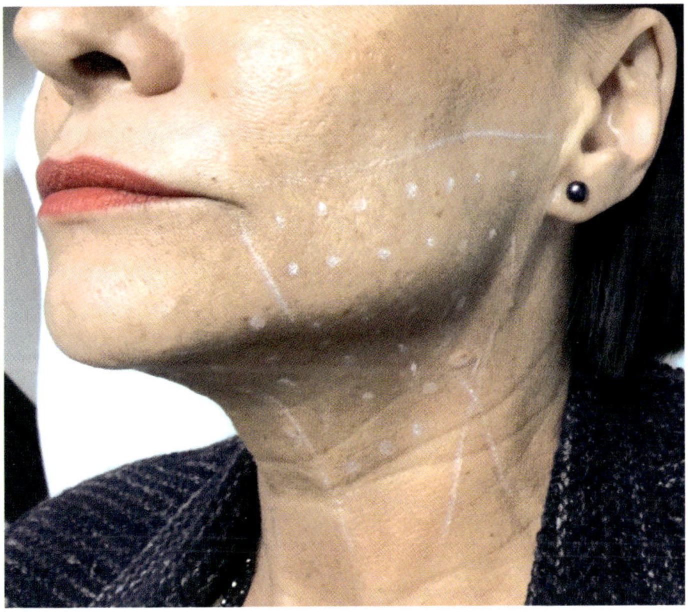

Figure 1 Microbotulinum: jawline and neck

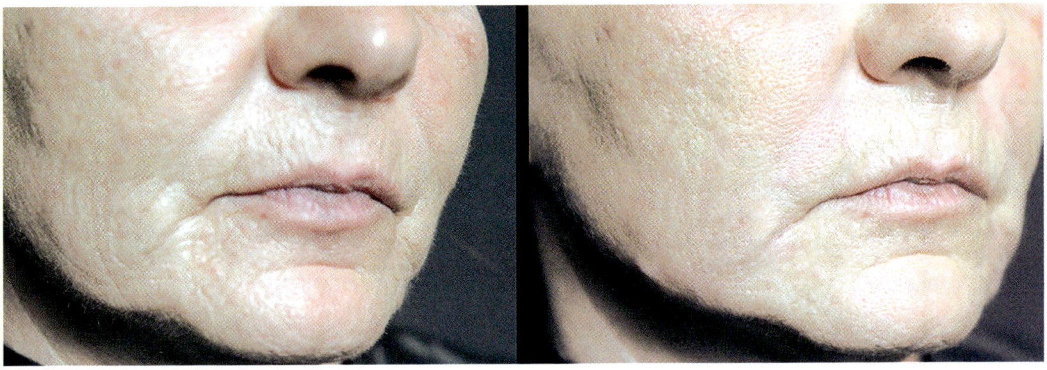

Figure 2 Microbotulinum: improvement of skin quality

The drug targets the superficial fibres of the facial muscles, weakened only at the level of their attachment to the dermis, which are responsible for the tonic component of fine wrinkles on the face and neck. The reduction in muscle strength exclusively in the part of the mimic muscles that penetrates the skin leads to the attenuation of wrinkles and fine lines, with maintenance of movement due to the action of the muscular region not affected by the diffusion of the drug [8].

The use of this technique on the forehead and in the eye area avoids the rigid and immobile appearance often obtained when injecting the solution at the traditional dilution.

It is possible to improve the quality of the skin on the lower part of the face and neck and, by reducing the activity of the superficial fibres of the platysma

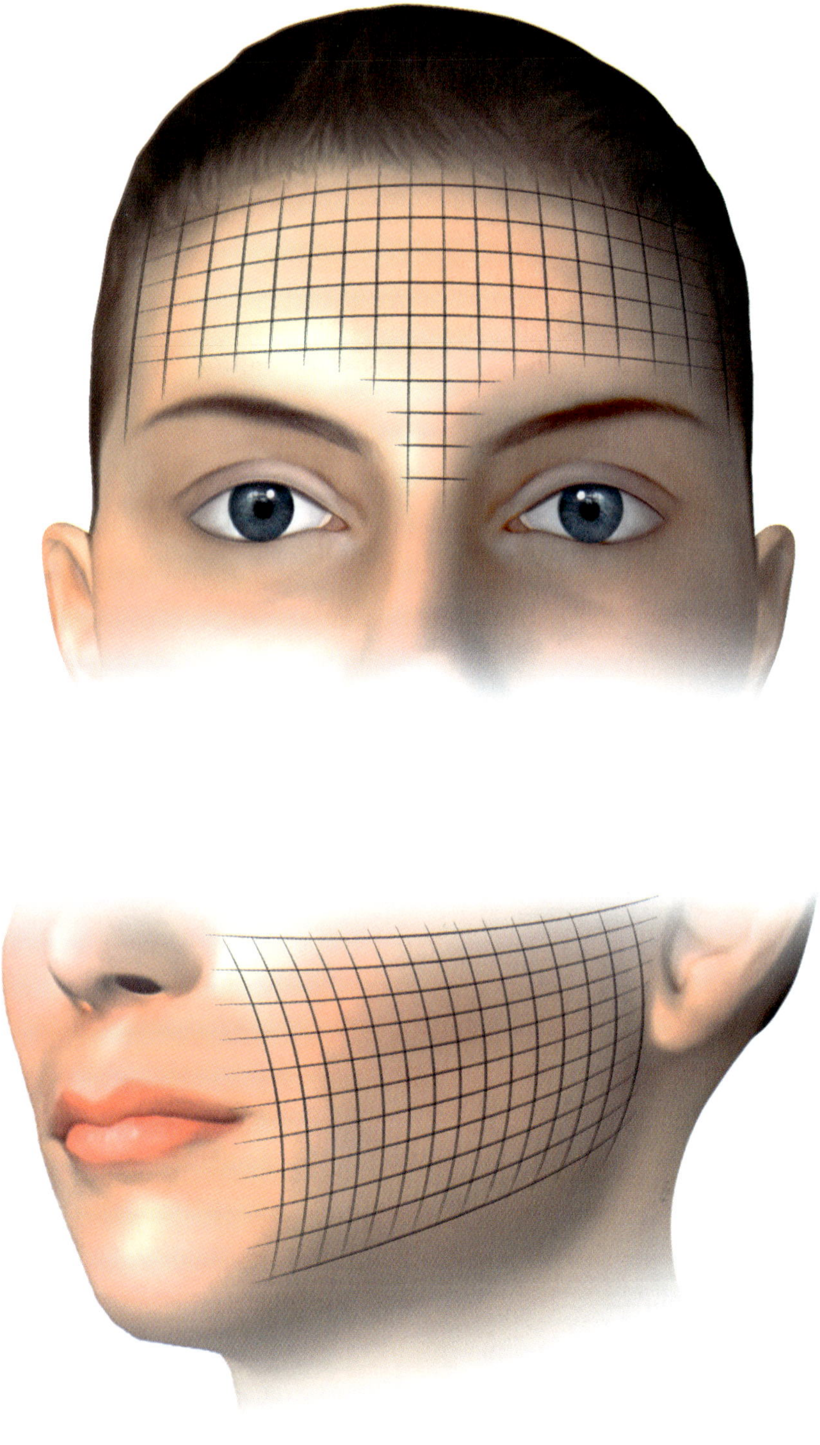

Figure 3 Injection planning grid

VIDEO 4.1

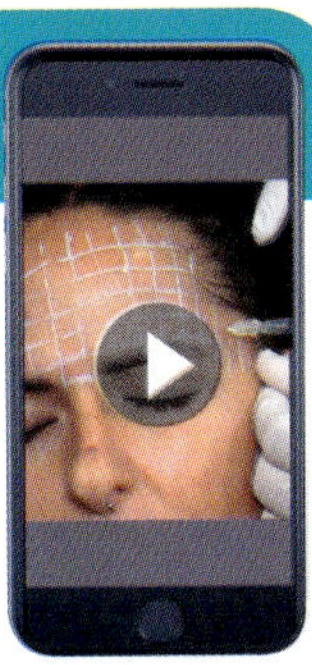

Microbotulinum

muscle, to enhance the profile of the jawline and close the cervical-mental angle, making it more defined [9].
Using abobotulinum to treat the face, a 125 U Speywood vial is reconstituted with 1.25 ml of saline solution. Then 0.5 ml (50 US) is aspirated into a 1 ml syringe and a further 0.5 ml of lidocaine (0.5%), or saline, if the patient is allergic to lidocaine, is added to the syringe for a final volume of 1 ml, with a concentration of 50 US/ml, 0.5 US in 0.01 ml.
When onabotulinum or incobotulinum is used, the 50 U Botox vial is reconstituted with 1.25 ml of saline solution. Then 0.5 ml (20 UB) are taken and combined with 0.5 ml of saline solution or an equal dose of lidocaine (0.5%) without adrenaline, creating a final quantity of 1 ml ready for injection.
The final concentration for each injection will, in this case, be 0.01 ml, which contains 0.2 UB, 20 UB/ml. For treatment of the neck, 0.7 ml is aspirated instead of the 0.5 ml mentioned [5].
During the injection procedure, the skin is kept taut by the non-dominant hand and the injections are performed over the entire area to be treated, spaced at regular intervals of 1 cm, using 32 G needles measuring 13 mm long (fig. 3). This length is optimal for controlling the depth of injection and limiting product loss.
The needle must penetrate the skin as superficially as possible, with the bevel up. When the plunger of the syringe is pressed with the correct technique, resistance to injection must be felt until a white papule forms on the skin: if the solution can be injected without resistance, the needle has been inserted too deeply into the subdermal or intramuscular layer (fig. 4) [10].
The best results are obtained in patients aged between 40 and 50 years of age, and it should be noted that their duration is more limited than that of the traditional intramuscular injection technique, which also requires a higher dose, with repetition of the injection after about three months for optimal maintenance of the clinical result [4].
Areas of the face to be injected with caution, or to be avoided by novice injectors, are the buccal area and the area below the oral commissure. Injections into the cheek should not be performed, to avoid weakening the zygomatic major and minor muscles, the altered action of which results in significant asymmetry of the mid-facial region, while those located caudally to the oral commissure, at the depressor anguli oris (DAO) and depressor labii inferioris (DLI) muscles, should be avoided, staying further to the side of these two muscles to avoid alterations in lip movement and also during speech.

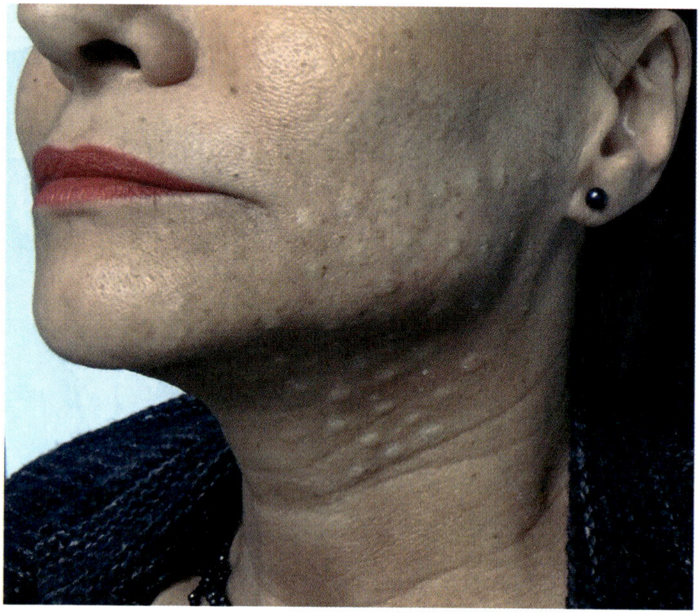

Figure 4 Injection technique with the needle bevel facing upwards: skin whitening and papule formation

Notes

Critics of this technique have argued that it is ineffective in improving skin quality, attributing any improvement to the collagen synthesis stimulated by the numerous superficial punctures rather than to the effect of the drug, as the intradermal plane does not offer any target, while the mechanical stress caused by the stretching of the tissue after injection of the solution contributes to the stimulation of fibroblastic activity [11].

To date, scientific literature proves the contrary, probably due to the evolution of diagnostic technologies which, in this field, must go beyond mere photographic observation.

This technique is undoubtedly more painful for the patient, but a topical anaesthetic can be applied before the session. The duration of action, which is often declared to be shorter than for intramuscular administration, is actually shorter, because a lower dose is injected: electromyographic studies confirm that, with the same number of units administered, the effect of the drug is not affected by the injection technique [10,12] and that doses can be increased to those used for intramuscular therapy without incurring side effects, if the technique is performed correctly [13].

Bibliography

1. Wu WTL. Microbotox of the lower face and neck: Evolution of a personal technique and its clinical effects. Plast Reconstr Surg. 2015;136(Suppl):92S–100S.
2. Jun JY, Park JH, Youn CS, Lee JH. Intradermal Injection of Botulinum

Toxin: A Safer Treatment Modality for Forehead Wrinkles. Ann Dermatol. 2018;30(4):458-461.
3. Lee SK. Multiple intradermal small bolus injection of botulinum toxin: the limit and the potentiality. J Cosmet Laser Ther. 2012 Dec;14(6):304-6.
4. Diaspro A, Calvisi L, Manzoni V, Sito G. Microbotulinum: A Quantitative Evaluation of Aesthetic Skin Improvement in 62 Patients. Plast Reconstr Surg. 2020 Nov;146(5):987-994.
5. Wanitphakdeedecha R, Ungaksornpairote C, Kaewkes A, Rojanavanich V, Phothong W, Manuskiatti W. The comparison between intradermal injection of abobotulinumtoxinA and normal saline for face-lifting: a split-face randomized controlled trial. J Cosmet Dermatol. 2016 Dec;15(4):452-457.
6. Petchngaovilai C. Midface lifting with botulinum toxin: intradermal technique. J Cosmet Dermatol. 2009 Dec;8(4):312-6.
7. Atwa EM, Nasr MM, Ebrahim HM. Evaluation of Intradermal Injection of Botulinum Toxin A for Facial Lifting. J Clin Aesthet Dermatol. 2020 Dec;13(12):22-26. Epub 2020 Dec 1.
8. Sapra P, Demay S, Sapra S, Khanna J, Mraud K, Bonadonna J. A single-blind, split-face, randomized, pilot study comparing the effects of intradermal and intramuscular injection of two commercially available botulinum toxin A formulas to reduce signs of facial aging. J Clin Aesthet Dermatol. 2017;10:34–44.
9. Awaida CJ, Jabbour SF, Rayess YA, El Khoury JS, Kechichian EG, Nasr MW. Evaluation of the microbotox technique: An algorithmic approach for lower face and neck rejuvenation and a crossover clinical trial. Plast Reconstr Surg. 2018;142:640–649.
10. Wanitphakdeedecha R, Yan C, Apinuntham C, Rojanavanich V, Cembrano KAG, Eimpunth S, Manuskiatti W. Intradermal Micro-Dosing of AbobotulinumtoxinA for Face-Lifting: How Long Does It Last? Dermatol Ther (Heidelb). 2020 Aug;10(4):779-789.
11. Kapoor R, Shome D, Jain V, Dikshit R. Facial rejuvenation after intradermal botulinum toxin: is it really the botulinum toxin or is it the pricks? Dermatol Surg. 2010 Dec;36 Suppl 4:2098-105.
12. Kim YJ, Lim OK, Choi WJ. Are There Differences Between Intradermal and Intramuscular Injections of Botulinum Toxin on the Forehead? Dermatol Surg. 2020 Dec;46(12):e126-e131.
13. Sirithanabadeekul P, Lapsomboonsiri S, Rungjang A, Thanasarnaksorn W. Split face comparison between common concentration vs double dilution of intradermal abobotulinum toxin type A (Dysport) injection for facial lifting in Asians. J Cosmet Dermatol. 2018 Jun;17(3):355-360.

CLINICAL CASES

CLINICAL CASE 1

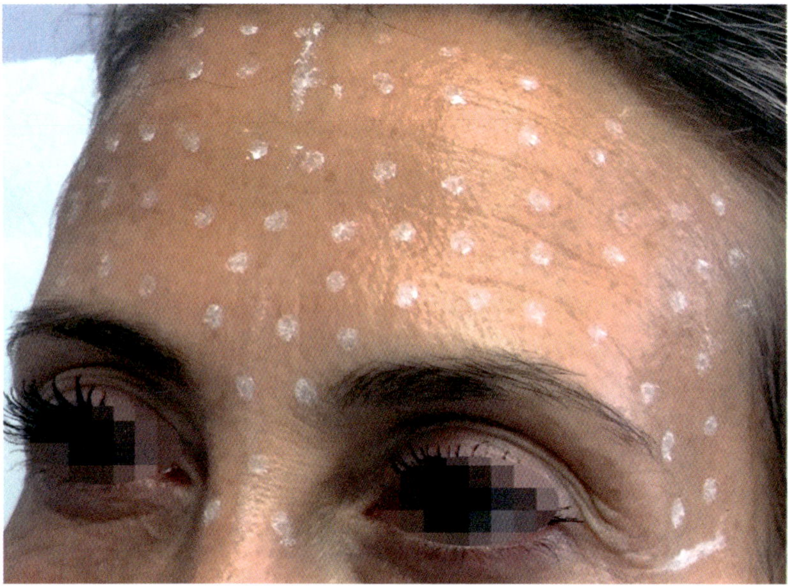

BEFORE

<

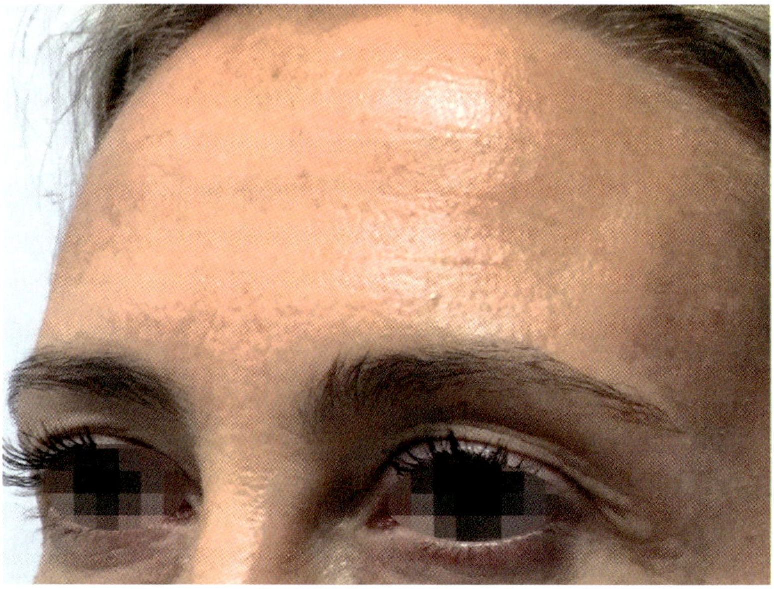

AFTER

>

Figure 5 Microbotulinum: forehead and eye area, pre and after-treatment pictures

5

BOTULINUM TOXIN IN DERMATOLOGY

Lucia Calvisi

Since its approval by the Food and Drug Administration in 2002 and by the Italian Drug Agency in 2004 for the correction of glabellar wrinkles, botulinum toxin has been widely used to treat dynamic facial wrinkles. For this reason, its use is considered generally but mistakenly to be exclusive to aesthetic medicine and surgery. Recent studies [1-3] support its use for the treatment of dermatological conditions such as acne, rosacea and hypertrophic scars, due to its pharmacological activity on various types of cells, such as fibroblasts, mast cells, sebocytes and endothelial cells.

Other promising and very recent uses of botulinum are in the treatment of androgenetic alopecia, post-herpetic neuralgia, Hailey-Hailey disease and chronic itching.

In androgenetic alopecia, botulinum acts by down-regulating TGF-β1 synthesis, which is usually increased by dihydrotestosterone [4,5]. Patients with androgenetic alopecia usually have a reduced oxygen supply to the affected area compared with the unaffected area. The use of botulinum relaxes the muscles, thereby allowing better vascularisation, converting testosterone into oestradiol and eliminating dihydrotestosterone from the affected area, resulting in a reduction in alopecia.

Post-herpetic neuralgia is a debilitating disease characterised by intense and continuous pain following an episode of herpes zoster. The risk of developing it increases with age. Botulinum toxin has been successfully used to treat several forms of migraine and headache caused by muscle tension, as it is able to inhibit not only the release of acetylcholine from neuromuscular endings, but also other mediators such as glutamate and substance P involved in the mechanism of pain transmission [6-11].

Hailey-Hailey disease, or chronic benign familial pemphigus, is a rare genetic bullous dermatosis first described by Hailey and Hailey in 1939. It is characterised by the formation of painful, foul-smelling blisters in skin folds and has a negative impact on patients' quality of life.

The way in which the botulinum toxin works is not fully known, but it probably reduces sweating, which results in the formation of fewer blisters [12].

Botulinum toxin and acne

Oily skin is a frequent complaint from patients who come to our clinic, and the treatments offered are often unsatisfactory. Oily skin is shiny and may be accompanied by enlarged pores on the nose, cheeks, forehead and chin. In addition, overproduction of sebum can cause skin problems such as acne and seborrheic dermatitis. Oily skin has a strongly negative impact on self-esteem and can lead to psychological consequences. Many people experience severe discomfort, frustration and embarrassment.

Sebum production is a physiological mechanism implemented by the skin to lubricate and moisturise, but when too much sebum is produced, it becomes pathological and causes acne.

The sebaceous gland is a holocrine gland located in the reticular dermis and is usually associated with the hair shaft. It releases its secretion in a holocrine manner onto the skin surface. In an adult, its production is approximately 1 mg/10 cm^2 every three hours. Sebaceous glands are usually concentrated mainly on the forehead.

The amount of sebum produced is related to numerous factors, such as the production of androgenous hormones, diet, age, gender, ethnicity and seasonal variations.

Androgenous hormones regulate sebum production and an increase in these hormones leads to an increase in sebocytes and lipid production. When the composition and quantity of food changes significantly, this can lead to a change in sebum secretion.

There is general agreement that sebum production is highest between the ages of 15 and 35, after which there is a decrease in both men and women. Sebum production is significantly higher in men than in women and this difference is maintained throughout life. Ethnically, black races have a higher sebum production than Caucasians. There are also studies showing that sebum production increases by 10% for every one degree rise in temperature. In conclusion, all of these factors explain why sebum production varies so much from individual to individual [13].

Sebum plays a key role in maintaining a healthy and vital epidermal barrier and preserving its integrity. However, when sebum production exceeds 1.5 mg/10 cm^2 every three hours, patients start suffering from oily skin, acne, enlarged pores and seborrheic dermatitis.

The effectiveness of botulinum toxin on oily skin was discovered quite by chance. When using it for aesthetic purposes, a reduction in pore size and the oily appearance of the skin was observed. We are not sure exactly how it works but, when injected intradermally, botulinum toxin appears to reduce sebum production due to its neuromodulator effect on the hair erector muscle and muscarinic receptors in the sebaceous gland (fig. 1).

The method of administration seems crucial to the success of the treatment and the toxin must be delivered into the dermis by inserting the needle into the skin at a 75-degree angle [14].

The studies reported in literature concern both Onabotulinum-ToxinA and Abobotulinum-ToxinA, especially on the oily skin [15] of the forehead region, and show an improvement in symptoms within the first week of administration of the drug. It is normally necessary to perform a touch up after 15 days to obtain effects that are usually maintained for four to six months.

According to the various studies mentioned in literature, the amount of product most frequently used is 30-45 U of Abobotulinum-ToxinA and 10-20 U of OnabotulinumtoxinA [13-20].

The microbotulinum technique has also given encouraging results: the face is divided into a grid and small quantities of the product are injected into the superficial intradermal area in such a way as to cover the area affected by the pathology, performing up to 100-150 microinjections. This treatment is clearly reserved for the most difficult cases or those which fail to respond to traditional treatments, but it is nevertheless a valid therapeutic alternative (fig. 3).

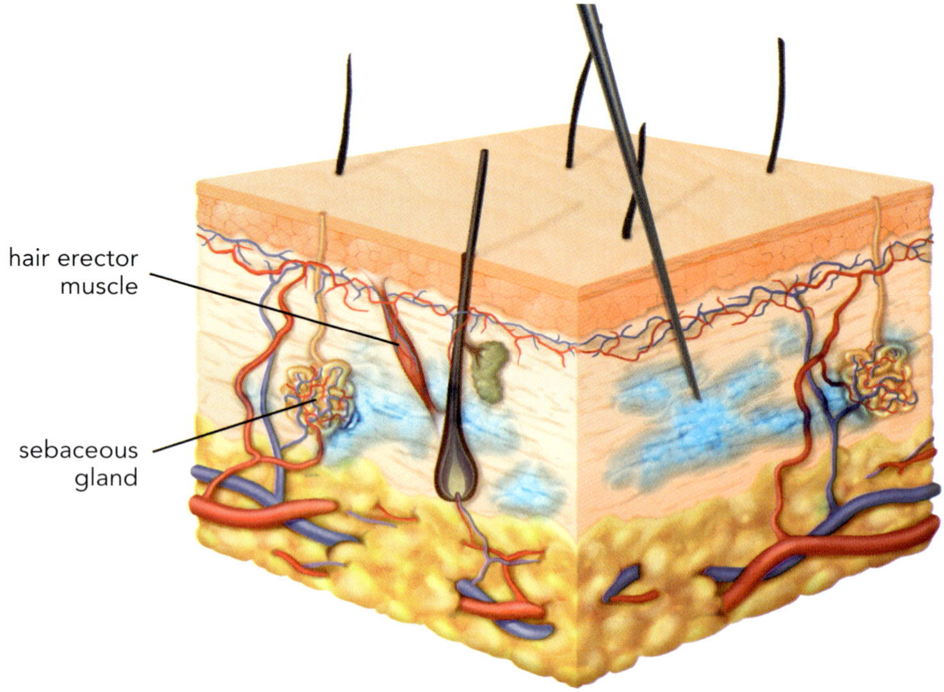

Figure 1 Hair erector muscle and muscarinic receptors in the sebaceous gland

Botulinum toxin and rosacea

Rosacea is a dermatosis characterised by persistent erythema, telangiectasias, papules, pustules and facial flushing. It is more common in women than men and the exact pathophysiological mechanism is still unknown.

Flushing (the first stage of rosacea) is a condition of episodic attacks of redness accompanied by heat and burning of the face, neck and, less frequently, the upper torso. It occurs more frequently in people with fair skin.

The term "flush" was first used in 1882 to indicate redness that can be episodic or constant. Repeated attacks result in permanent erythema, telangiectasias and a cyanotic facial background.

An increase in facial telangiectasias is a common condition in fair-skinned people and can be triggered by several factors, such as washing with water that is too hot or too cold, spicy foods, exercise or hot drinks.

Facial flushing can be divided into two categories:

- mediated by the autonomic nervous system (moist);
- mediated by direct vasodilation (dry).

Vasodilator-mediated flushing can, in turn, be subdivided into a group with dysesthesia and a group without dysesthesia.

It is very important to collect an accurate patient history to exclude diseases such as pheochromocytoma or carcinoid syndrome.

In primary forms not associated with other diseases, as the disease progresses, permanent erythema, inflammatory papules and pustules occur, with phimatous changes especially in the nose, and

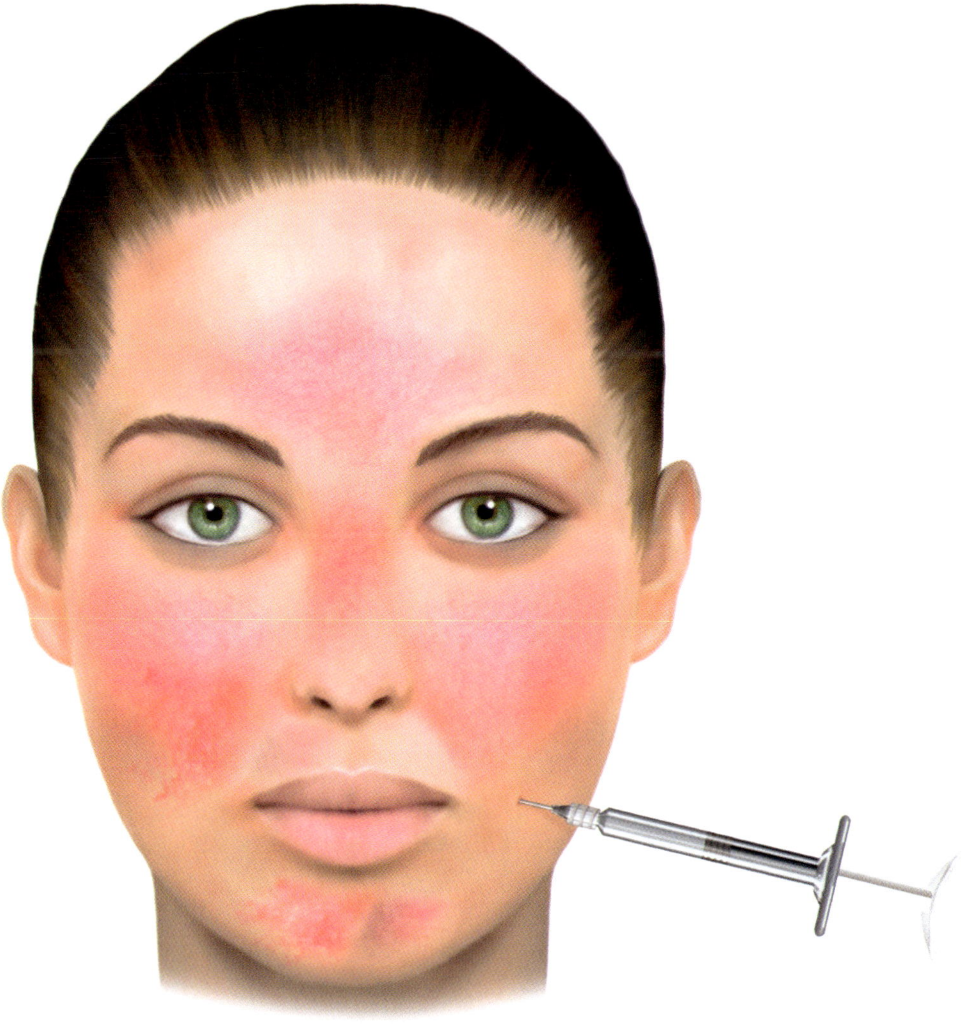

Figure 2 Botulinum toxin treatment for the reduction of facial flushing

signs and symptoms in the eyes.

The pathogenesis is complex and not completely clear: abnormal neurovascular signals, dysregulation of the neurovascular system and dysmicrobialism, triggered by factors such as alcohol, heat, exercise and spicy food, play a key role, supporting the neurogenic inflammation already present.

Traditional topical and systemic therapies are often unsuccessful in treating this skin condition, which creates considerable psychological distress for the patient suffering from it, not least because of the fact that it progressively worsens. The treatment of rosacea is variable and depends on the severity of the clinical situation; it can range from changes in lifestyle to the use of appropriate skincare products to systemic therapies. Laser therapies with both KTP laser and IPL (Intense Pulsed Light) are particularly effective for the vascular component.

The use of botulinum to treat flushing has also been recently proposed. Botulinum improves the symptoms of rosacea by blocking the release of acetylcholine [21]. Botulinum toxin also inhibits the release of inflammatory mediators such as substance P, preventing mast cell degranulation [22]. Studies reported in literature show that patients who have botulinum toxin treatment experience a reduction in skin flushing, resulting in improved quality of life (fig. 2).
The dosages reported in literature are variable. Park et al. report the use of 15 U of Onabotulinum-ToxinA, Odo et al. used 6.2 U of Abobotulinum-ToxinA in each site [21-24].
Yuraitis et al. report the following treatment: OnabotulinumToxinA reconstituted with 5 cc of saline solution to obtain a final dilution of 2 U per 0.1 cc. 10 U (0.5 cc) of product is then injected intradermally into the cheeks where the problem is most acute. Within two weeks of treatment the patient notices an improvement in erythema, both at rest and during flushes.

Botulinum toxin and scars

Scars are the marks that remain after a wound heals following surgery or trauma; they can be a cause for concern for the patient, especially when located on the face or neck.
The wound healing process is a complicated procedure that consists mainly of three steps: an inflammatory phase, tissue granulation and scar formation. If the scar formation is pathological, it results in the formation of hypertrophic and keloid scars.
The prevalence of hypertrophic and keloid scars is the same in both sexes, but keloids are more frequent among Asians and African Americans [25]. There is often confusion between hypertrophic and keloid scars. Hypertrophic scars are usually raised, but rarely more than 4 mm above the skin surface. They are reddish or pinkish in colour and have margins within the wound. Keloids, on the other hand, are bigger and typically extend beyond the wound margins.
The treatment of both hypertrophic scars and keloids remains problematic due to their uncertain aetiology. Current treatments include surgical and non-surgical methods such as compression, silicone sheets, cryotherapy, laser, intralesional corticosteroid injections, intralesional 5-fluorouracil injections and botulinum toxin.
The theory of using botulinum toxin in scars was first published in 2000. We know that the most important factor that determines the final aesthetic result of a scar is the tension that occurs at the wound edges during the healing process. Tension at the wound edges can lead (directly mechanically or indirectly chemically) to an abnormal healing process. The tension applied perpendicularly to the edges of the wound places the muscles in such conditions as to cause the formation of significant scars. Repeated micro-trauma, caused by continuous muscular activity around the wound, induces a prolonged inflammatory response with deposition of collagen and glycosaminoglycans, resulting in hypertrophic and keloid scars.
When botulinum toxin is injected lo-

cally, it causes temporary paralysis of the wound muscles, reducing perpendicular tension and promoting the healing process.
Botulinum toxin works both to prevent the formation of keloids and hypertrophic scars and to treat them. The determining factor in the wound healing process is the tension created between the edges of the wound, which affects the aesthetic outcome, leading to hypertrophy and visibility. By blocking the release of the neurotransmitter acetylcholine at peripheral nerve ending level, botulinum allows the almost complete elimination of the tension that has an influence on the healing process; this is associated with inhibition of TGF-β1 at myofibroblast level, as shown in numerous studies [25].
Botulinum also acts on hypertrophic scars and keloids, by regulating the abnormal scarring process with dysregulated growth and excessive production of collagen. Numerous studies have shown the effectiveness of botulinum on this type of scar, especially on hypertrophic scars, thanks to interference with the activity of fibroblasts. Botulinum also seems to suppress the expression of TGF-β1, collagen I and III, smooth muscle actin and myosin in keloid fibroblasts. The dosages used differed according to the clinical studies reported in literature: in one study, botulinum injections (2.5 UI/cm^3 of OnabotulinumtoxinA) were performed once a month for three months; in another study the effectiveness of botulinum (5 UI/cm^3 of OnabotulinumtoxinA), repeated every four weeks, was compared to that of kenacort, where botulinum yielded a more significant reduction in symptoms associated with hypertrophic scars such as itching and inflammation (fig. 4) [26].
Another study demonstrates the successful use of botulinum as a preventative measure against significant scar formation. 0.2 ml of saline were injected with 15 U of OnabotulinumtoxinA into the edges of a surgical wound in one group of patients and this group was compared with another group of patients injected with saline alone. The patients treated with botulinum showed a statistically and clinically significant improvement compared to the placebo-only group.
In conclusion, the use of botulinum looks very promising in the treatment of scars, both in the prevention of significant scars and in the treatment of scars once they have formed.

Bibliography

1. Schlessinger J, Gilbert E, Cohen JL, Kaufman J. New Uses of AbobotulinumtoxinA in Aesthetics. Aesthet Surg J. 2017 May1;37(suppl_1):S45-S58.
2. Feily A, Fallahi H, Zandian D, Kalantar H. A succinct review of botulinum toxin in dermatology; update of cosmetic and noncosmetic use. J Cosmet Dermatol. 2011 Mar;10(1):58-67.
3. Freeman MD, Margulies IG, Sanati-Mehrizy P, Burish N, Taub PJ. Nonaesthetic Applications for Botulinum Toxin in Plastic Surgery. Plast Reconstr Surg. 2020 Jul;146(1):157-170.
4. Shon U, Kim MH, Lee DY, Kim SH, Park BC. The effect of intradermal botulinum toxin on androgenetic

alopecia and its possible mechanism. J Am Acad Dermatol. 2020 Dec;83(6):1838-1839.
5. Carloni R, Gandolfi S, Postel F, Bertheuil N, Pechevy L. Reply to: "The effect of intradermal botulinum toxin on androgenetic alopecia and its possible mechanism". J Am Acad Dermatol. 2020 Dec;83(6):e435-e436.
6. Sandrini G, De Icco R, Tassorelli C, Smania N, Tamburin S. Botulinum neurotoxin type A for the treatment of pain: not just in migraine and trigeminal neuralgia. J Headache Pain. 2017 Dec;18(1):38.
7. Wei J, Zhu X, Yang G, Shen J, Xie P, Zuo X, Xia L, Han Q, Zhao Y. The efficacy and safety of botulinum toxin type A in treatment of trigeminal neuralgia and peripheral neuropathic pain: A meta-analysis of randomized controlled trials. Brain Behav. 2019 Oct;9(10):e01409.
8. Wei J, Zhu X, Yang G, Shen J, Xie P, Zuo X, Xia L, Han Q, Zhao Y. The efficacy and safety of botulinum toxin type A in treatment of trigeminal neuralgia and peripheral neuropathic pain: A meta-analysis of randomized controlled trials. Brain Behav. 2019 Oct;9(10):e01409.
9. Shackleton T, Ram S, Black M, Ryder J, Clark GT, Enciso R. The efficacy of botulinum toxin for the treatment of trigeminal and postherpetic neuralgia: a systematic review with meta-analyses. Oral Surg Oral Med Oral Pathol Oral Radiol. 2016 Jul;122(1):61-71.
10. Fischoff DK, Spivakovsky S. Botulinum toxin for facial neuralgia. Evid Based Dent. 2018 Jun;19(2):57-58.
11. Sotiriou E, Apalla Z, Panagiotidou D, Ioannidis D. Severe post-herpetic neuralgia successfully treated with botulinum toxin A: three case reports. Acta Derm Venereol. 2009;89(2):214-5.
12. Bar-Ilan E, Koren A, Shehadeh W, Mashiah J, Sprecher E, Artzi O. An enhanced transcutaneous delivery of botulinum toxin for the treatment of Hailey-Hailey disease. Dermatol Ther. 2020 Jan;33(1):e13184.
13. Sayed KS, Hegazy R, Gawdat HI, Abdel Hay RM, Ahmed MM, Mohammed FN, Allam R, Fahim A. The efficacy of intradermal injections of botulinum toxin in the management of enlarged facial pores and seborrhea: a split face-controlled study. J Dermatolog Treat. 2020 Jan 3:1-7.
14. Shuo L, Ting Y, KeLun W, Rui Z, Rui Z, Hang W. Efficacy and possible mechanisms of botulinum toxin treatment of oily skin. J Cosmet Dermatol. 2019 Apr;18(2):451-457.
15. Rose AE, Goldberg DJ. Safety and efficacy of intradermal injection of botulinum toxin for the treatment of oily skin. Dermatol Surg. 2013 Mar;39(3 Pt 1):443-8.
16. Degouy A, Aubin A, Aubin F, Monnier G, Humbert P. La toxine botulique en dermatologie [Botulinum toxin in dermatology]. Ann Dermatol Venereol. 2000 Jun-Jul;127(6-7):638-42. French.
17. Messikh R, Atallah L, Aubin F, Humbert P. La toxine botulique dans les maladies dermatologiques invalidantes [Botulinum toxin in disabling dermatological diseases]. Ann Dermatol Venereol. 2009 May;136 Suppl 4:S129-36. French.

18. Böni R, Kreyden OP, Burg G. Revival of the use of botulinum toxin: application in dermatology. Dermatology. 2000;200(4):287-91.
19. Diamond A, Jankovic J. Botulinum toxin in dermatology - beyond wrinkles and sweat. J Cosmet Dermatol. 2006 Jun;5(2):169.
20. Giordano CN, Matarasso SL, Ozog DM. Injectable and topical neurotoxins in dermatology: Indications, adverse events, and controversies. J Am Acad Dermatol. 2017 Jun;76(6):1027-1042.
21. Choi JE, Werbel T, Wang Z, Wu CC, Yaksh TL, Di Nardo A. Botulinum toxin blocks mast cells and prevents rosacea like inflammation. J Dermatol Sci. 2019 Jan;93(1):58-64.
22. Philipp-Dormston WG. Botulinum toxin in der Dermatologie [Botulinum toxin in dermatology]. Hautarzt. 2014 Feb;65(2):133-43; quiz 144-5. German.
23. Park KY, Hyun MY, Jeong SY, Kim BJ, Kim MN, Hong CK. Botulinum toxin for the treatment of refractory erythema and flushing of rosacea. Dermatology. 2015;230(4):299-301.
24. Eshghi G, Khezrian L, Alirezaei P. Botulinum Toxin A in Treatment of Facial Flushing. Acta Med Iran. 2016 Jul;54(7):454-7.
25. Kasyanju Carrero LM, Ma WW, Liu HF, Yin XF, Zhou BR. Botulinum toxin type A for the treatment and prevention of hypertrophic scars and keloids: Updated review. J Cosmet Dermatol. 2019 Feb;18(1):10-15.
26. Calvisi L, Diaspro A, Sito G. Microbotulinum: a quantitative evaluation of dermatological skin improvement in 50 patients. J Cosmet Laser Ther. 2020. In press.
27. Calvisi L, Diaspro A, Sito G. Microbotox: a quantitative evaluation of dermatological improvement in patients with mild to moderate acne and erythematoteleangectatic rosacea. J Cosmetic Dermatol. In press.

CLINICAL CASES

CLINICAL CASE 1

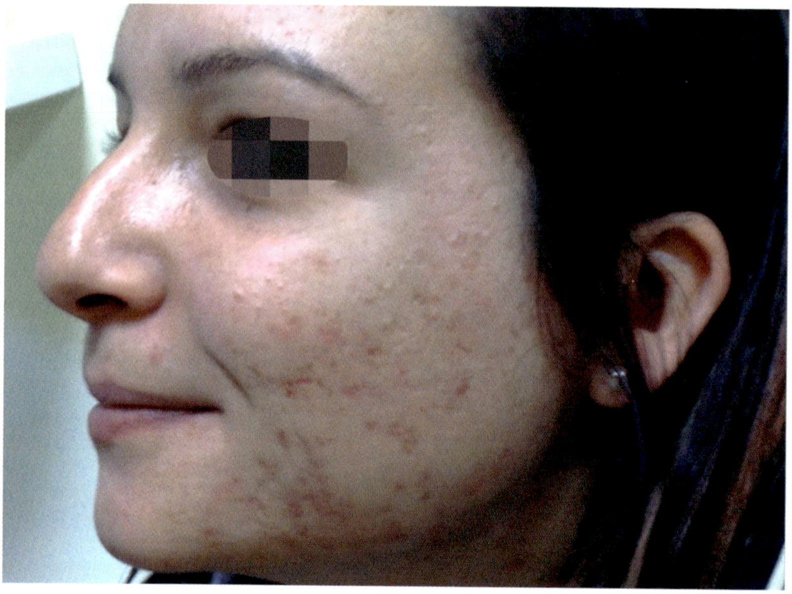

BEFORE

<

AFTER

>

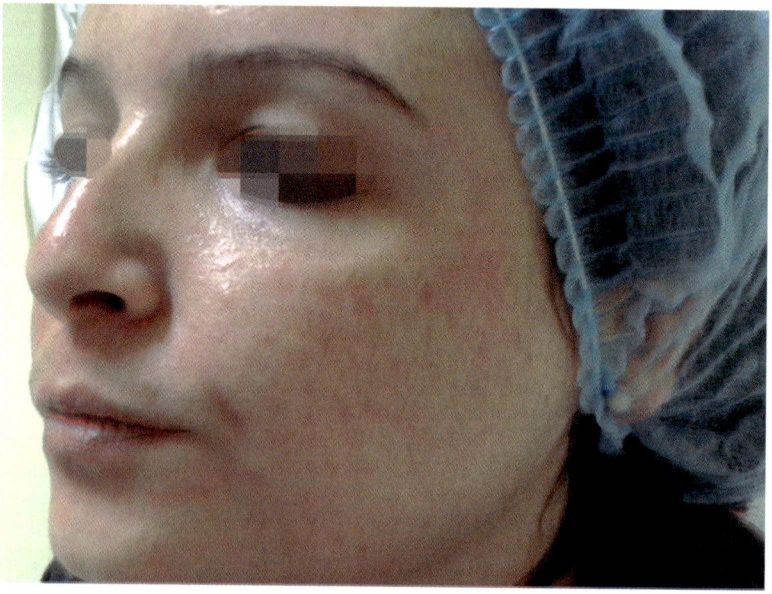

Figure 3 Patient treated with the microbotulinum technique. Pictures before and 15 days after treatment

CLINICAL CASES

CLINICAL CASE 2

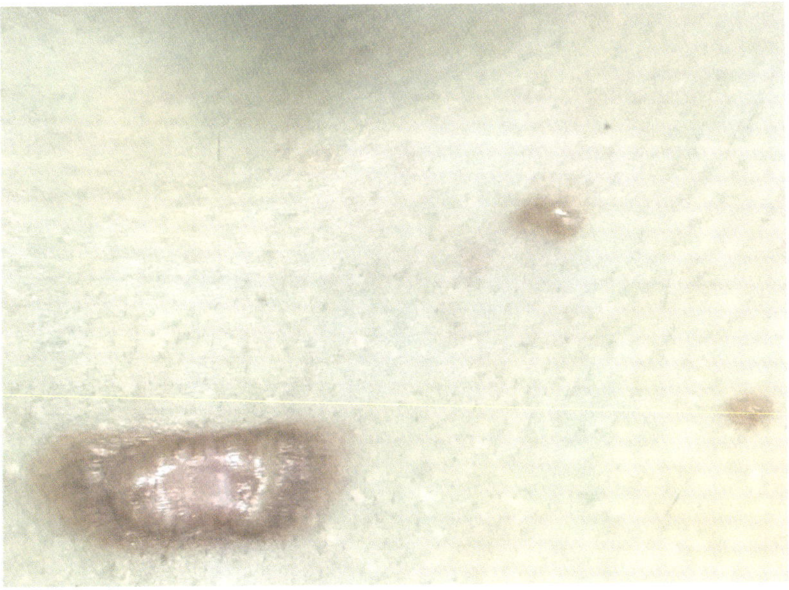

BEFORE <

AFTER >

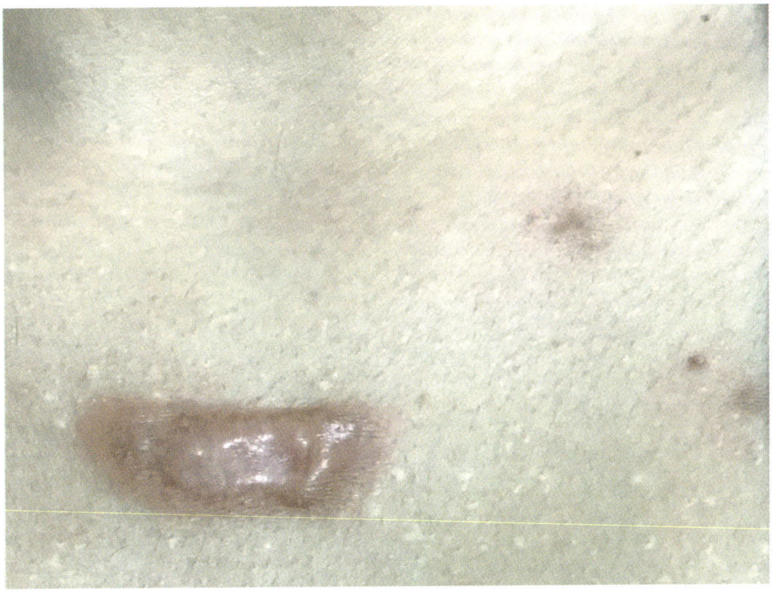

Figure 4 Keloid lesions before and after infiltration of 15 U of botulinum toxin. Note how the smaller lesions in the upper part of the cleavage have completely disappeared, while the larger one has shrunk in size

6

BOTULINUM TOXIN IN THE TREATMENT OF HYPERHIDROSIS

Lucia Calvisi, Giuseppe Sito

Hyperhidrosis is defined as an overactivity of the eccrine sweat glands [1,2]. It affects between 1 and 3% of the population and is mostly (90%) primary, i.e.: idiopathic, and typically affects the armpits, palms of the hands, soles of the feet and craniofacial region. It can be hereditary and usually occurs during adolescence but can occur as early as childhood. Primary hyperhidrosis does not usually occur during sleep. More than one-third of people with hyperhidrosis report the condition as unbearable and highly influential on their normal daily activities; more than two-thirds of patients report a family history of the condition, suggesting a genetic predisposition.

The causes of primary hyperhidrosis are not fully understood. The eccrine sweat glands, which are distributed throughout the body but are more concentrated on the palms of the hands, soles of the feet, armpits and face, are innervated by autonomous nerve fibres stimulated by the neurotransmitter acetylcholine.

To diagnose primary hyperhidrosis, the patient must have been sweating excessively for at least six months, without any other secondary causes.

Secondary causes of hyperhidrosis include alcohol abuse, acute respiratory failure, congestive heart failure, certain endocrine diseases such as diabetes, thyrotoxicosis, skin tumours or the intake of certain drugs. In the event of sudden onset of hyperhidrosis, it is always necessary to exclude other primary causes which, as we have seen, can be much more serious and may be masked by the onset of hyperhidrosis.

The clinical characteristics that help distinguish between the two forms of hyperhidrosis are the age of onset, the way sweating occurs and the associated symptoms. Secondary hyperhidrosis usually has a later onset (after the age of 25) than primary hyperhidrosis. Patients with primary hyperhidrosis frequently tend to have a unilateral or asymmetric distribution of the problem, which tends to be generalised rather than focal and also typically occurs at night. Secondary hyperhidrosis is less frequently associated with familiarity [3].

The mechanism of action is to block the release of acetylcholine, although sweat glands should not be affected by acetylcholine, at the neuromuscular junction, with a fully reversible effect lasting an average of 4-6 months [4-8].

Eccrine glands

Let's look at the anatomy and function of the eccrine glands (fig. 1). They are merocrine-secreting tubular glands, varying in number from two million to four million, and are present in virtually every part of the body. They are, however, most abundant on the palms of the hands and the soles of the feet, and in the armpits and groin. There is no difference in number between males and females, but they are more numerous in African Americans, probably due to genetic factors.

The secretion of the glands is a sterile solution of electrolytes containing bicarbonate, potassium and sodium chloride. There is also a minority presence of glucose, pyruvate, cytokines, immunoglobulins, antimicrobial pepti-

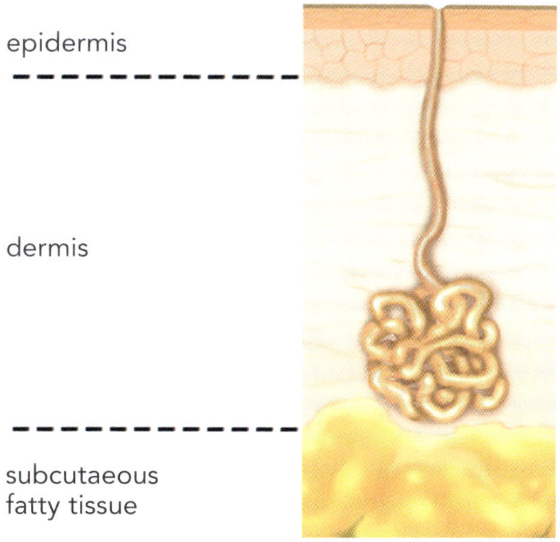

Figure 1 Eccrine glands

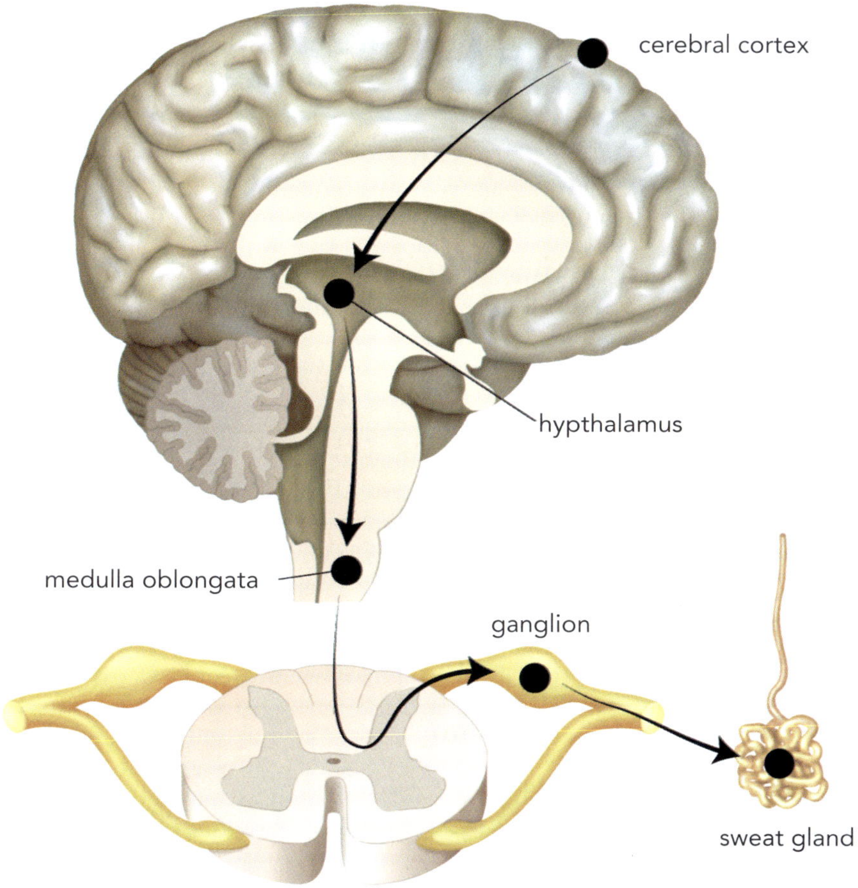

Figure 2 Stress sweating

des and many other substances.
The sweat glands perform the following functions:
- thermoregulation;
- solute secretion;
- formation of the hydrolipid film.
The physiological secretion of the sweat glands is mediated by cholinergic innervation, with acetylcholine as the main mediator. Heat is the main stimulus for sweating, but there are also other factors, such as stress for example.
It is thought that, in patients with hyperhidrosis, there is an alteration in signal transmission, as follows: 1) from the cerebral cortex to the hypothalamus; 2) from the hypothalamus to the medulla; 3) fibres that cross the medulla and travel in the lateral horns of the vertebral column; 4) from the lateral horns to the sympathetic ganglia; 5) from the sympathetic ganglia to the sweat glands as postganglionic C fibres (fig. 2).

Patient assessment

Primary hyperhidrosis is a condition of great discomfort for the patient. Defining what constitutes excessive sweating is not easy, but a level that affects quality of life seems to be a good definition.
The first step is the differential diagnosis between primary and secondary hyperhidrosis, based on age of onset, exclusion of drug intake and secondary disease, and bilaterality in one or more sites. Many patients have a positive family history or complain of at least one episode per week.
Indications that a patient suffers from secondary hyperhidrosis are widespread hyper-sweating, especially at night, the use of drugs, with their

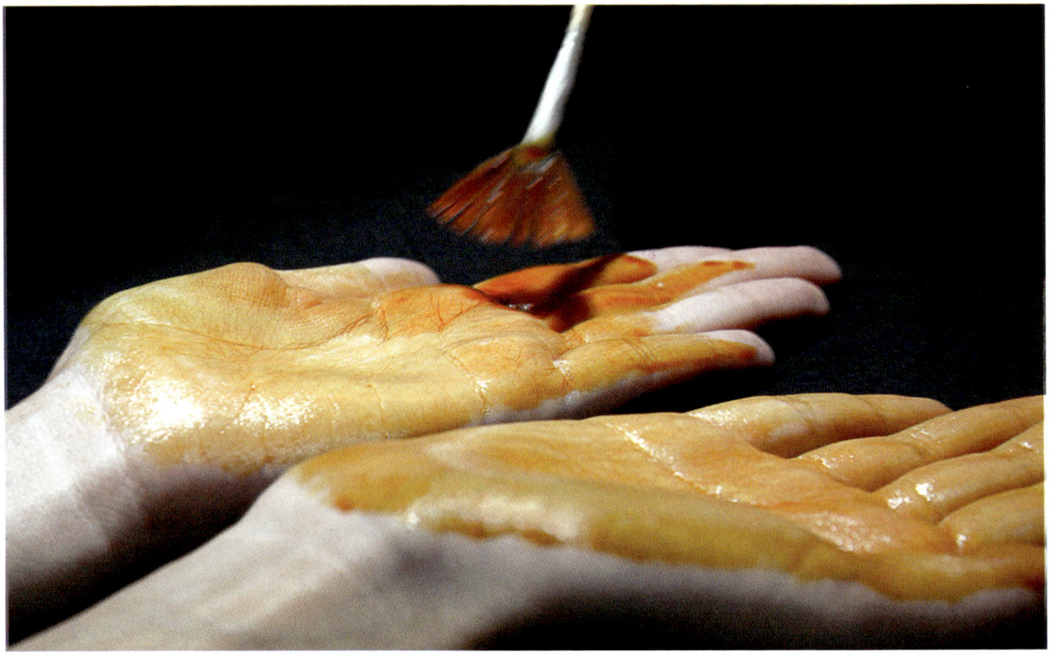

Figure 3 Minor test: application of an iodine solution

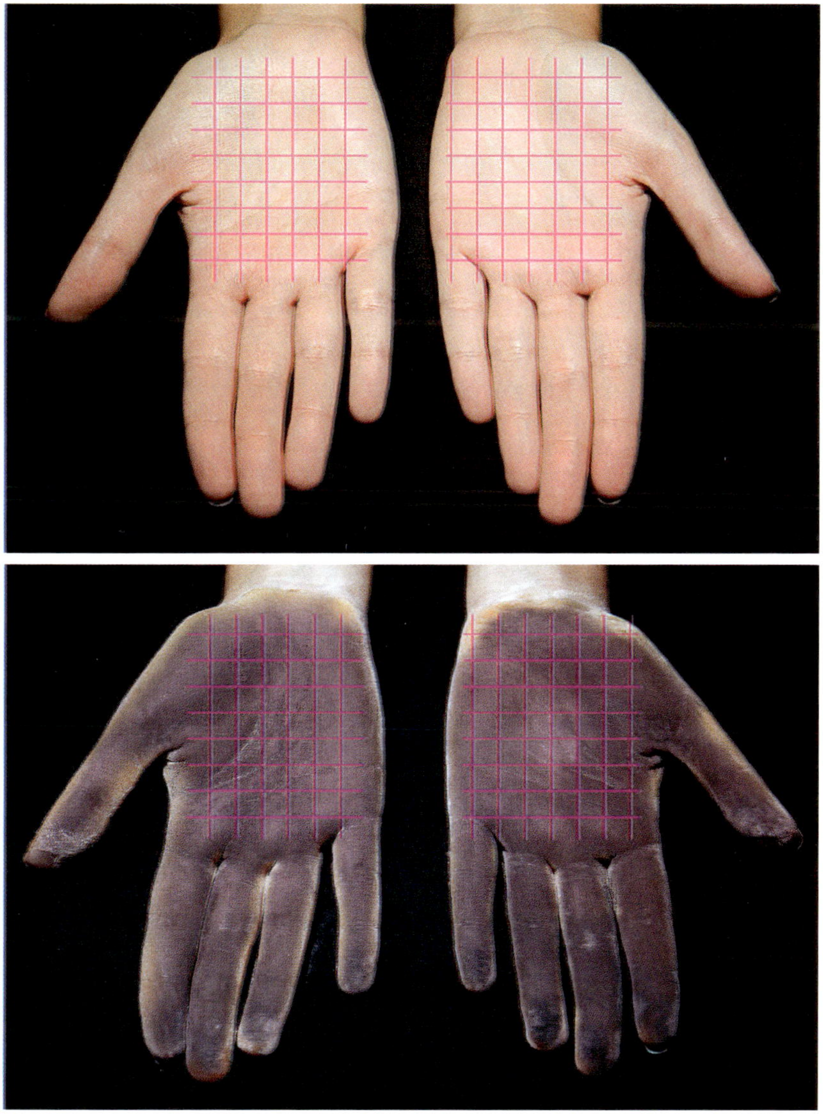

Figure 4 Minor test: if the area is affected by hyperhidrosis it turns dark blue-black

side effects, weight loss (suggesting cancer) or palpitations (linked to thyrotoxicosis). In short, the presence of other symptoms that may be related to other pathologies.

The Minor test (fig. 3), also known as the starch test, is useful to identify the area in which to inject the toxin. It involves applying an iodine solution to the area affected by hyperhidrosis, followed by the application of starch powder. If the area is affected by hyperhidrosis, it will turn a dark blue-black colour (fig. 4).

The Minor test is also very useful after treatment, to assess its effectiveness, or to consider the need for retreatment or retouching.

For patients who are allergic to iodine,

red ponceau dye is a good alternative, as it develops a pink colour when mixed with starch powder.

Recommended treatments

In addition to botulinum toxin, which is the treatment of choice, a number of other treatments can be offered to treat primary hyperhidrosis.

Topical agents (anticholinergics, astringents, perfumes, antiperspirants) are all used without particular success and can irritate the skin.

As far as oral treatments are concerned, the most commonly used drugs are anticholinergics, which inhibit the release of acetylcholine by binding to the muscarinic receptor (they have an affinity for the M3 receptor in glandular tissue).

Injection technique and dilution

There are four types of botulinum toxin A approved by the FDA for use in the United States, and each of these has an equivalent in Europe: OnabotulinumtoxinA (Vistabex 50-100 U) IncobotulinumtoxinA (Xeomin 100 U-Bocoture 50 U), AbobotulinumtoxinA (Dysport 375 U-Azzalure 125 U) and RimabotulinumtoxinA (Myobloc-Neurobloc).

The only toxin approved for use in hyperhidrosis in Italy is OnabotulinumtoxinA, although international literature takes the other three toxins extensively into consideration.

The 50-unit vial is used, diluted with 2.5 ml of saline solution, and approximately three 1 cc syringes are prepared, with a 32 G needle and a length of 13 mm. The injection should be performed intradermally, at a 45 degree angle to ensure that it is in the dermis.

Axillary hyperhidrosis

At this point, a grid made up of square segments measuring one centimetre per side can be drawn in the area to be treated and the toxin can be into each segment. An average of 24-28 squares each measuring 1 cm are usually drawn (figs. 5-6).

Small amounts of product are injected intradermally until small bumps form. The amount of product per bump is usually 0.1-0.2 ml. 50 IU are usually required per side, but a larger area may require more product.

Possible side effects may include bruising, pain, headache, muscle weakness, itching, hives and compensatory sweating. The patient should always be advised not to apply pressure under the armpit for a couple of hours [9-11].

Palm hyperhidrosis

As this is a very painful area, sometimes topical anaesthesia with lidocaine is inadequate, and the ulnar and median nerve must be blocked.

The block is performed with the elbow flexed at 30 degrees. 3-5 ml of anaesthetic is injected into the subcutaneous tissue, under the muscle fascia between the medial condyle and the olecranon. The needle is positioned parallel to the direction of the nerve.

As far as blocking the median nerve is concerned, we palpate the brachial artery and inject 5-7 ml of anaesthetic under the antecubital fold.

If the patient is cooperative and motivated and has a good pain threshold,

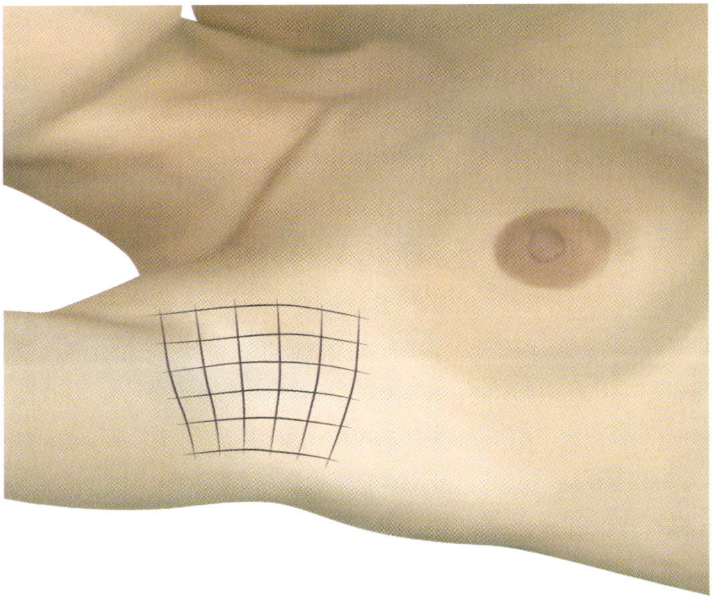

Figure 5 Grid for axillary botulinum injection

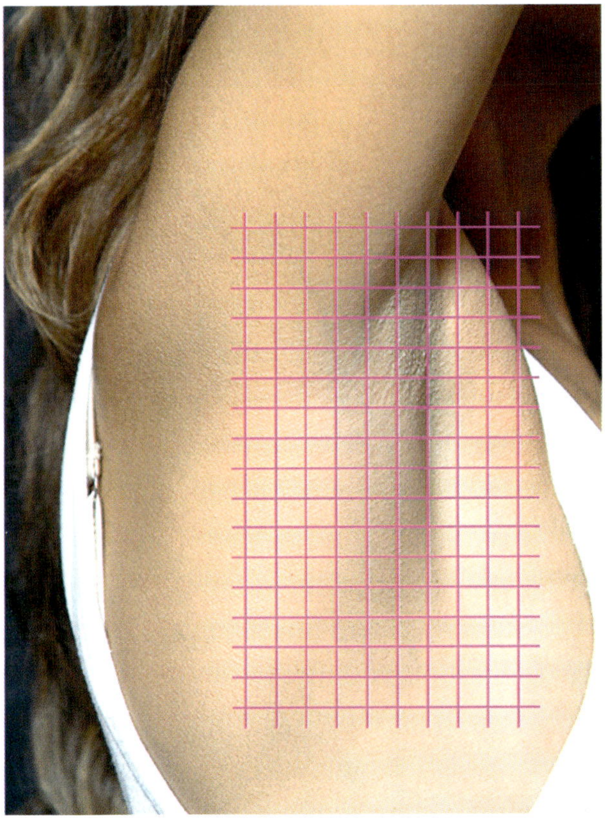

Figure 6 Grid for axillary botulinum injection

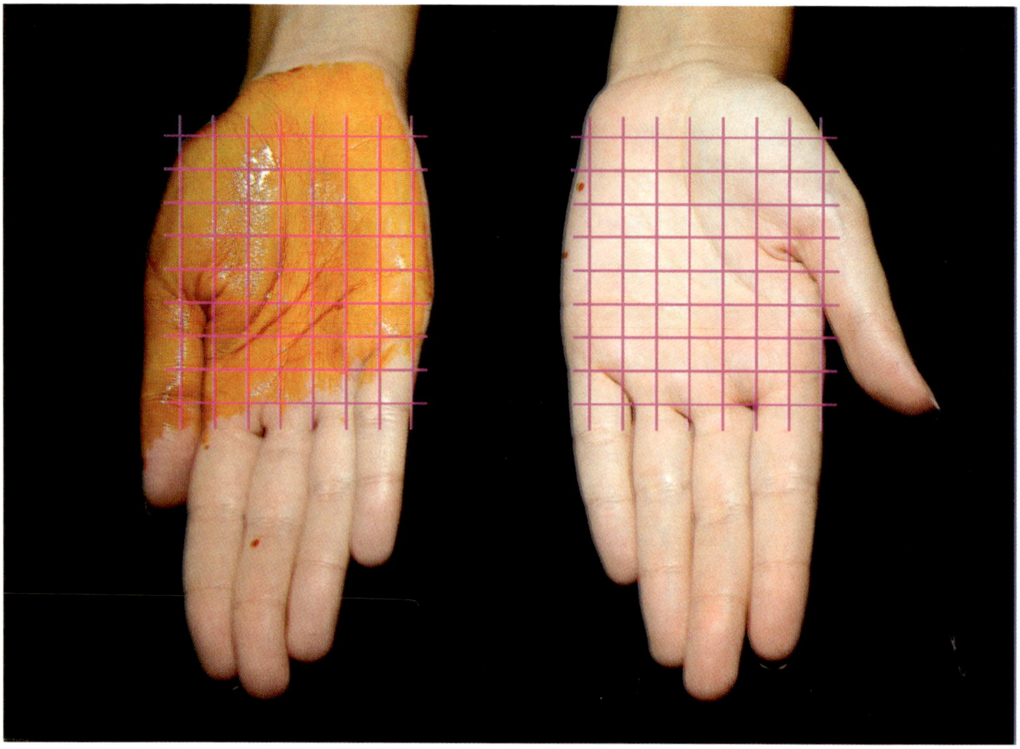

Figure 7 Grid for palmar botulinum injection

freezing sprays can be used to reduce the sensation of pain, although they make injection more difficult.
The amount of product used is 0.05-0.1 ml, which corresponds to approximately two units injected 1-1.5 cm apart, for a total of 50 IU per hand (fig. 7).
Possible side effects include pain, which can be severe, requiring anaesthesia in some cases, a weak grip, paraesthesia and bruising. It is always better to advise against driving and carrying heavy shopping bags for a couple of hours to prevent the substance from migrating to the neighbouring prehensile muscles [12].

Sole hyperhidrosis

To inject the anaesthesia, the patient lies supine with the leg rotated externally. The needle is inserted behind the tibial artery until it touches the bone, after which it is slightly retracted and 5 ml of anaesthetic is injected.
In this case, the amount of product used is always 50 IU per foot, distributed in micro doses at a distance of 1-1.5 cm from each other.
Freezing sprays can be used in this case too [12].
Possible complications are the same as for the palm, with the addition of difficulty in walking.

Bibliography

1. McConaghy JR, Fosselman D. Hyperhidrosis: Management Options. Am Fam Physician. 2018 Jun 1;97(11):729-734.
2. Fujimoto T. Pathophysiology and Treatment of Hyperhidrosis. Curr Probl Dermatol. 2016;51:86-93.
3. Nawrocki S, Cha J. The etiology, diagnosis, and management of hyperhidrosis: A comprehensive review: Therapeutic options. J Am Acad Dermatol. 2019 Sep;81(3):669-680.
4. Nawrocki S, Cha J. Botulinum toxin: Pharmacology and injectable administration for the treatment of primary hyperhidrosis. J Am Acad Dermatol. 2020 Apr;82(4):969-979.
5. Wechter T, Feldman SR, Taylor SL. The Treatment of Primary Focal Hyperhidrosis. Skin Therapy Lett. 2019 Jan;24(1):1-7.
6. Maillard H, Lecouflet M. Prise en charge d'une hyperhidrose [Management of hyperhidrosis]. Ann Dermatol Venereol. 2015 Apr;142(4):252-61.
7. Singh S, Davis H, Wilson P. Axillary hyperhidrosis: A review of the extent of the problem and treatment modalities. Surgeon. 2015 Oct;13(5):279-85.
8. Wang JV, Saedi N, Zachary CB. Hyperhidrosis and Aesthetics. Handb Exp Pharmacol. 2021;263:161-170.
9. Lynch OE, Aherne T, Gibbons J, Boland MR, Ryan ÉJ, Boyle E, Egan B, Tierney S. Five-year follow-up of patients treated with intra-dermal botulinum toxin for axillary hyperhidrosis. Ir J Med Sci. 2020 Aug;189(3):1023-1026.
10. Heckmann M. Hyperhidrosis of the axilla. Curr Probl Dermatol. 2002;30:149-55.
11. Benson RA, Palin R, Holt PJ, Loftus IM. Diagnosis and management of hyperhidrosis. BMJ. 2013 Nov 25;347:f6800.
12. Glaser DA, Galperin TA. Botulinum toxin for hyperhidrosis of areas other than the axillae and palms/soles. Dermatol Clin. 2014 Oct;32(4):517-25.

CLINICAL CASES

CLINICAL CASE 1

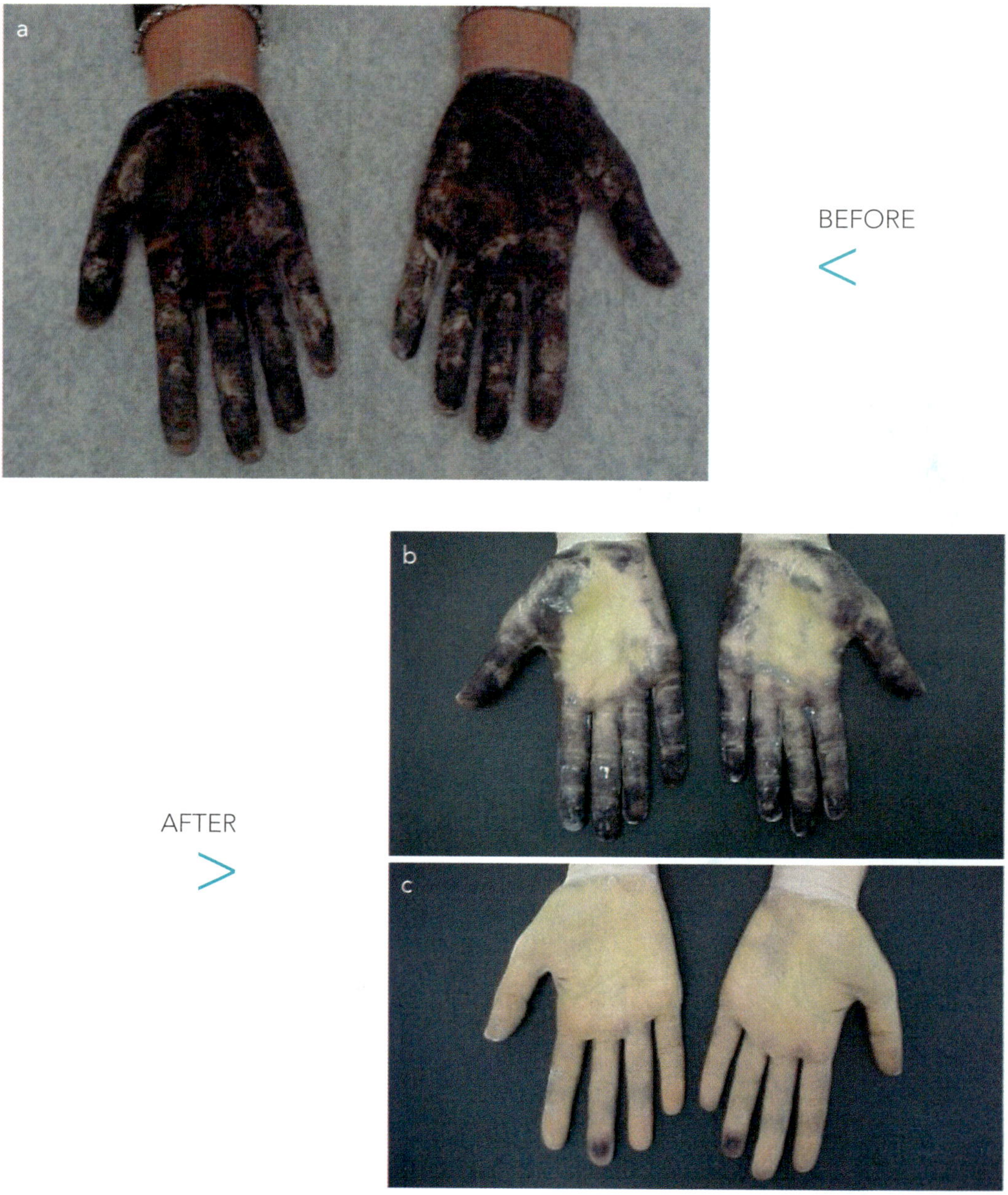

Figure 8 Palmar hyperhidrosis. Minor test after botulinum toxin injection: basal conditions (a), after 50 units (b), after 100 units (c). Note the reduction in staining

7

BOTULINUM TOXIN AND GENDER

Giuseppe Sito, Maria Vittoria Giatti

More and more men have recently begun seeking plastic surgery and aesthetic medical treatments, including botulinum toxin. We always have to consider the age of the patient in order to preserve the typical characteristics of beauty at every stage of life, as well as gender-related differences, in order to guarantee a very natural and individually tailored result. These differences are mainly anatomical, morphodynamic, physiological and psycho-social, and we have to be aware of them. Most importantly, we have to respect them when we are preparing to perform a botulinum toxin treatment [1-3].

In terms of morphodynamic anatomy, the following differentiations must be considered (figs. 1-2):

- skeletal, the ideal male facial skeleton has a broader, more prominent chin, a well-defined and square jaw, a higher and wider forehead, and a more pronounced orbital rim; in women, on the other hand, the contours appear softer and more convex, with gentler and less prominent bone structures;
- muscular, the muscle fibres in men are more evident, with stronger and more hypertrophic mimic muscles (e.g.: the frontalis muscle and the masseter);
- general aesthetics, in men, the eyebrows are thicker, running horizon-

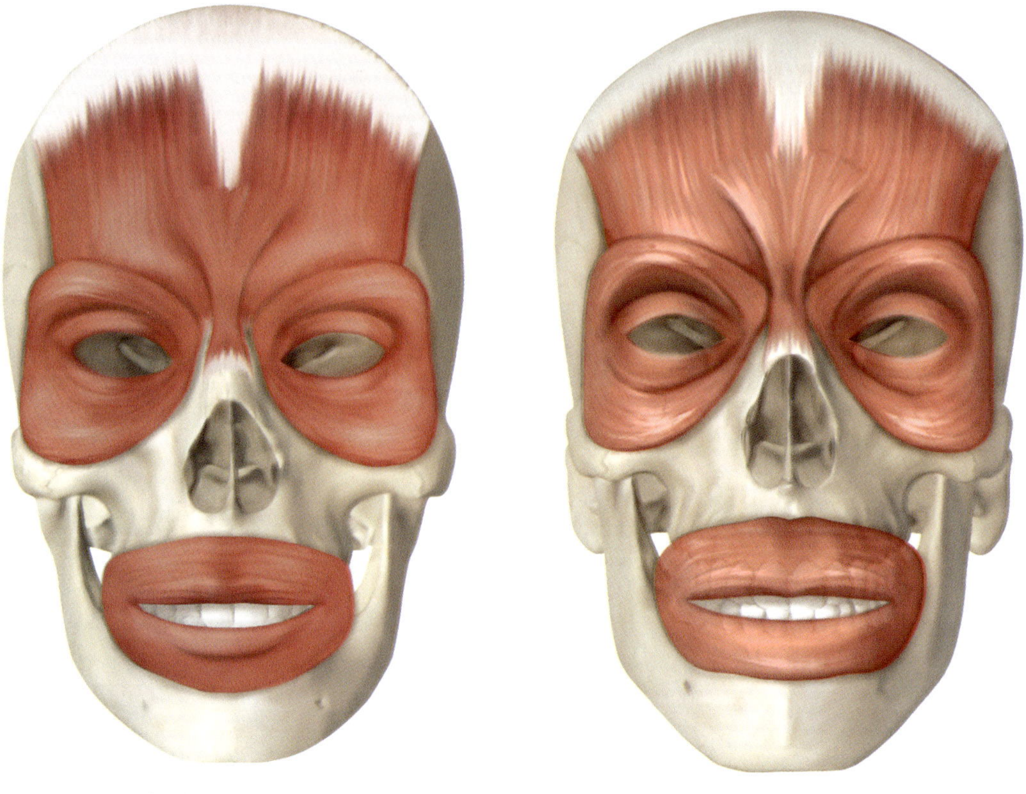

Figure 1 Gender-based anatomical differences: woman (on the left) and man (on the right)

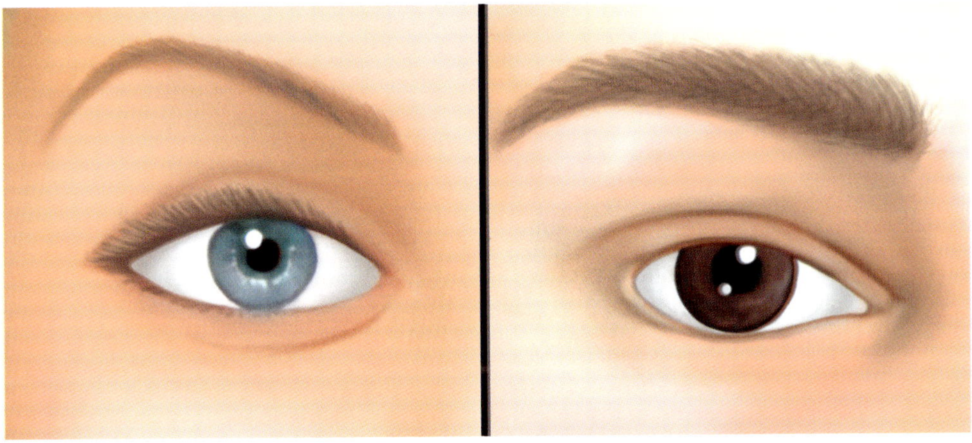

Figure 2 Gender-based differences in eyebrow shape: woman (on the left) and man (on the right)

tally and positioned on or just above the orbital rim, whereas in women, they are positioned above the orbital rim and are thinner and arched, with a delicate gull-wing shape, much appreciated and sought after by women in general, with the end (tail) slightly higher than the medial part (head of the eyebrow);

- dynamic, increased muscular representation and consequent greater tension result in more pronounced facial expressions in men, putting greater strain on the skin.

The physiological differences are due to the influence of different sexual hormones: primarily oestrogen and progesterone in women and androgens in men. Testosterone and dihydrotestosterone are responsible for the greater presence and characteristic and thicker distribution of hair (armpits, pubis, torso, limbs, moustache, beard) in men, along with an increased number and volume of sebaceous glands with consequent greater excretion of sebum (oilier skin, enlarged pores, greater tendency to develop acne), increased sweating and a tendency to have a more pronounced odour that sometimes results in bromhidrosis, due to the greater quantity of lactic acid and consequent greater acidity of the pH, increased skin thickness and greater skin vascularisation.

Gender-related differences also affect ageing: in men, the dense lamina at the dermo-epidermal junction appears to be more substantial than in women, resulting in a more undulating dermo-epidermal junction and consequently a firmer anchorage of the epidermis to the dermis, which is more resistant to the effects of ageing [4]. Men have a thicker dermis, higher collagen density and thicker skin, all of which translate into slower ageing, with wrinkles appearing later but then becoming deeper (especially on the forehead and around the eyes) (fig. 3). Moreover, ageing in men does not accelerate the way it does in women with the onset of

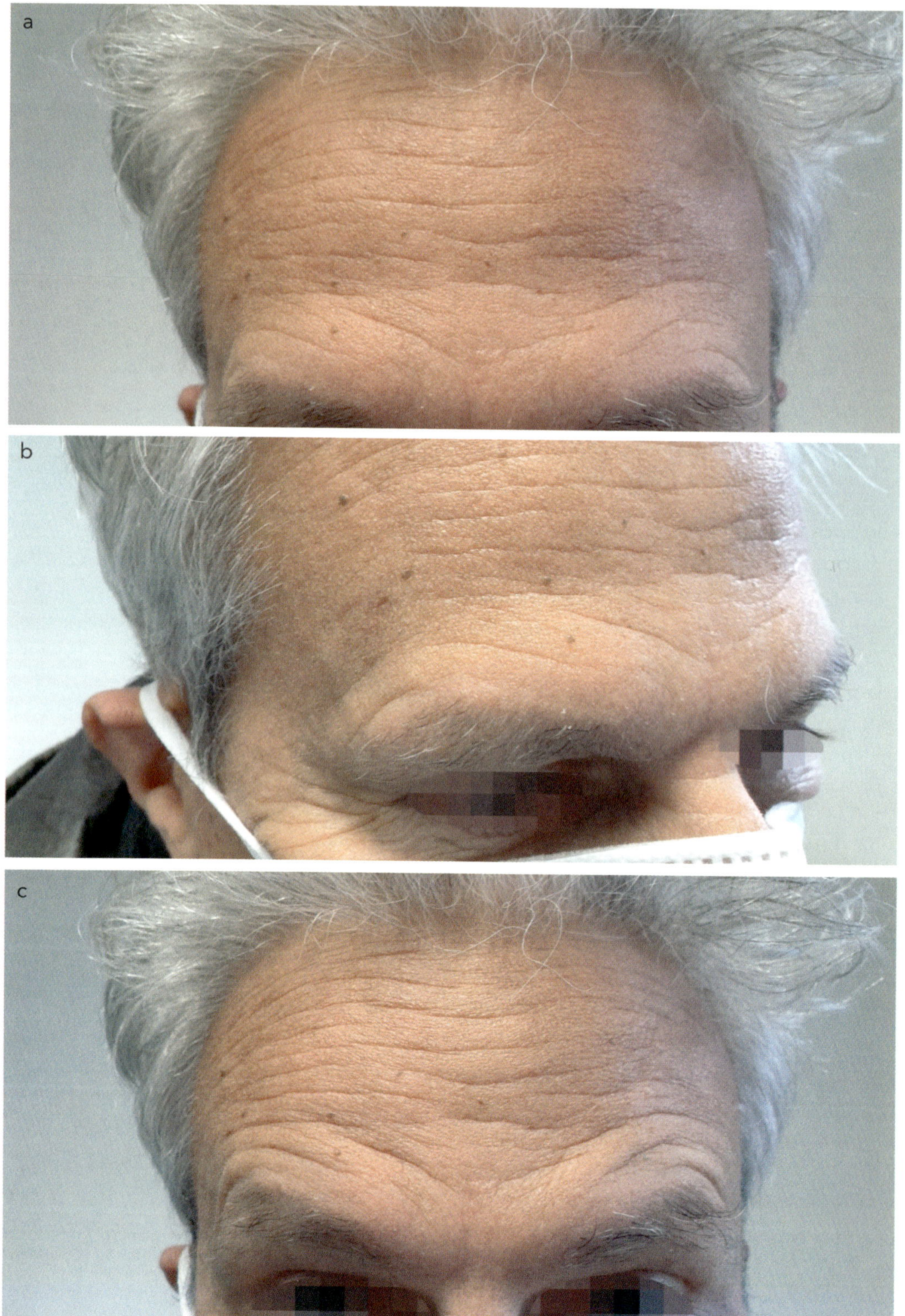
a
b
c

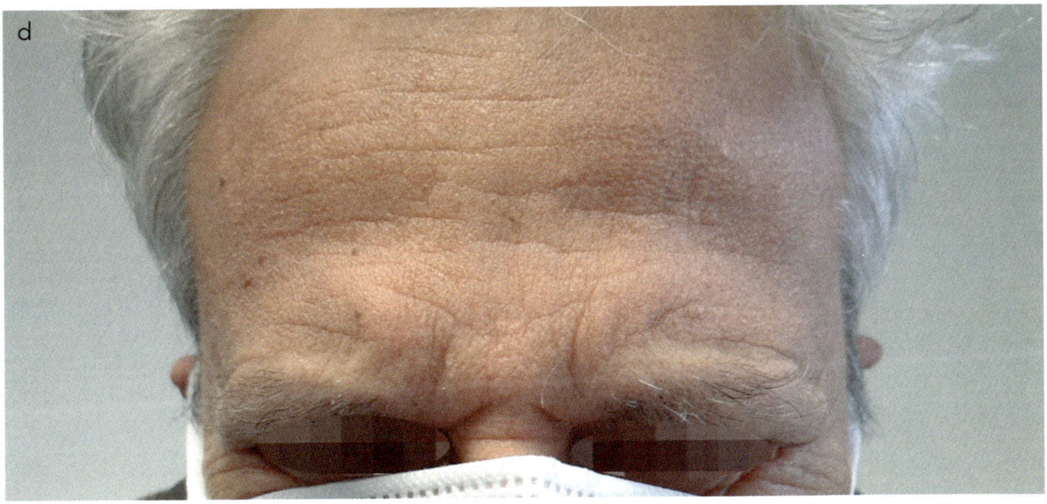

Figure 3 Wrinkles in men. Forehead lines when resting (a), lines around the eyes when resting (b), forehead lines during movement (c), glabellar lines during movement (d)

menopause and hormone reduction, but seems slower and more constant.

At psychosocial level, men tend to ask for a more subtle enhancement, while women often request a more decisive modulation. The reasons that lead men to seek treatment with botulinum toxin are that they want to look younger and more attractive, to improve their relational prospects, to maintain a competitive and efficient image in their social and professional spheres, to counteract skin ageing and a tired appearance in a quick, painless, non-invasive way, with no downtime, or simply because someone (usually wives or girlfriends) suggests it. However, men are often afraid that undergoing medical aesthetic treatment will make them look different and feminise their face, resulting in a loss of the virility and masculinity that identify them socially.

From these gender-based considerations, it is clear that the approach to medical treatment with botulinum toxin in men is different. Treatment in men [5] often requires more injection sites and higher doses (especially in the glabellar and forehead regions). Results may be less effective and long-lasting, requiring more closely scheduled sessions. Some authors suggest halving the amount of saline solution used to reconstitute the botulinum toxin (although this will create some technical problems) as an effective means of reducing the injection volume while doubling the doses needed to treat male patients, especially those with particular muscle hypertonia. In any case, it is always advisable to calibrate the dosage of botulinum correctly, avoiding feminising the face (taking particular care not to create eyebrows with an exaggerated gull-wing shape) and sometimes preferring under-correction: men better tolerate the presence of dynamic wrinkles after treatment, as these preserve a gre-

ater degree of virility, than the more extreme corrections requested by women. It is essential to clarify all these aspects during the first consultation, to avoid dissatisfaction on the part of the patient (who may see more effective and lasting results in his wife who has had the same medical treatment).
The treatments with botulinum toxin most frequently requested by men are the correction of dynamic wrinkles on the forehead and around the eyes, the treatment of hyperhidrosis, and microbotulinum treatment to improve oily and acne-prone skin.
Treatment with botulinum toxin should always be modulated, whether performed in men or women, to suit the age of the patient, considering the "ages of beauty" and respecting the characteristics of each season of life.

Bibliography

1. Dao H, Kazin R. Gender differences in skin: a review of the literature. Gend Med. 2007 Dec;4(4):308-28.
2. De Goursac C. L'esthétique au masculin. Soins, cosmétique, chirurgie. Paris. Ellébore 2012.
3. Verschoore M. Le Guide de la beauté au masculin. À la pointe de la recherche et de l'innovation. 2016 Janvier. Odile Jacob.
4. Tidman M, Eady R. Ultrastructural morphometry of normal human dermal-epidermal junction. The influence of age, sex and bodt region on laminar and non laminar components. J. Invest. Dermatol. 1994;83: 448-453.
5. Keaney TC, Alster TS. Botulinum toxin in men: review of relevant anatomy and clinical trial data.Dermatol Surg. 2013 Oct;39(10):1434-43.

8

COMBINED TECHNIQUES FOR A GLOBAL APPROACH

Maria Vittoria Giatti

To ensure that our treatments are even more effective and long-lasting in the third millennium, it is essential to take a global approach to the patient, designing an aesthetic path that includes synergistic treatments in the same session or at different times. Combining different procedures can optimise the results and increase patient satisfaction (thereby increasing patient loyalty) and that of the doctor too. The best results can only be achieved with an adequate knowledge of the anatomophysiology of ageing and the different levels at which it is necessary to intervene, and with a broader 4D vision that also considers the dynamism of beauty, focusing on the face as a set of interrelated aesthetic units in harmony with each other rather than just on individual wrinkles or blemishes to be corrected.

Various methods can be combined before, during or after the botulinum toxin treatment to optimise the results. Several areas can also be treated simultaneously, using combined techniques within the same session, to ensure the best possible result in terms of harmony and naturalness. It is therefore essential to draw up a correct treatment plan during the first consultation, assessing the patient's requests, their real needs in terms of biotype, degree of ageing, anatomical and physiological characteristics, gender specificity

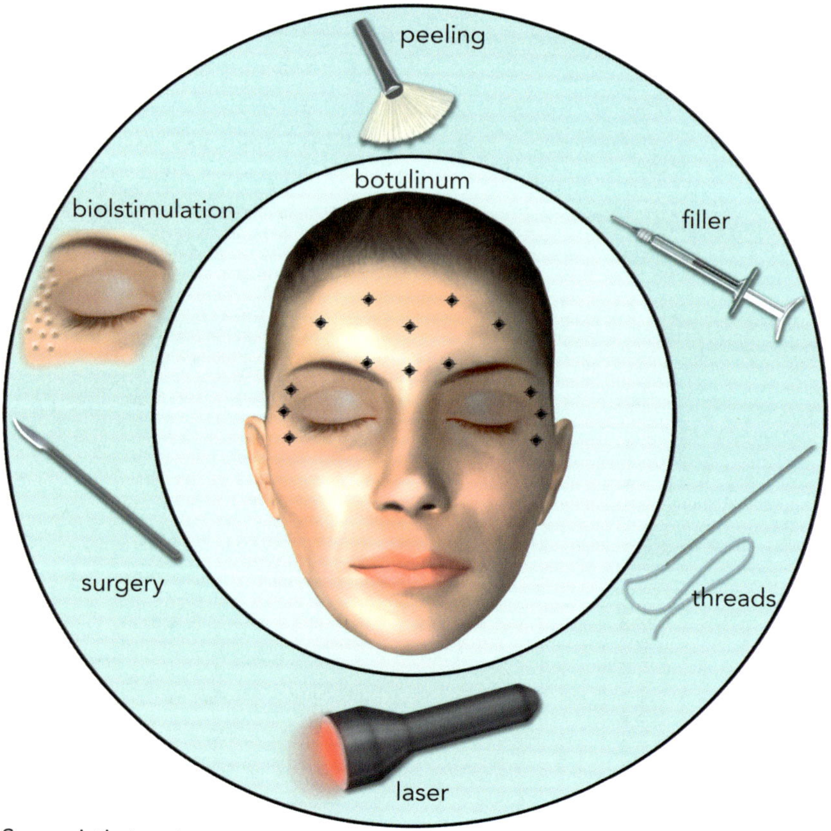

Figure 1 Synergistic treatments

and psychosocial aspects, in order to suggest the most suitable and personalised clinical procedure.
Botulinum toxin plays a central role before certain aesthetic methods by reducing the action of the underlying muscles, or in association with them to achieve synergistic and more lasting results. It can also be used as a complementary finishing technique after others. Aesthetic medical treatments that are often combined with botulinum toxin sessions are fillers, biostimulation, chemical peels, threads, lasers, plastic surgery, etc. (fig. 1). Combination with HiFu (High-intensity Focused Ultrasound), needling, radiofrequency, dermabrasion and micro-hydrodermabrasion, carboxytherapy, pulsed light and Prp is also very common.

Filler

The methods most frequently combined with botulinum toxin treatments involve the use of fillers, especially hyaluronic acid. Fillers can be used as part of the combined treatment of other aesthetic areas in the same session (e.g.: treatment of the upper third of the face with botulinum toxin and correction of the middle and lower thirds with fillers) for all-round correction. It can also be used subsequently to perfect the correction of dynamic wrinkles, especially in patients with muscular hypertone (e.g.: in the glabellar, eye and lip areas); in this case, it is advisable to wait at least two weeks after the injection of botulinum toxin, so that the underlying mimic muscles have already been weakened, allowing the filler to yield better results [1,2]. Cutting edge dynamic fillers with excellent stretch and adaptability to the underlying mobile areas are recommended for this purpose, guaranteeing natural-looking results even during movement. In patients with deep glabellar wrinkles, sometimes memory of these remains even after treatment with botulinum toxin, so from the beginning they should be informed that sequential and synergistic treatment with botulinum toxin followed by filler will guarantee better results and greater satisfaction; this can easily be assessed before treatment by stretching the skin between the eyebrows: if the lines fail to disappear completely during this manoeuvre, combined treatment is necessary (fig. 2).
For the lip area, particularly the vertical lines above the upper lip that we call the "bar code" (which often occur in hyperkinetic patients or those who make repeated sucking movements, such as smokers), the "blanching technique" can be used. This involves the very shallow injection of high resilience fillers using very fine needles (32 or 33 G) with an almost tangential inclination to the line and the delivery of the product in adjacent micro-bumps in the superficial dermis, often with the help of electronic injectors; the temporary whitening that occurs (which does not indicate ischaemia but only overstretching of the skin) and which gives the technique its name, disappears after massaging, which helps distribute the filler evenly. To complete the rejuvenation of the eye area, especially in the medical brow lift, about two weeks after treatment of this area

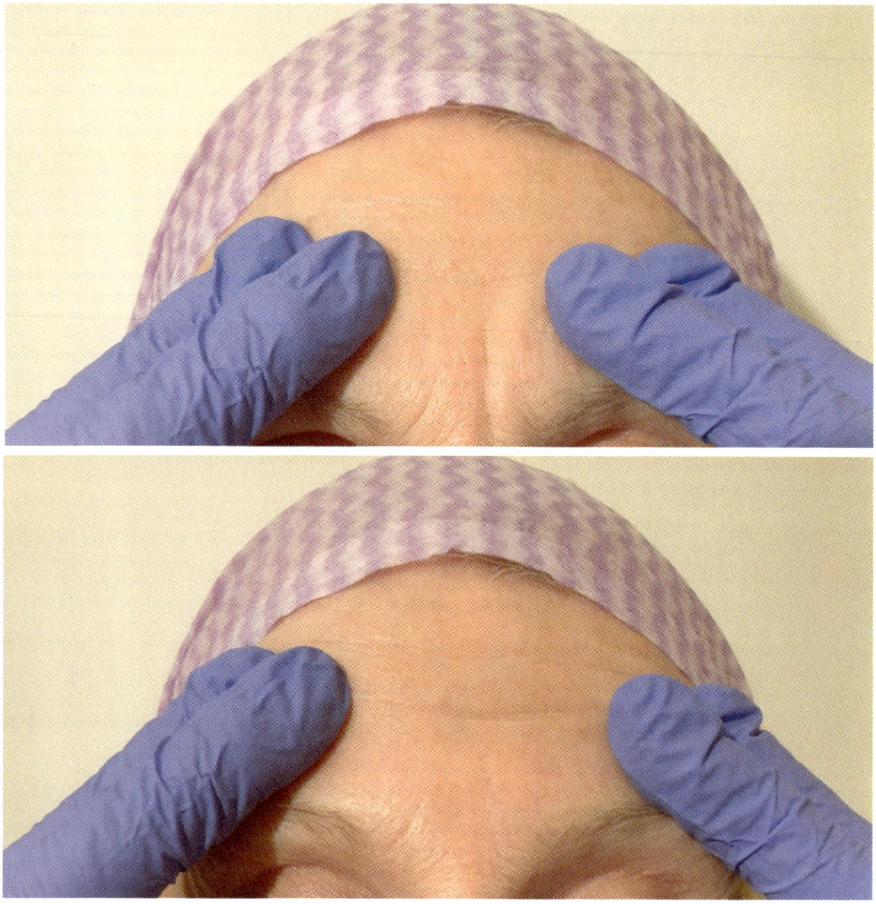

Figure 2 Manoeuvre to distend the glabellar region

with botulinum toxin, an additional correction with hyaluronic acid may be carried out using a cannula technique, in a fan shape, just below the lower outer edge of the eyebrow hairline (fig. 3). Filler can be used after botulinum toxin with deep injection and slow retrograde release at the base of the columella to complete the elevation of the tip of the nose. It can also be used to complete the correction of gummy smile, where the activity of the muscles that raise the upper lip has been reduced using botulinum. The filler is injected using a long, fine needle (30 G/13 mm) deep into the to the side of the nasal alar (in the most cranial portion of the nasolabial fold, about 3 mm to the side of the alar cartilage); by weakening the muscle fibres of the levator labii superioris and the nasal alar, the compression of the filler modulates and diminishes their contractile response [3].

Filler is also used after botulinum toxin to treat marionette lines (with the microcannula and fan technique) or horizontal neck lines (with dynamic filler and the linear retrograde technique) (fig. 4).

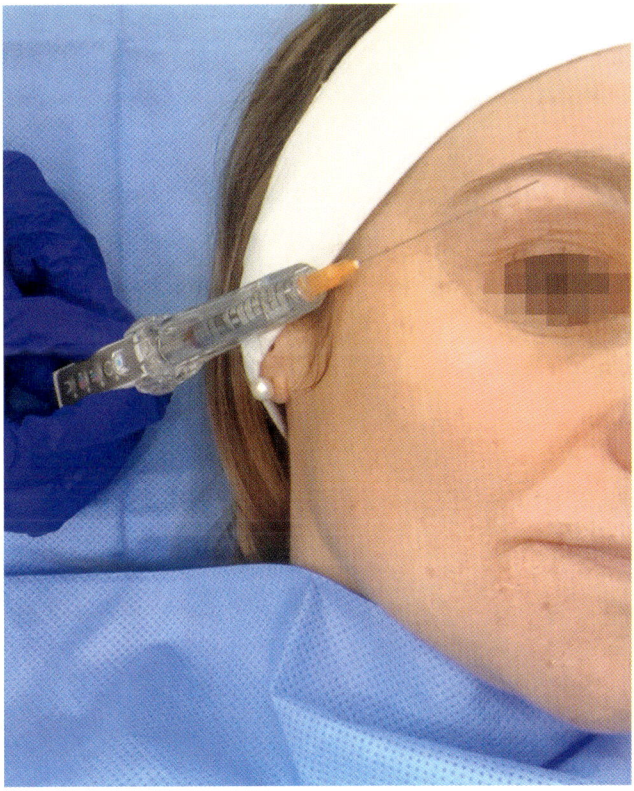

Figure 3 Brow filler

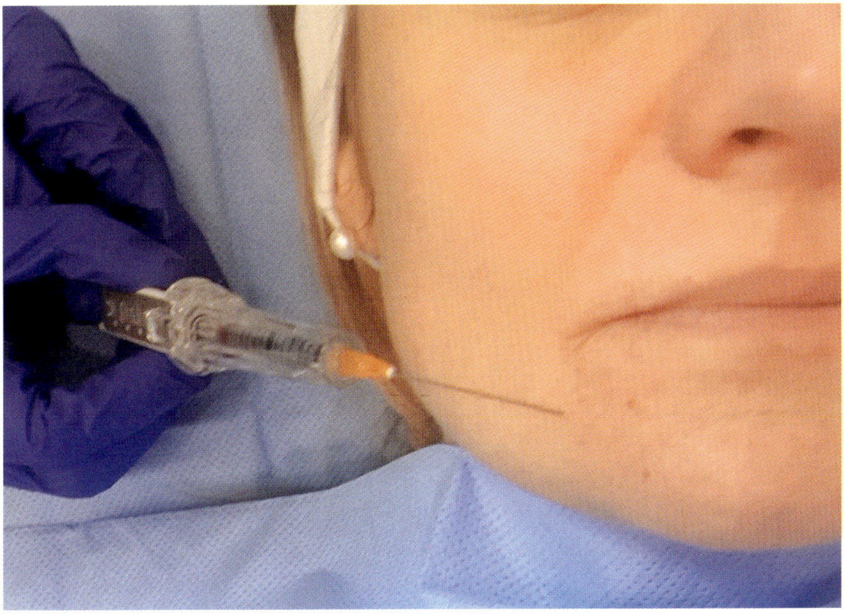

Figure 4 Marionette line filler

Biostimulation

Biostimulation can be combined in a synergistic sequential manner with botulinum toxin during the same session without any difficulty (fig. 5). Botulinum toxin can also be combined with bio-revitalizing substances in a single vial and this method is called meso-botulinum (or also biobotulinum). This consists of two combined therapies: hyperdiluted botulinum (known as microbotulinum, which is discussed in the specific chapter) with biostimulation. This treatment is preferable when the patient's skin does not present any particular problems, only requiring improvement from a qualitative point of view. Unlike traditional botulinum toxin treatment, which targets a specific muscle, very large areas of the mesoderm can be treated with mesobotulinum, particularly hypotonic areas such as the face, neck and cleavage, using superficial microinjections with very small needles (32 or 33 G). Bio-stimulants containing hyaluronic acid with a particular molecular weight, collagen precursors, vitamins, antioxidants and biomimetic peptides are chosen. The cocktail of these ingredients acts in synergy with botulinum toxin to improve skin hydration, luminosity, texture, micro-wrinkles and sagging. Remember that botulinum toxin also has the capacity to induce the formation of collagen.

Chemical peeling

Botulinum toxin, and particularly micro-botulinum toxin, can be combined with various types of peeling agents (salicylic acid, glycolic acid, trichloroacetic acid, mandelic acid, pyruvic acid, etc.) to achieve the synergistic correction of micro-wrinkles, hyperseborrhea and acne, with a redensifying

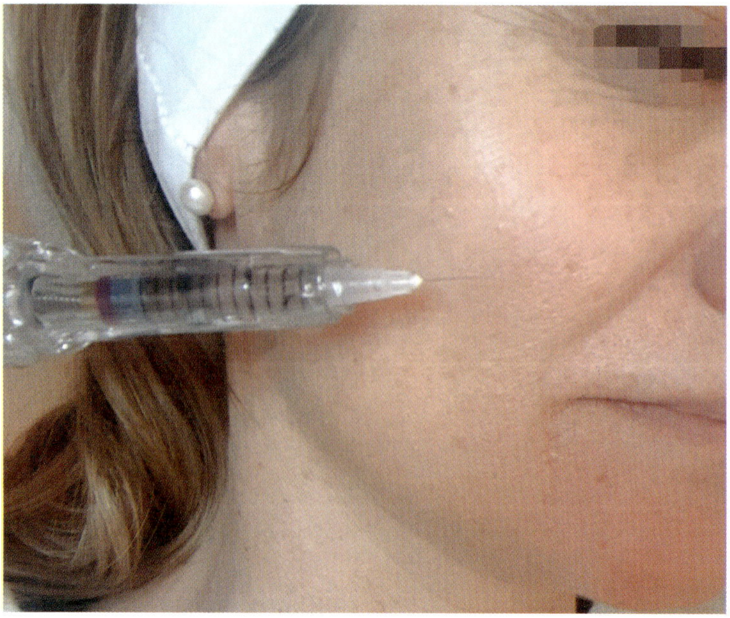

Figure 5 Biostimulation with electronic injector

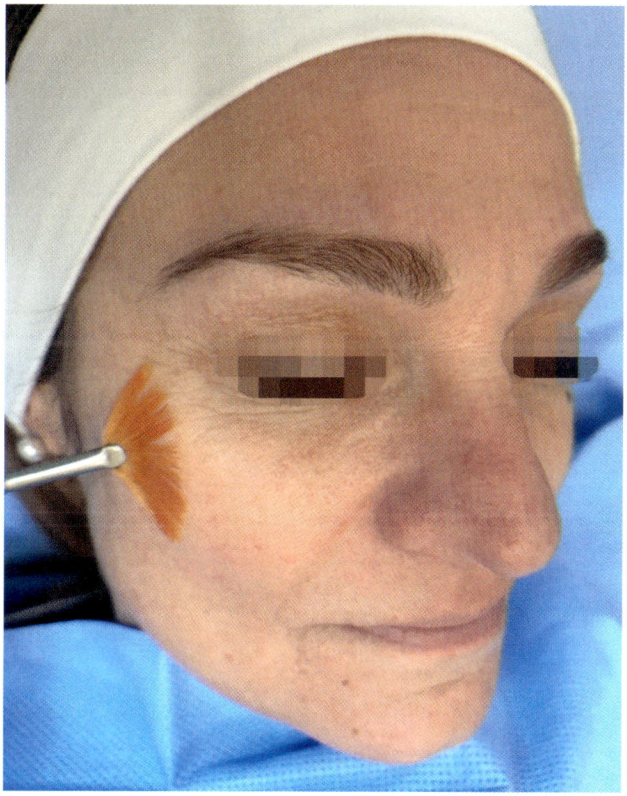

Figure 6 Chemical peeling

and sebum-regulating effect, to improve radiance and skin texture. Peeling can be scheduled in alternating sessions with botulinum toxin or even during the same session, taking care to perform it before injecting botulinum to avoid rubbing or manipulating areas that have just been treated with the toxin (fig. 6).

Threads

Treatment with threads (made of polylactic acid, polycaprolactone, polydioxanone, etc.) can also be combined with botulinum toxin. It is advisable to schedule a treatment two to three weeks after injection with botulinum, to ensure optimal muscle relaxation, allowing more effective upward traction and repositioning of the tissues and longer lasting results. Suspension threads are often used to improve the brow area after botulinum toxin, especially as part of a medical brow lift.

Laser

Various types of lasers (ablative lasers, fractional lasers, vascular lasers, laser endolifting, etc.) are combined with botulinum toxin treatments with the aim of helping to correct rhytides (particularly those caused by photoageing), with an anti-ageing effect and also improving skin texture and uniformity. They are often used synergistically in the eye and lip areas.

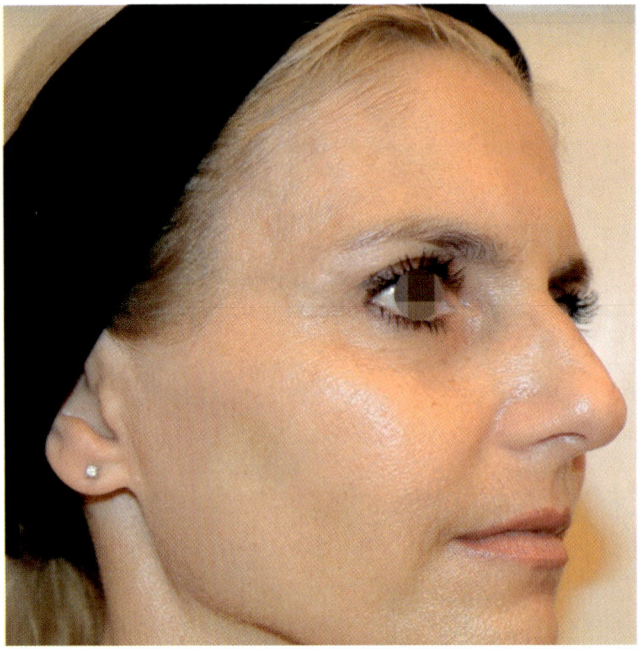

Figure 7 Results of upper lid blepharoplasty

Plastic surgery

Botulinum toxin can also be a complementary and refinement technique in various aesthetic plastic surgery procedures such as blepharoplasty (fig. 7), brow lift, neck and face lift, and lipofilling. It is also useful as part of other therapies to correct symmetry and malfunctioning or paralysis of the facial nerve [4]. Its use in wound healing is also significant.

Bibliography

1. Carruthers J, Glogau R, Blitzer A. Advances in facial rejuvenation: botulinum toxin type a, hyaluronic acid dermal fillers, and combination therapies-consensus recommendations. Plast Reconstr Surg. 2008 May;121(5 Suppl):5S-30S.
2. Sundaram H, Liew S, Signorini M, Vieira Braz A, Fagien S, Swift A, De Boulle K, Raspaldo H, Trindade de Almeida A, Monheit G. Global Aesthetics Consensus: Hyaluronic Acid Fillers and Botulinum Toxin Type A-Recommendations for Combined Treatment and Optimizing Outcomes in Diverse Patient Populations. Plast Reconstr Surg.2016 May;137(5):1410-1423.
3. Diaspro A, Cavallini M, Piersini P, Sito G. Gummy Smile Treatment: Proposal for a Novel Corrective Technique and a Review of the Literature. Aesthet Surg J. 2018 Nov 12;38(12):1330-1338.
4. Lovice D. Botulinum toxin use in facial plastic surgery. Otolaryngol Clinic North Am. 2002 February; 35(1): 171-186.

9

COMPLICATIONS: AVOIDING AND HANDLING THEM

Giuseppe Sito

Despite being a neurotoxin that induces muscle paralysis, leading in extreme cases to death, botulinum toxin (mainly type A) is currently used in aesthetic medicine, with millions of cases treated. Compared with surgical methods capable of achieving the same effects, it is safe, minimally invasive and sometimes even more effective [1]. Nevertheless, certain factors, such as dilution, migration of the substance, anatomic variability, technical errors and, last but not least, the inexperience of the injector, can sometimes result in the occurrence of side effects.
It should be noted from the outset that the side effects of botulinum toxin never become permanent and usually disappear as the toxin is metabolised, within a reasonably short space of time. Some, as we will see in this chapter, can be easily alleviated or eliminated using other methods. However, without this appearing contradictory, serious and long-lasting events have been reported. These include dysphagia, which can occur (very rarely) due to migration during injection of the platysma bands, respiratory impairment, again for the same reason, very rare generalised muscular weakness, severe bilateral ptosis, pseudoaneurysm of the frontal branch of the temporal artery, necrotising fasciitis, sarcoid granuloma, Fournier's gangrene [2,3]. Some fatalities have been attributed to the onset of botulism or anaphylactic shock, although the direct correlation with the injection of botulinum toxin has never been proven. However, the authors are in agreement that these events, if serious, can be attributed mainly to the therapeutic use of the toxin, while there are no such cases in cosmetic use. Complications that we might describe as common or relatively common are much more frequent. These are:
- brow ptosis;
- upper eyelid ptosis;
- mild, transient headache;
- asymmetries and Mephistophelian eyebrow;
- lower eyelid oedema;

Rare side effects are:
- fatigue;
- itching;
- mild nausea;
- necrotising fasciitis;
- diplopia.

Common side effects are usually caused by overdose, injection in inappropriate points, excessive dilution of the toxin with migration to the adjacent muscles. Let's look at them in detail.

Brow ptosis

Brow ptosis is usually caused by excessive immobilisation of the infero-lateral portion of the frontalis muscle, which, left "free", is drawn downwards by the action of the orbicularis and/or corrugator muscle, which then causes the brow to droop. This can occur during the treatment of wrinkles on the forehead or around the eyes, and of glabellar lines. It is an undesirable but transient effect that is quickly reversible. It is frequent in those who have a pre-existing ptosis, even if only of slight entity, and can be treated by successively blocking the brow with a few units of toxin, injecting it in two places: the first in the caudal portion of the brow, more superficially, and the second deeper,

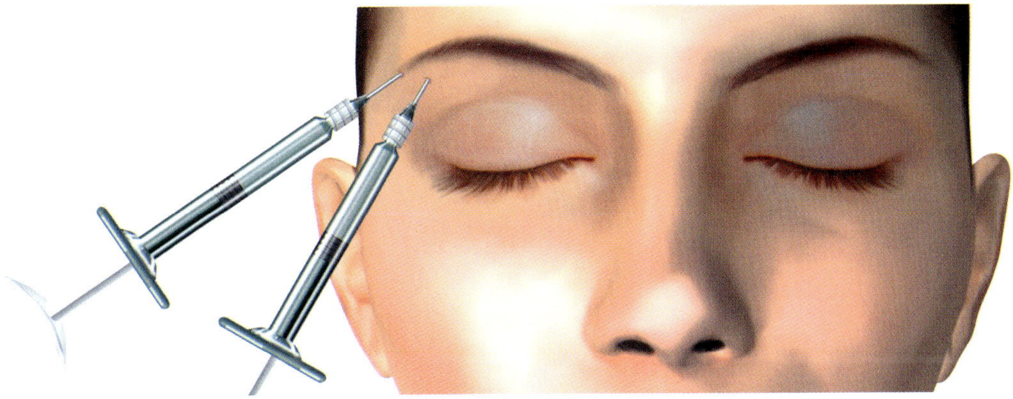

Figure 1 Injection points to correct brow ptosis

again in the caudal portion, under the medial margin (fig. 1).

Brow ptosis can be prevented as follows:

- by injecting more than 1 cm away from the upper edge of the eyebrow;
- by not using dilutions higher than those normally used;
- by not treating patients with very pronounced wrinkles, who can lower their eyebrows by more than 2-3 mm.

It is also necessary to respect the mapping that must always precede injection, and it is advisable to perform injection into the subdermal plane, which, due to its proximity, will have the same effect as the muscular plane, which is hard to find.

Mild, transitory headache

A small percentage of patients complain of headaches after treatment. As this almost always occurs after the first injection and rarely after subsequent treatments, it is thought by some to be due to the state of tension that always accompanies these procedures. Some suggest that headache can also occur due to contact between the tip of the needle and the periosteum. A paper published by Carruthers states that the headache appears mostly following injection by inexperienced practitioners.

Upper eyelid ptosis

Upper eyelid ptosis occurs due to paralysis of the levator palpebrae superioris and is usually observed 7-14 days after treatment. It is typically unilateral, varies from 1 to 3 mm and lasts from two to four weeks (fig. 2).

It is caused by the migration of the toxin due to overdose or excessive injection in the treatment of glabellar lines. Its prevention consists in careful injection of toxin into the targeted areas with the lowest possible dilution and dose. It may be helpful to avoid massaging the area for the subsequent two hours and to refrain from wearing a motorbike helmet, for example, for the subsequent two hours.

The correction of eyelid ptosis, which actually disappears on its own if mild, can be speeded up with the administration of medication. In mild cases,

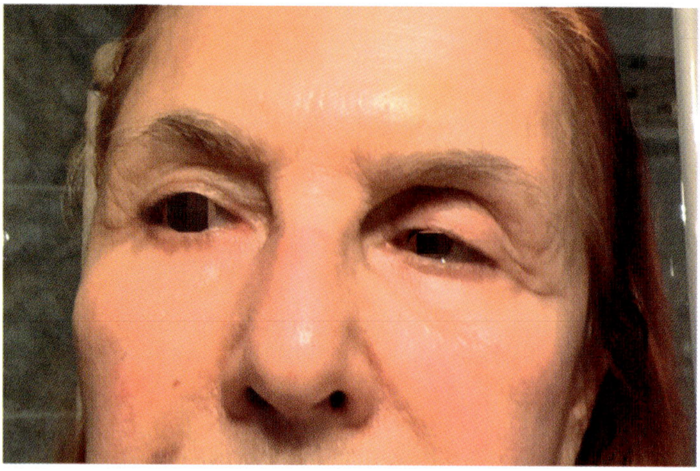

Figure 2 Left eyelid ptosis

one to three drops per eye 3-4 times a day of eyedrops containing nafazolin nitrate and thonzylamine hydrochloride can be used with some success and a complete absence of side-effects. In more severe cases, and with a slight degree of risk, one drop three times a day of apraclonidine 5% (iopidine 0.5%), an α-adrenergic agonist, which causes contraction of the Müller muscle and opens the eyelid, thereby correcting the ptosis, can be used. These are eyedrops routinely used to treat glaucoma and should therefore be used with extreme caution. Overdosage results in dry eye, blurred vision and eyelid oedema. If any of these symptoms occur, stop use immediately [5].

Asymmetrical eyebrows

Asymmetrical eyebrows are among the most common side effects and can occur due to asymmetry in the injection sites on the side of the forehead. They can be corrected by injecting 1-2 U just above the wrinkle produced by the lateral muscle of the forehead. Sometimes the classic Mephistophelian effect (fig. 3), on one or both sides, can occur due to inadequate and incomplete treatment of the lateral fibres of the frontalis muscle. There is a semiotic manoeuvre that we can perform to assess the possibility of Mephistophelian eyebrow. Press firmly against the glabellar muscle group with a thumb and then ask the patient to raise their forehead. In the case of susceptibility to Mephistophelian eyebrow, this is immediately noticeable and extra care should be taken with injection along the lateral fibres (fig. 4). The treatment consists in injecting a few units along a line indicating the maximum projection of the eyebrow.

Lower eyelid oedema

The subpalpebral and peri-zygomatic areas are known to be rich in lymphatic vessels, which, despite not having acetylcholine-mediated innervation, are particularly sensitive to botulinum

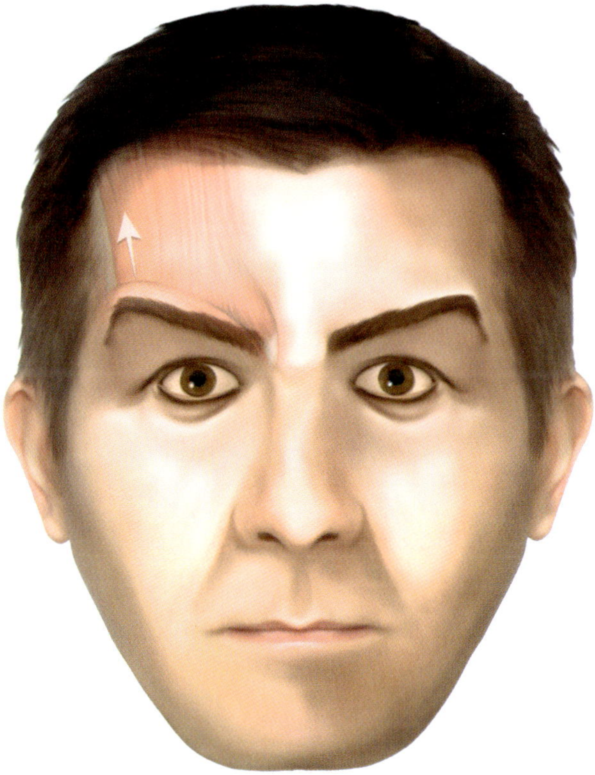

Figure 3 Mestiphelian eyebrow due to incomplete correction of the lateral fascia of the muscle

toxin. This is why oedema of the region sometimes occurs, but only rarely. In this case it is sufficient to massage several times a day and wait for spontaneous remission.

Diplopia

This is considered to be a rare side effect and depends on accidental injection of the toxin or migration into the external rectus muscle. It occurs 4-5 days after treatment and its duration depends on the number of units delivered into the muscle. Its resolution cannot be speeded up and we must wait until the toxin has been metabolised. Prevention consists in injecting the wrinkles around the eyes as laterally as possible, perhaps pointing the tip of the needle towards the hairline.

Necrotising fasciitis

This is considered a very serious and very rare side effect. Only one case of this complex problem has been described in recent years [6]. The diagnostic assumption is that certain debilitating diseases, such as diabetes, alcoholism and polymyositis, can be considered as predisposing factors for necrotising fasciitis. The fact that this infection spread to a subfascial plane was probably due to the immobilisation caused by the toxin, used for non-aesthetic purposes. Of course, this is a condition that can affect immunocompromised individuals.

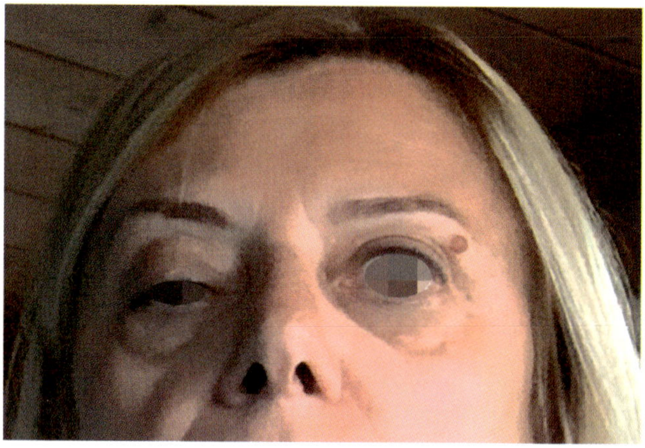

Figure 4 Right eyelid ptosis

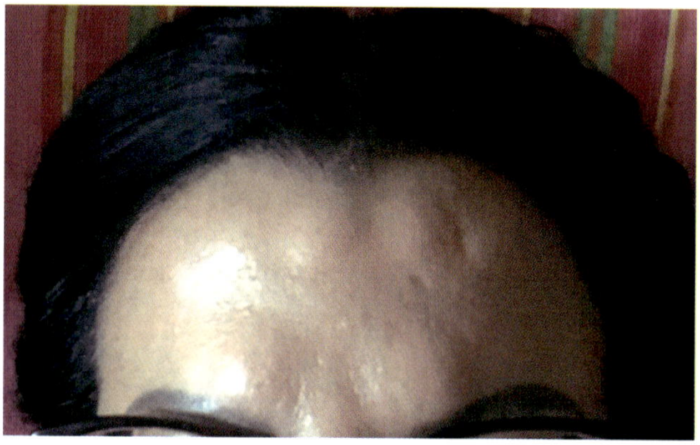

Figure 5 Persistence of bumps (incorrect injection volume)

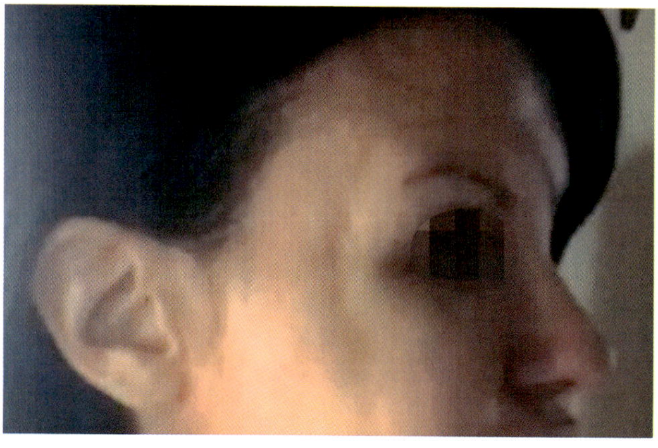

Figure 6 Scleroderma-like appearance a few days after injection with botulinum toxin for unknown reasons

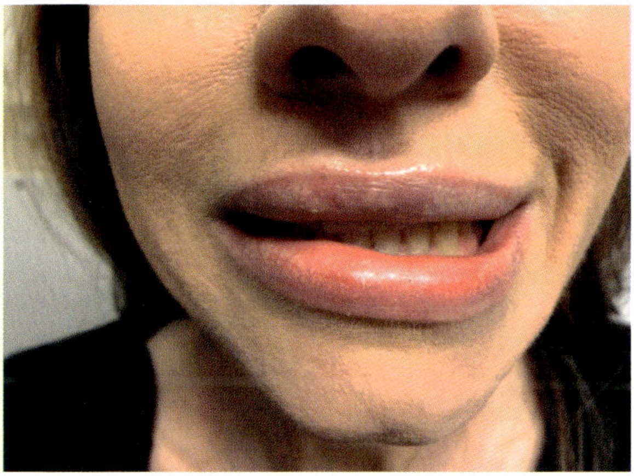

Figure 7 Involvement of the DAO and levator labii on the left, after microbotulinum therapy

The case described involved an 80-year-old patient who had received botulinum toxin injections for bilateral blepharospasm three days earlier. The day after the injections, the patient had noticed redness and progressive oedema in the area treated. The blepharospasm had been diagnosed eleven years previously and treated with injections of botulinum toxin every three months, with no apparent problems. The patient had a history of well-compensated chronic myeloid leukaemia treated with drugs. After the episode she was admitted to hospital with mild periorbital cellulitis on the right side and antibiotics were administered immediately. Despite this, her condition deteriorated rapidly and progressively over the next four days, also affecting the right half of the lower middle third of her face and both sides of her neck. After four more days, a rectangle of necrosis developed, coinciding with the point where the toxin had been injected, on the right. It became impossible for her to open her eye and when it was opened manually, there was significant conjunctival chemosis. Necrotising fasciitis was diagnosed on the right side, while the left side of the face appeared normal. The patient underwent surgical debridement of the area. The skin, subcutis and muscles of the right side of the face were removed until healthy tissue was identified. The diagnosis of group A beta haemolytic Streptococcus necrotising fasciitis, sensitive to penicillin and erythromycin, which was immediately treated, was confirmed by examination of the tissue that was removed. However, the patient continued to deteriorate, and it was necessary to enucleate the eyeball and extend debridement to the corner of the mouth. Further debridement was necessary, and a flap was made with the rectus abdominis, part of which suffered dehiscence but then healed, allowing the patient to return home after three months.

As we have seen, side effects of botulinum toxin are not frequent and they are not stable. They can sometimes be

remedied with other injections and sometimes with drugs.
The technical timeframe for litigation is therefore very short, because the effect of the toxin itself is short and the side effect will disappear quickly. It is not, however, possible to rule out civil or criminal proceedings so it is good practice to have the patient sign an Informed Consent form. There are several types of these, with each company supplying a different one. I submit the form shown in Appendix. Always remember that the best way to prevent legal problems is to follow the rules for botulinum toxin injection to the letter.

Bibliography

1. Chen S, Long J. [Adverse events of botulinum toxin A in facial injection: Mechanism, prevention and treatment]. Zhong Nan Da Xue Xue Bao Yi Xue Ban. 2019 Jul 28;44(7):837-844.
2. Yiannakopoulou E. Serious and long-term adverse events associated with the therapeutic and cosmetic use of botulinum toxin. Pharmacology. 2015;95(1-2):65-69.
3. Sorensen EP, Urman C. Cosmetic complications: rare and serious events following botulinum toxin and soft tissue filler administration. J Drugs Dermatol. 2015;14(5):486-491.
4. Jia Z, Lu H, Yang X, et al. Adverse Events of Botulinum Toxin Type A in Facial Rejuvenation: A Systematic Review and Meta-Analysis. Aesthetic Plast Surg. 2016;40(5):769-777.
5. Kontis TC, Lacombe VG. Iniezioni di Tossina Botulinica e Filler in Medicina Estetica. Edizioni Piccin.
6. Latimer PR, Hodgkins PR, Vakalis AN, Butler RE, Evans AR, Zaki GA. Necrotising fasciitis as a complication of botulinum toxin injection. Eye (Lond). 1998;12 (Pt 1):51-53.
7. De Boulle K et al. Phase 3 Study of OnabotulinumtoxinA Distributed Between Frontalis, Glabellar Complex, and Lateral Canthal Areas for Treatment of Upper Facial Lines. Dermatol Surg. 2018;44(11): 1437-1448.

10

NOTES ON THE USE OF BOTULINUM TOXIN IN NEUROLOGY

Claudia Ledda, Alberto Diaspro

BOTULINUM TOXIN IN NEUROLOGY

Claudia Ledda

Botulinum toxin is an effective treatment for many neurological conditions, such as blepharospasm, spasticity, cervical dystonia, facial hemispasm, oromandibular dystonia, writer's cramp and musician's dystonia [1]. Many of the conditions described above are forms of dystonia, a group of pathologies characterised by involuntary contractions of a group of muscles, intermittent or sustained, that cause abnormal posture. For many dystonia patients, certain movements or tactile stimulation can attenuate the dystonic contraction (antagonistic gesture). Dystonia can be made worse by strong emotional stimuli, stress and fatigue, and is absent while sleeping. Dystonias are characterised according to clinical traits (age of onset, physical distribution, temporal pattern and associated characteristics) and aetiology (pathology of the nervous system, hereditary or acquired) [2].
Some of the most common uses in neurology are described in detail below.

Blepharospasm

Blepharospasm is one of the conditions commonly known as focal dystonia and is characterised by chronic, intermittent or persistent involuntary spasmodic contraction of the periorbital muscles. Dystonia is almost always bilateral and synchronous and involves the orbicularis oculi muscle. It is also frequently associated with contraction of the procerus muscle and the corrugator supercilii [3]. The antagonistic gesture is present in 87% of the affected population and often consists in tactile stimulation of the face or eyelid, singing, speaking or murmuring [4].
Blepharospasm can be idiopathic or caused by the use of drugs (e.g.: antipsychotics), stroke, trauma or neurodegenerative conditions.
The prevalence is of 1.3-13 people per 100,000, the age of onset is between 50 and 60 and it is more common in women than in men [3]. It usually begins with an increase in the frequency of blinking and can gradually progress to the point of persistent eyelid closure caused by tonic spasms of the muscle resulting in functional blindness [3-5]. It manifests less commonly as clonic spasms or apraxia of the opening of the eyes. Spontaneous remission occurs in 10% of cases and is often followed by relapse [4].
Botulinum toxin is considered the first-line treatment for this condition, leading to improvement in more than 90% of those treated. The average duration of the effect is 2.5-2.8 months [5] and most studies show a good clinical response even in the long term [3]. The muscles treated with botulinum toxin are the orbicularis oculi muscles bilaterally and, in about one third of cases, the corrugator supercilii and the procerus (tab. 1). The orbicularis oculi muscle can be divided anatomically into two portions: palpebral and orbital. The palpebral portion contains the pretarsal and preseptal are-

TABLE 1 - MUSCLES TREATED IN BLEPHAROSPASM

Muscle	Dosage	Injection points	Needle length	Treatment protocol
Orbicularis oculi	1.25-5 Xeomin 1.25-5 Botox/ Vistabex 3.75/5-15/20 Dysport	3-5 points	20 mm (27-30 G)	Subcutaneous injection of the upper (medial and lateral) and lower (medial and lateral) pretarsal portion, bilaterally
Corrugator supercilii	2.5-5 Xeomin 2.5-5 Botox/ Vistabex 7.5/10-15/20 Dysport	1-2 points	20 mm (27-30 G)	One or two points on each side are identified; it is usually performed at one point unilaterally. Frequently treated together with the procerus muscle
Procerus	2.5-5 Xeomin 2.5-5 Botox/ Vistabex 7.5/10-15/20 Dysport	1-3 points	20 mm (27-30 G)	The injection points are identified depending on the clinical indication. However, injection is often performed in one central point only. The injection can be performed proximodistally or dystoproximally

as. Many studies have shown that treatment of the pretarsal portions results in greater efficacy, reduced incidence of side effects and longer duration. The interval between treatments is usually three months.

Injection is performed with a 30 G needle. The recommended toxins are onabotulinumtoxinA (onaBoNTA, Botox) and incobotulinumtoxin-A (incoBoNTA, Xeomin) (evidence class B, i.e.: probably effective) and abobotilunmtoxinA (aboBoNTA, Dysport) (evidence class C, i.e.: possibly effective) [6]. OnaBoNTA and incoBoNT-A can be diluted to a concentration of 5 U/0.1 cc, 2.5 U/0.1 cc or 1.25 U/0.1 cc, while aboBoNTA is diluted to 20 U/0.1 cc.

The initial dose for each inoculation site is 1.25 to 2.5 U, and the injection sites are usually 3-4 per eye [3]. The orbicularis oculi is treated subcutaneously in the superior, medial and lateral, and inferior, medial and lateral tarsal portions (fig. 1). In the upper eyelid area, injection is directed towards the nose when injecting the medial point and towards the orbital ridge when injecting the lateral point, staying away from the eye. To avoid the

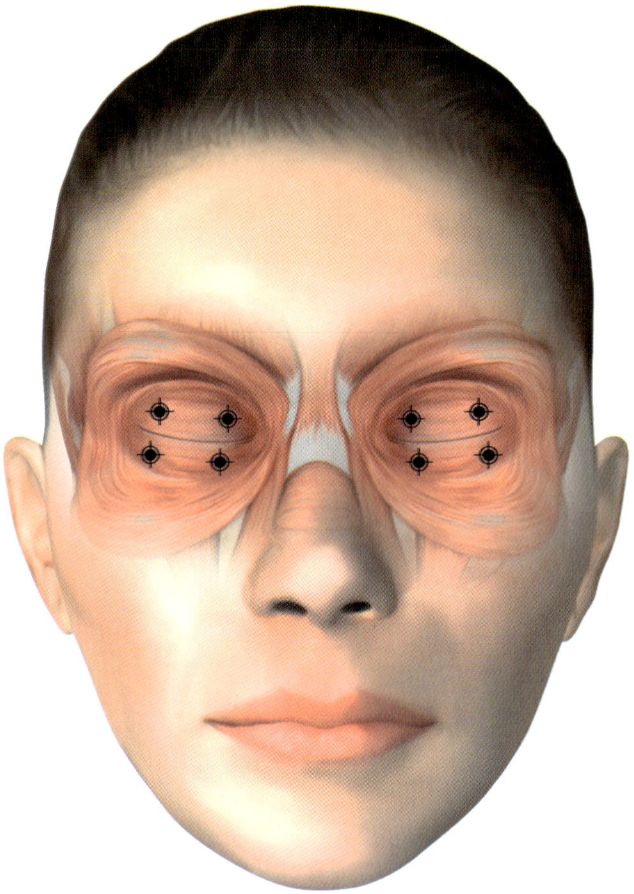

Figure 1 Injection points in the orbicularis oris (pretarsal portion) in blepharospasm

occurrence of side effects, it is important to avoid injection near the outer corner of the eye, in the central portion of the eyelid (risk of injecting the levator palpebrae superioris) or too close to the lower margin of the eyelid. The injections of the medial part of the lower eyelid may cause lacrimation disorders, due to difficulty in emptying the tear sac, and diplopia, due to involvement of the inferior oblique muscle or the inferior rectus muscle [1].
Side effects occur in 3-5% of cases and the most commonly reported are lacrimation, ptosis, dry eyes, diplopia, lagophthalmos, ectropion and photophobia [3,5].

Hemifacial spasm

Hemifacial spasm is characterised by synchronous involuntary tonic or clonic contractions of the muscles innervated by the facial nerve [5]. It is considered a peripheral myoclonic movement disorder and not dystonic [4]. Hemispasm is almost always unilateral, occurring bilaterally in only 2% of cases [3]. The prevalence is of approximately 10 per 100,000 people and occurs more frequently in women, with a peak occurrence between the ages of 40 and 60 [5,7]. It usually begins with spasms of the lower eyelid and then spreads

TABLE 2 - MUSCLES TREATED IN FACIAL HEMISPASM

Muscle	Dosage	Injection points	Needle length	Treatment protocol
Orbicularis oculi	1,25-5 Xeomin 1,25-5 Botox/ Vistabex 3,75/5-15/20 Dysport	3-5 points	20 mm (27-30 G)	Subcutaneous injection of the upper (medial and lateral) and lower (medial and lateral) pretarsal portion, unilaterally
Zygomaticus major	1,25-2,5 Xeomin 1,25-2,5 Botox 3,75/5-7,5/10 Dysport	1-2 points	10-20 mm (27-30 G)	Intramuscular injection, with the needle slightly tangent to the skin surface
Corrugator supercilii	2,5-5 Xeomin 2,5-5 Botox/ Vistabex 7,5/10-15/20 Dysport	1-2 points	20 mm (27-30 G)	It is usually injected at a point in conjunction with the procerus muscle
Frontal part of the occipito-frontalis muscle	1,25-5 Xeomin 1,25-5 Botox 3,75/5-15/20 Dysport	4-8 points	20 mm (27-30 G)	The unaffected side can be treated to reduce the asymmetry caused by injection of the muscle ipsilateral to the hemispasm. It is important to consider functional aspects of facial expression and aesthetics
Procerus	2,5-5 Xeomin 2,5-5 Botox/ Vistabex 7,5/10-15/20 Dysport	1-3 points	20 mm (27-30 G)	Injection is frequently performed at a single point in the centre. Injection may be performed proximodistally or dystoproximally

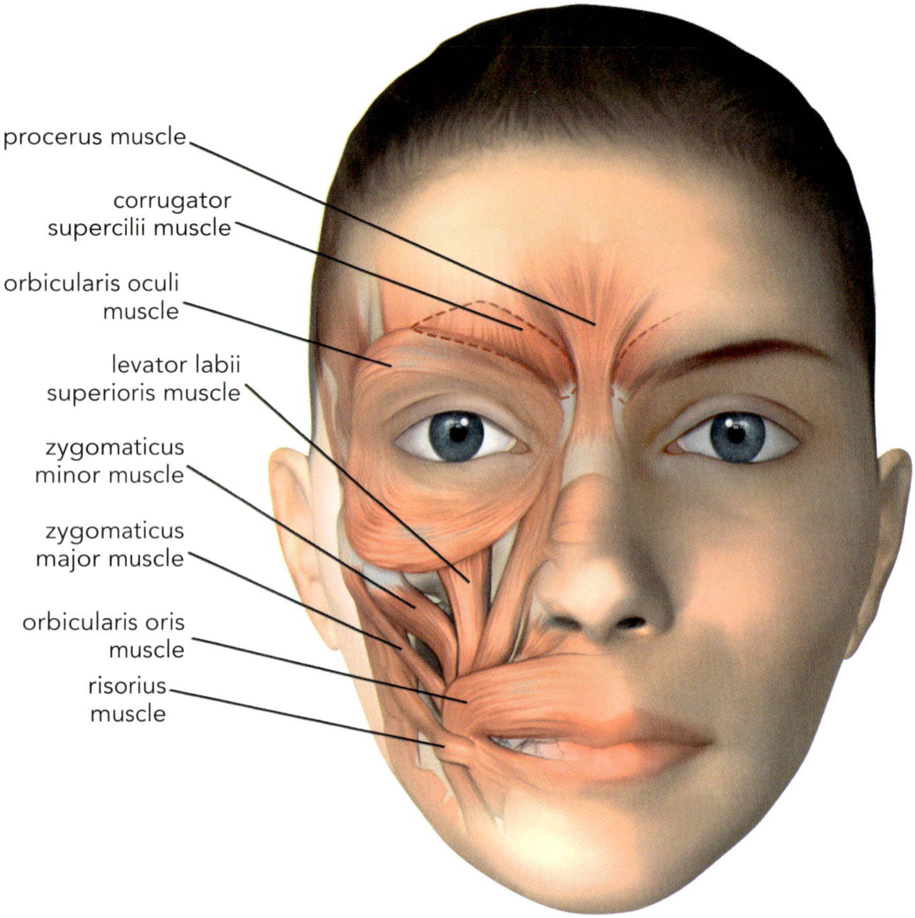

Figure 2a Topographical anatomy of the facial muscles involved in hemifacial spasm

to other facial muscles of the ipsilateral hemiface [5,7].

There is a primary form, which is much more frequent, and a secondary form, which is related to facial nerve damage along its course from the pontocerebellar angle to the parotid gland [7]. Botulinum toxin is considered to be a first-choice therapy in this condition, with an efficacy of 76% to 100% [5,8]. The effect lasts about three months and the latency of efficacy lasts about seven days [5]. It starts with injection of the orbicularis oculi, favouring the pretarsal portion, as already mentioned for blepharospasm (tab. 2) [8]. There are two primary serotypes of botulinum toxin commercially available for use in facial hemispasm, BTX-A and BTX-B. BTX-A is that most commonly used and includes onabotulinumtoxin-A (onaBoNT-A, Botox), abobotulinumtoxin-A (aboBoNT-A, Dysport) and incobotulinum toxin-A (incoBoNT-A, Xeomin). The standard dose ranges from 10 to 20 units of aboBoNT-A and 2.5-5 units of onaBoNT-A, injected at 2-10 sites [7]. IncoBoNT-A and onaBoNT-A are typically diluted to a concentration of 5 U/0.1 cc, aboBoNT-A to 20 U/0.1 cc [3].

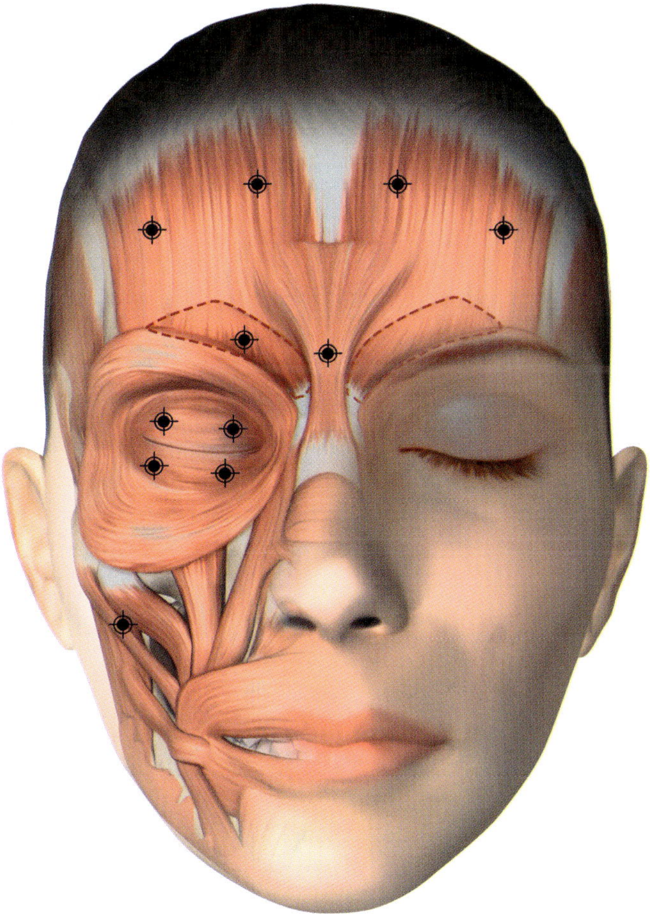

Figure 2b Most common injection points in hemifacial spasm

The subcutaneous facial muscles can be identified using superficial landmarks, while the injection of deeper muscles can be performed correctly using ultrasound or electromyographic guidance. The injection points always include the orbicularis oculi and then, depending on the hyperactive sites in the patient, the zygomaticus major, corrugator supercilii, frontalis and procerus muscles as appropriate (tab. 2, fig. 2) [7].

Techniques for injecting the orbicularis oculi are similar to those for blepharospasm (fig. 1) [3].

Reported side effects include ptosis, diplopia, blurred vision, dry eyes, dysphagia, swelling or bruising of the eyelid, nausea, conjunctival redness and facial asymmetry [5,8]. The latter can become more pronounced with treatment of the zygomaticus muscle, particularly when smiling, causing problems in the retraction of the lip; injection of the contralateral zygomaticus muscle can counterbalance the asymmetry [3,7].

Cervical dystonia

Cervical dystonia, also known as spasmodic or spastic torticollis, is the most common form of focal dystonia. It is characterised by involuntary contraction of the neck muscles resulting in abnormal postures and/or movements of the neck, often associated with pain and tremor [5]. Several head postures can be observed in cervical dystonia: rotacollis, laterocollis, retrocollis and anterocollis (fig. 3).

Rotacollis is the most common form and consists of the twisting of the chin towards the shoulder so that the head rotates laterally; the ipsilateral head splenius, contralateral trapezius, ipsilateral semispinalis capitis, contralateral sternocleidomastoid, ipsilateral levator scapulae and scalene muscles are often involved in its genesis. Laterocollis is the inclination of the head to one side and the sternocleidomastoid, splenius capitus, levator scapulae, scalene, trapezius and semispinalis muscles may be involved ipsilaterally. Retrocollis is the inclination of the head backwards, in which the splenius and semispinalis muscles of the head and neck, trape-

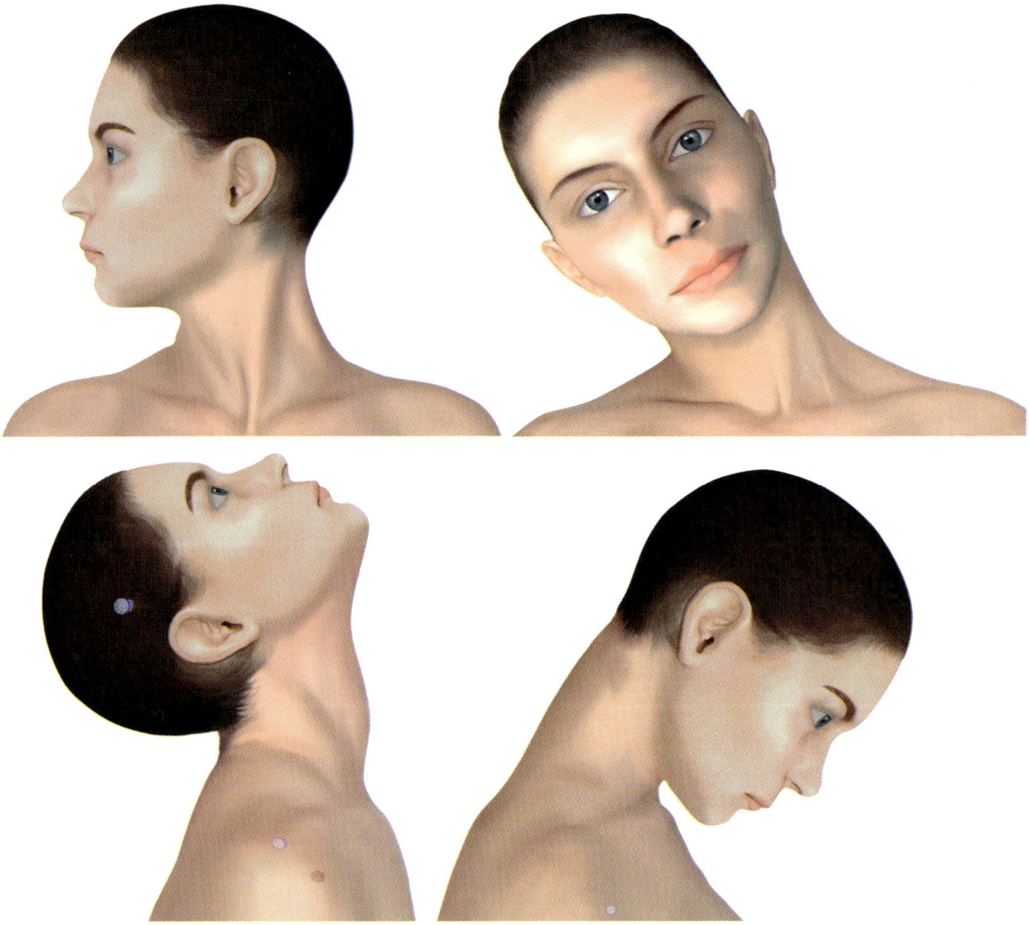

Figure 3 Postures of the head in cervical dystonia: rotacollis, laterocollis, retrocollis and anterocollis

TABLE 3 - MUSCLES MOST COMMONLY TREATED IN CERVICAL DYSTONIA

Muscle	Dosage	Injection points	Needle length	Treatment protocol
Splenium capitis	10-100 Xeomin 10-100 Botox 30/40-300/400 Dysport Neurobloc	1-3 points	40 mm	The injection site is posterior to the insertion of the sternocleidomastoid muscle and anterior to the trapezius. The inoculation angle is 60-90°, directly into the muscle belly
Trapezius, descending part	5-20 Xeomin 5-20 Botox 15/20-60/80 Dysport	2-4 points	20-40 mm	The injection site is at the limit between the neck and shoulder in a vertical direction or according to the orientation of the muscle bundles. If the injection site is too deep, there is a risk of infiltrating the levator scapulae muscle, if it is too lateral, the supraspinatus muscle. Vertical and deep injection pose a risk of pneumothorax
Semispinalis capitis	20-100 Xeomin 20-100 Botox 60/80-300/400 Dysport Neurobloc	1-3 points	40 mm	The muscle is overlapped by the trapezius and the splenium capitis. The injection site is posterior and 1-2 cm lateral to the transverse processes with an injection angle of 60-90°. The muscle can be easily palpated when the head is extended against resistance
Scalenus anterior, median and posterior	5-25 Xeomin 5-25 Botox 15/20-75/100 Dysport Neurobloc	1-3 points	20-40 mm	Injection is made into the muscle belly perpendicular to the skin. The most easily palpable muscle should be infiltrated. Particular care should be taken to avoid the jugular vein, carotid artery,

>>

>> **TABLE 3**

Muscle	Dosage	Injection points	Needle length	Treatment protocol
				subclavian vein, brachial plexus and subclavian artery which run in the interscalene space
Levator scapulae	5-60 Xeomin 5-60 Botox 15/20-180/240 Dysport	1-2 points	40 mm	Injection is performed through the trapezius muscle. The muscle is located and injected between the sternocleidomastoid muscle and the trapezius, 3-4 cm above and 1-2 cm lateral to the upper angle of the scapula
Sternocleido-mastoid	5-50 Xeomin 5-50 Botox 15/20-150/200 Dysport Neurobloc	1-3 points	20-40 mm	Grasp the muscle between the thumb and index finger and inject between the two fingers. Injection should preferably be performed in the upper half of the muscle body
Platysma	1,25-5 Xeomin 1,25-5 Botox 3,75/5-15/20 Dysport Neurobloc	2-3 points per side	10-20 mm	Ask the patient to contract the muscle and inject into the subcutaneous tissue. In the case of deep injection there is a risk of infiltrating the underlying muscles

zius, longissimus and posterior scalene muscles are involved bilaterally. Lastly, anterocollis is the most difficult form to treat, in which the head inclines forward and is characterised by bilateral involvement of the sternocleidomastoid, anterior and medial scalene, suprahyoid, longissimus and occasionally the platysma muscles [1].

The prevalence is approximately 5.7-400 per 100,000 people and the age of onset is around 40. Some people go into remission about five years after onset, but the frequency of recurrence is significant.

Botulinum toxin is the first-line tre-

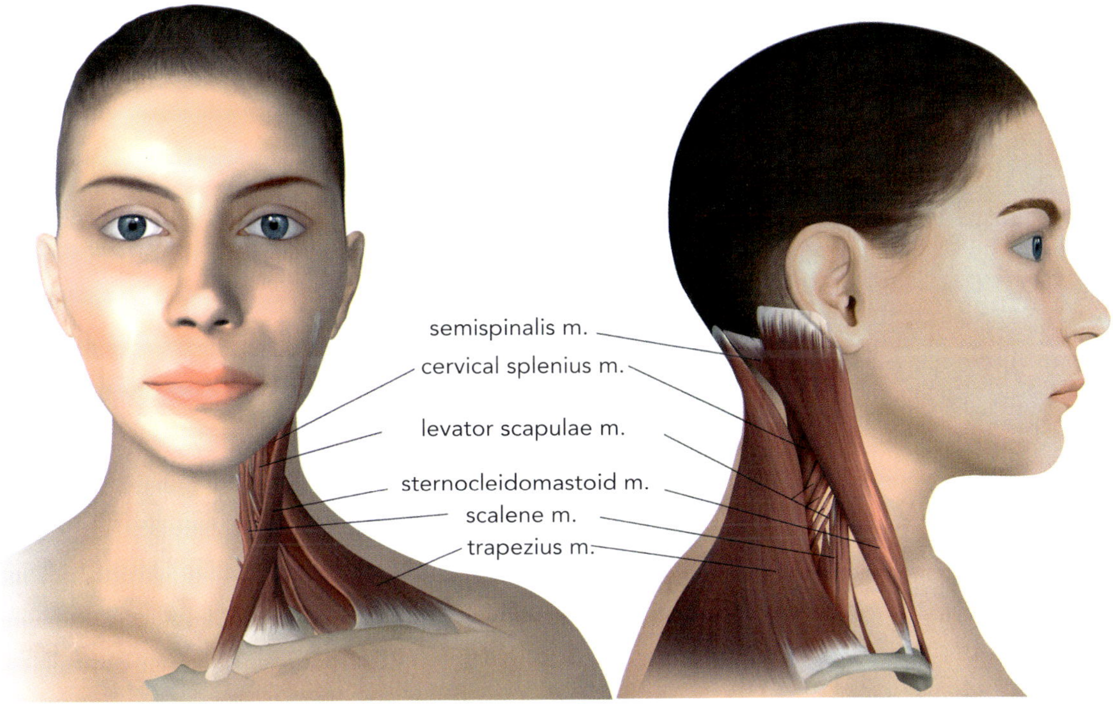

Figure 4 Graphic anatomy of the cervical region

atment for this condition. Injection into the deep cervical muscles benefits from the use of ultrasound and electromyographic guidance [5]. The muscles treated most frequently are the paravertebral nuchal muscles (cervical splenius muscle and semispinalis muscle), splenius capitis muscle, sternocleidomastoid, levator scapulae, scalene and trapezius (descending part) (tab. 3, fig. 4). Sometimes the platysma, suprahyoid and deep muscles of the neck are also treated [9].

The abobotulinum toxin-A (aboBoNTA, Dysport) and rhinobotulinum toxin-B (rimaBoNTB, Neuro-Bloc/Myobloc) formulations are approved for use with evidence type A (i.e.: effective) and the onabotulinum toxin-A (onaBoNTA, Botox) and incobotulinum toxin-A (incoBoNTA, Xeomin) formulations are approved for use with evidence type B (i.e.: probably effective). The total dosages used range from 150 U to 500 U of onaBoNTA, 120 U to 240 U of incoBoNTA, and 250 U to 1,000 U of aboBoNTA [6]. There is no medical evidence from randomised clinical trials to draw definitive conclusions about optimal treatment intervals and doses, the usefulness of injection guidance techniques or the duration of the treatment [10]. The most frequently reported side effects are dysphagia, generalised weakness and weakness of the neck [5,10].

Oromandibular dystonia

Oromandibular dystonia may involve involuntary, intermittent or persistent

contraction of the facial, masticatory, pharyngeal and lingual muscles. This form of dystonia can impair speech, chewing and swallowing and can therefore be particularly disabling [3,4].
Oromandibular dystonia may or may not be associated with blepharospasm, spasmodic dysphonia or cervical dystonia. When accompanied by blepharospasm it is also called Meige syndrome or craniofacial dystonia [4,11].
Oromandibular dystonia is often classified according to the primary direction of jaw deviation: open, closed, deviated. The muscles commonly involved in closure of the mandible are the masseter, temporalis and medial pterygoid. Those involved in the opening of the mandible are the lateral pterygoid and the digastric, and those involved in the deviation of the mandible are the contralateral lateral pterygoid and the ipsilateral temporalis [3]. The genioglossus muscle is involved in the protrusion of the tongue [4]. Triggers for spasm are bright lights, driving, watching television, talking, reading and chewing; it can also occur only when performing certain specific tasks. The consequences of this disorder can be dysarthria, dysphagia, difficulty breathing, weight loss, temporomandibular joint dysfunction, pain and cutaneous lesions of the oral mucosa, lips or tongue. The origin may be primary or secondary to neurodegenerative diseases, such as neuroacanthocytosis and Wilson's disease, or to anoxic damage, tumours or infections. When dystonia predominantly involves the lips, it may be tardive dyskinesia, neuroacanthocytosis or Lesch-Nyhan syndrome. Primary and secondary forms can be distinguished on the basis of age of onset, progression, pharmacological history and the presence of other neurological symptoms. The prevalence is approximately 6.9 cases per 100,000, it is more common in women and the age of onset of primary forms is around the sixth decade [3].
Differential diagnosis should be made with chorea, myoclonus, facial muscle myokymia and hemifacial and hemimasticatory spasms [3]. It is important that these patients undergo dental, oral and barium oesophageal assessment to evaluate oropharyngeal swallowing function [3]. Logopaedic rehabilitation sessions may also be useful. Medications used for oromandibular dystonia include benzodiazepines, anticholinergic drugs, levodopa, baclofen, lithium, gabapentin and zolpidem. In addition, in the absence of extensive studies, deep brain stimulation of the inner pallid globe has been found to be a useful treatment in resistant forms of cranial dystonia. However, the first-line treatment continues to be botulinum toxin. About two-thirds of patients report a moderate benefit from the treatment, lasting about 3-6 months.
The selection of the muscles to be treated must be specific to each patient. The patient must be assessed at rest with the eyes closed and open, and actions that cause the disorder to worsen must be determined, so the patient must also be assessed while speaking and chewing. The tongue should be observed at rest within the oral cavity and protruding outside the mouth and when speaking. Injection can be

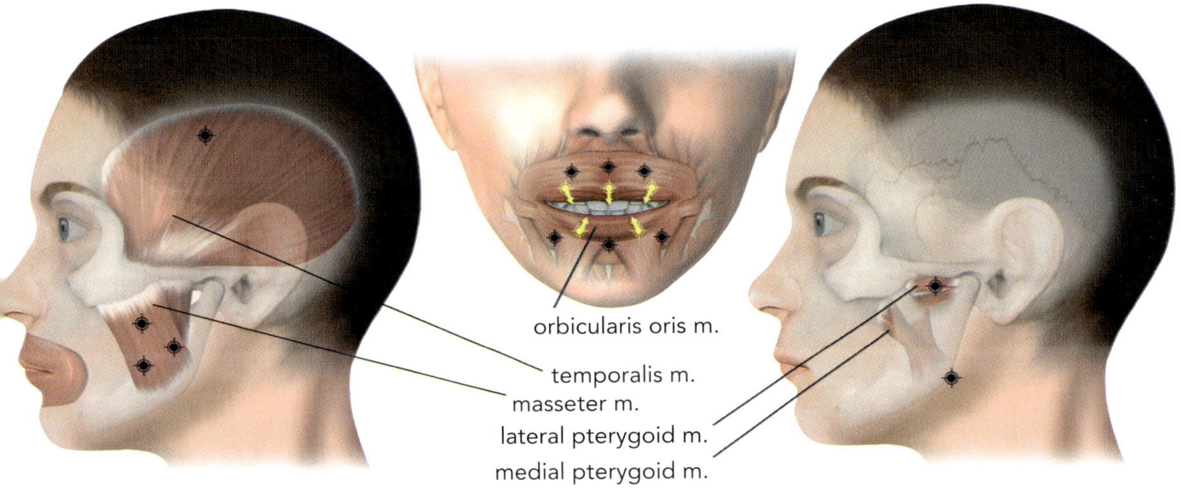

Figure 5 Graphical anatomy of the masticatory muscles and common injection points in oromandibular dystonia

performed using ultrasound or electromyographic guidance; some muscles can be approached either percutaneously or trans-orally [3].

OnabotulinumtoxinA (onaBoNTA) and abobotulinumtoxinA (aboBoNTA) are approved for use in oromandibular dystonia with a type C level of evidence (possibly effective), while incobotulinumtoxinA (incoBoNTA) and rimabotulinumtoxinB (rimaBoNTB) are approved with a type U level of evidence (insufficient evidence) [6].

The indications are to use the lowest dosage useful for the patient to avoid side effects. IncoBoNTA and onaBoNTA should be diluted with 0.9% saline solution at a dilution of 1 ml per 100 U. More superficial muscles can be injected with a 30 G needle, while deeper muscles, such as the pterygoid and genioglossus muscles, are injected with a 27 G needle. The needle is directed perpendicular to the skin. In most cases, the masseter muscle is treated; it is important to avoid injecting the parotid gland, which could cause xerostomia. The lateral pterygoid muscle can be approached trans-orally or externally, in the mandibular incisura (2-4 cm anterior to the external auditory canal at the level of the tragus and 1 cm inferior to the margin of the zygomatic arch). To limit protrusion of the tongue, the genioglossus muscle can be treated by means of a submandibular approach, approximately 2.5-3 cm posterior to the chin, lateral to the midline, medial to the digastric muscle, at a depth of at least 1 cm. Treatment of the orbicularis oris muscle in cases of dystonia of the lips can cause asymmetry of the mouth, difficulty in drinking and drooling (fig. 5) [4].

Adverse effects related to treatment with botulinum toxin may be weakness of the injected muscles resulting in possible worsening or appearance

TABLE 4 - MUSCLES MOST COMMONLY TREATED IN OROMANDIBULAR DYSTONIA

Muscle	Dosage	Injection points	Needle length	Treatment protocol
Masseter	5-15 Xeomin 5-15 Botox 15/20-45/60 Dysport	1-3 points	20 mm	The superficial part of the muscle is easily palpable. Excessively deep injection poses a risk of infiltrating the pterygoid muscles, and if directed too posteriorly there is a risk of the toxin migrating to the parotid gland. The external route is easier. The masseter is involved bilaterally in closure of the mouth. The initial dose is usually 50 U (Dysport)
Medial pterygoid	5-20 Xeomin 5-20 Botox 15/20-60/80 Dysport	1 point	40 mm	The use of electromyographic guidance is useful. The injection is performed posteriorly and in the direction of the mandibular angle. However, trans-oral injection is preferred. The medial pterygoid m. is involved in closure of the mouth and the initial dose is usually 20 U (Dysport)
Lateral pterygoid	5-25 Xeomin 5-25 Botox 15/20-75/100 Dysport	1 point	40 mm	The muscle should be injected 3 cm in front of the tragus on an imaginary line joining the tragus and the infraorbital margin, at a depth of about 15-25 mm. The muscle is involved in opening the mouth and the initial dose is usually 20 U (Dysport)

>>

>> **TABLE 4**

Muscle	Dosage	Injection points	Needle length	Treatment protocol
Temporalis	5-10 Xeomin 5-10 Botox 15/20-30/40 Dysport	1-4 points	20-40 mm	Injection is performed over the temporal fossa, 5 cm above the insertion of the muscle in its thickest part. The muscle belly can be identified by palpation. Particular care must be taken to avoid injecting the temporal artery. The muscle is involved in closure (bilaterally) and deviation (ipsilaterally) of the mouth and the initial dose is usually 40 U (Dysport)

of dysarthria, dysphagia, difficulty in chewing, or xerostomia in cases of accidental injection of the parotid gland [3].

The treatment of sialorrhea

Sialorrhea is a disabling symptom resulting in reduced quality of life and can lead to complications such as aspiration pneumonia, oral cavity infections, dehydration, malnutrition, tooth decay and skin problems in the surrounding areas [12,13]. Sialorrhea is caused by the presence of excessive saliva in the oral cavity leading to drooling from the mouth. It can be caused by increased saliva production or by the absence or malfunction of mechanisms that remove saliva from the oral cavity. Sialorrhea is considered to be a normal phenomenon in children up to the age of four [13].

Sialorrhea is commonly seen in some neurological disorders, such as Parkinson's disease (MP), amyotrophic lateral sclerosis (ALS) and muscular dystrophies [12,13]. Swallowing is a complex neuromuscular activity that requires a voluntary oral phase and an involuntary pharyngeal and oesophageal phase; in neurological diseases the disorder is frequently caused by an inability to eliminate secretions rather than by their increased production [13].

Approximately 1-1.5 l of saliva is produced by the salivary glands in the oral cavity during a single day. The main glands are the parotid gland, which is the largest, and the submandibular and the sublingual glands. The parotid gland extends from the lower margin of the zygomatic arch to the anterior

TABLE 5 - SITES OF INJECTION OF THE SALIVARY GLANDS MOST INVOLVED IN SIALORRHEA

Muscle	Dosage	Injection points	Needle length	Treatment protocol
Parotid	20-50 Xeomin 20-50 Botox 60/80-150/200 Dysport	1-4 points per side	20 mm	Injection in two points is usually sufficient. It should be performed in the upper and lower half of the gland body or can be performed under ultrasound guidance. The facial nerve runs through the body of the gland and can be injured accidentally. Excessively deep injection can injure the masseter muscle
Sub mandibular	20-50 Xeomin 20-50 Botox 60/80-150/200 Dysport	1-4 points per side	20 mm	Injection in one point is usually sufficient. It is hard to localise in the absence of ultrasound guidance. Injection can be performed in a direction parallel to the excretory duct

margin of the sternocleidomastoid muscle and horizontally from the mastoid process to the masseter muscle; secretions pass through the parotid duct, which passes through the buccinator muscle and enters the oral vestibule. The submandibular gland is located below the mylohyoid muscle, on the inner surface of the mandible. The sublingual gland is located in the mucosa of the oral floor. The parotid gland is responsible for producing 25% of the total saliva, while the submandibular gland is responsible for producing 75% of the saliva generated during the day. The production of saliva is important for carbohydrate metabolism, lubrication of the chyme and control of bacterial biofilm growth. Saliva secretion is regulated by the autonomous system, in particular by postganglionic sympathetic fibres that reach the salivary glands via the 10th cranial nerve and parasympathetic fibres that reach the salivary glands via the 7th and 9th cranial nerves.

Treatment of sialorrhea includes relearning how to swallow, with motor exercises or palate training devices, dietary changes, intervention with drugs such

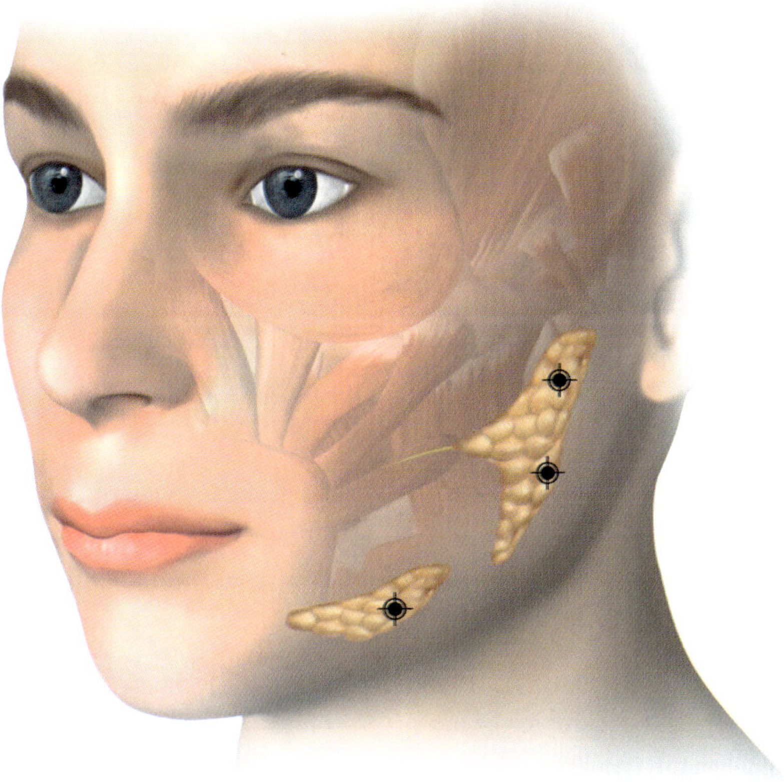

Figure 6 Topographical anatomy and salivary gland injection points in the treatment of sialorrhea

as atropine, scopolamine, benztropine and glycopyrrolate, surgery, such as submandibular duct relocation or salivary duct ligation, radiotherapy and, lastly, injection with botulinum toxin [13,14].

Botulinum toxin is safe and effective; older age seems to be associated with the longer lasting effect of the toxin, and sufferers of Parkinson's disease seem to have a better safety-effectiveness ratio than patients with amyotrophic lateral sclerosis, with fewer side effects and longer duration [12]. Botulinum toxin injections are able to temporarily reduce salivary flow [12,13]. The toxin rimabotulinumtoxinB (rimaBoNTB) has been approved in the United States but not in Europe, whereas incobotulinumtoxinA (incoBoNTA, Xeomin) is approved in Europe for chronic sialorrhea, without restrictions based on the underlying pathology. The recommended dose is 100 U, 30 U of which for each parotid gland and 20 U for the two submandibular glands (tab. 5, fig. 6) [14].

Injections are usually performed transcutaneously directly into the salivary glands; most studies agree on the usefulness of treating the parotid and submandibular glands simultaneously. Ultrasound-guided treatment is very useful to avoid the accidental migration of the toxin to the adjacent muscles and to check for anatomical variations, especially in the submandibular gland. The use of a linear ultrasound probe placed on the mandibular angle and progressively moved to find the position to locate the largest diameter of the gland is recommended. The best site for injection of the parotid gland is midway between the tragus and the mandibular angle, while for the submandibular gland it is about 1 cm from the mandibular angle, in the distal third between the mandibular angle and the apex of the chin. The salivary glands are easily visible due to their homogeneous echogenicity and clear demarcation from the surrounding tissues.

Side effects may include xerostomia and dysphagia [14].

Prophylaxis of chronic migraine

The 2015 *Lancet Global Burden of Disease Study* classified migraine as the seventh cause of disability in the world. Migraine is a primary headache characterised by unilateral, pulsating attacks of moderate to severe intensity, aggravated by routine exercise (e.g.: climbing stairs), associated with nausea and/or vomiting, photophobia and/or phonophobia, lasting 4-72 hours. 15% of the population is affected by this pathology.

Chronic migraine is a headache (migraine or tension-type headache) that occurs 15 or more days in a month for more than three months, with at least eight of those days being characterised by migraine headache (International Classification of Headache Disorders). Chronic migraine is a debilitating disorder that affects about 2% of the general population [15].

In 2010, following incidental discovery in patients being treated with botulinum toxin for cosmetic purposes, the possible role of the toxin in the treatment of this condition was investigated. Consequently, in 2010, two multicentre randomised clinical trials were conducted, demonstrating the efficacy of botulinum toxin (onabotulinumtoxinA, Botox) treatment in the prophylaxis of patients with chronic migraine: Phase 3 Research Evaluating Migraine Prophylaxis Therapy (PREEMPT). OnabotulinumtoxinA has not proven effective in the treatment of patients with episodic migraine and tension-type headaches. Although the treatment has been approved by the European Drug Agency (EMA) and the US Food and Drug Administration (FDA) for the prophylaxis of chronic migraine, no European guidelines on the use of the toxin are available, so in 2018 the European Headache Federation published guidelines based on the scientific evidence available and the opinion of a panel of experts [15].

The mechanisms of action of botulinum toxin in migraine patients have long been studied and are still not fully understood. Efficacy does not appear to be limited to local effects but may include action on anatomically connected areas thanks to axonal transport of the toxin. Efficacy may be the result of the blockage of peripheral nociceptive signals to the central nervous system, leading indirectly to a reduction in sensitivity to pain at central level. Moreover, central afferent input from the meninges is considered to be an important source of pain in headache, and the toxin seems capable of inhibiting the activation of meningeal nociceptors. It is well known that peripheral pain receptors are sensitised by inflammatory mediators and that these, in turn, cause the sensitisation of central receptors and persistent pain. Botulinum toxin has been shown to inhibit not only the release of acetylcholine, but also that of neurotransmitters involved in headache, such as serotonin, glutamate, noradrenaline, γ-aminobutyric acid (GABA), calcitonin gene-related peptide (CGRP) and substance P (SP). In addition, botulinum toxin seems to inhibit the expression of certain nociceptors, such as TRPV1, TRPM8, TRPA1, P2XR and GABA-A, while acting as an agonist on μ-type opioid receptors [16].

The guidelines of the European Headache Federation concluded that onabotulinumtoxinA is recommended for the treatment of patients with chronic migraine and is an effective and well-tolerated treatment. Before treatment is proposed, at least two or three treatments for prophylaxis of migraine episodes must have failed (due to ineffectiveness or intolerable side effects), unless the patient has multiple comorbidities that mean that it is not possible to attempt treatment with these drugs. In patients who make excessive use of painkillers, it would be preferable to precede the botulinum toxin treatment with a detoxification protocol. The recommended injection protocol is the one used in the PREEMPT studies, as it is the only one supported by scientific evidence to be effective [15]. The PREEMPT protocol envisages a fixed dosage in fixed injection sites (the "fixed dose, fixed site" method), with a total of 155 U of onabotulinumtoxinA to be injected into 31 sites in seven muscle groups: the corrugator supercilii, the procerus, the frontalis, the temporalis, the occipitalis, the cervical paravertebral muscles and the trapezius (tab. 6, fig. 7). In addition, during the PREEMPT clinical trial an additional 40 U were allowed to be injected into three muscle groups where the patient reported the most pain ("follow the pain" method). The US Food and Drug Administration has approved the PREEMPT "fixed dose, fixed site" protocol for the treatment of chronic migraine. However, in other countries, a total dosage of 195 U has been approved, allowing the addition of injections into the temporalis, occipitalis and trapezius muscles according to the "follow the pain" method. The cycle is repeated every 12 months [17].

Patients receiving botulinum toxin should continue to be monitored using headache diaries and treatment should be discontinued in those who do not benefit from treatment (<30% reduction in headache days) after 2-3 cycles of treatment; discontinuation is also recommended in patients who have achieved a reduction of up to less than 10 headache days per month for at least three months. However, the in-

TABLE 6 - "FIXED DOSE, FIXED SITE" INJECTION PROTOCOL USED IN PREEMPT STUDIES

Muscle	Dosage	Injection point	Treatment protocol
Corrugator supercilii	5 U Botox per injection site bilaterally (total 20 U)	2 points per side	The corrugator muscle is located on the medial part of the orbital rim and can be located by asking the patient to wrinkle their forehead. It should be palpated and pinched between the index finger and thumb and then injected with the needle angled at 90°, remaining just above the periosteum
Procerus	5 U Botox	1 point	Injection of the procerus is performed at a single site midway between the two eyebrow corrugator injections. The injection must be positioned superficially in the muscle belly at a 90° angle
Frontalis	5 U Botox per injection site bilaterally (total 40 U)	4 points per side	The injection sites can be identified by visually drawing a line from the medial edge of the supraorbital margin upwards. The muscle is injected in the upper third, at least one or two fingers above the corrugator injection site. The other injection areas are parallel, approximately 1.5 cm lateral to the medial injection site
Temporalis	5 U Botox per injection site bilaterally (total 40 U)	4 points per side	The first injection site is approximately 3 cm above the tragus on a line drawn visually from the tragus upwards. The second site can be located by moving approximately 1.5-3 cm upwards from the first injection site, remaining on this vertical line. The third site is approximately 3 cm anterior to the vertical line, midway between the two previous injection sites. The fourth site is 1.5 cm posterior to the second injection site, in line with the helix of the ear. All the injections are performed at a 45° angle

>>

>> **TABLE 6**

Muscle	Dosage	Injection point	Treatment protocol
Occipitalis	5 U Botox per injection site bilaterally (total 30 U)	3 points per side	The first injection site is in the middle of a line running from the inion of the occipital bone to the mastoid process, just above the nuchal crest. The second site is about 1.5 cm diagonally upwards and towards the helix of the ear. The third is about 1.5 cm diagonally upwards and medially. The injections are performed at an angle of 45° and upwards, above the nuchal crest
Paraverte-bral cervical muscles	5 U Botox per injection site bilaterally (total 20 U per side)	2 points per side	The first injection site is 1 cm lateral to the midline and approximately 3 cm below the occipital protuberance. The second site is approximately 1.5 cm upwards diagonally at 45° towards the helix of the ear from the first injection site
Trapezius	5 U Botox per injection site bilaterally (total le 30 U)	3 points per side	The first injection site can be identified by visually dividing the upper part of the trapezium in half, from the inflection point of the neck to the acromio-clavicular joint: the injection should be at the midpoint. The second point is at the midpoint between the first injection site and the acromion. The third point is at the midpoint between the first injection site and the neck inflection point. Injections should be made into the supraclavicular portion of the trapezius muscle, medial to the deltoid and acromioclavicular joint and should be horizontal and shallow

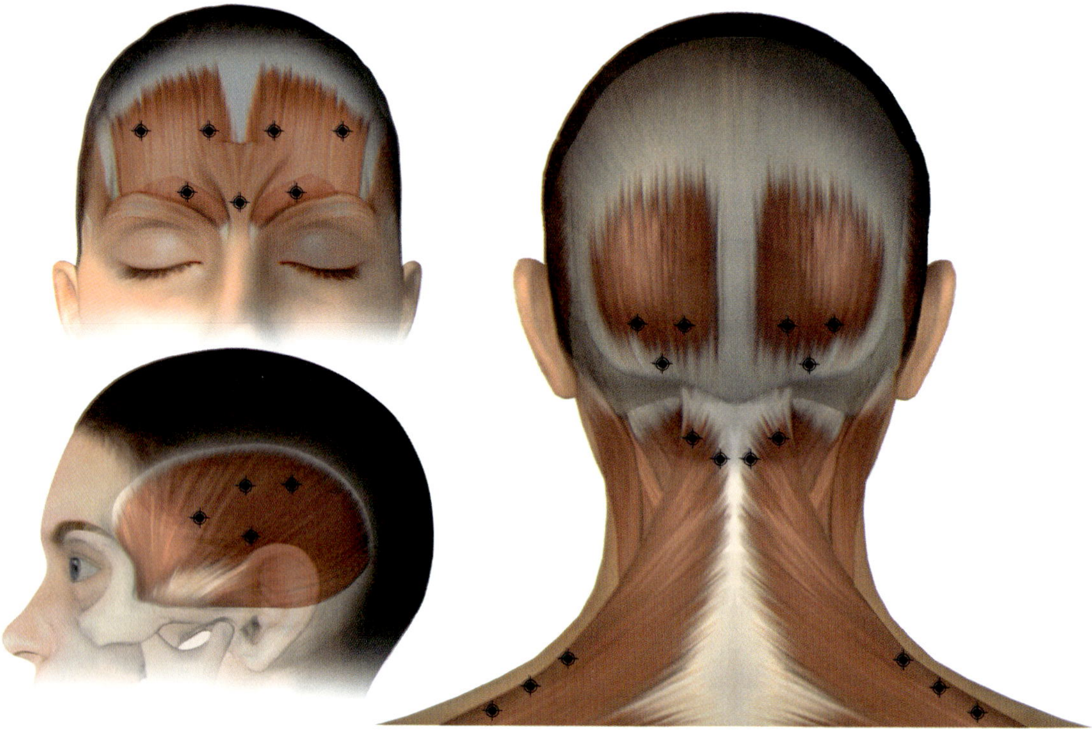

Figure 7 Injection points of the PREEMPT fixed dose, fixed site protocol

tensity of the headache, the disability caused to the patient and the patient's own preferences must also be considered. The patient should be re-assessed 4-5 months after discontinuation of treatment with botulinum toxin to ensure that they have not regressed to a state of chronic migraine [15].
Reported side effects are neck pain, muscle weakness and ptosis. To avoid post-injection headache, it is important always to remain above the periosteum. [17].

BRUXISM

Claudia Ledda, Alberto Diaspro

Bruxism is considered a parafunctional activity of the masticatory muscles that can lead to headaches, muscle pain, wearing of the teeth and temporomandibular joint disorders. It is divided into sleep bruxism (SB), which is a stereotyped oromandibular muscle activity characterised by rhythmic or non-rhythmic grinding and clenching of the teeth, and awake bruxism (AB), which is a muscle activity characterised by repetitive or prolonged contact between the teeth and/or continuous jaw movements.

The former is considered part of the phenomena of sleep micro-awakenings, with a prevalence of 7.4% in the adult population, while the latter is associated with other motor disorders, or determined by psychosocial factors, and is reported in 22.1-31% of the adult population [18].

Bruxism in healthy individuals is considered an attitude that determines a dental risk factor for tooth wear and the appearance of temporomandibular joint disorders, rather than a pathology in itself; however, it can also be due to the use of drugs or be associated with neurological pathologies and psychiatric disorders (so-called secondary bruxism). The common goal of therapies is muscle relaxation and different options have been considered for this, including the use of botulinum toxin A (BTXa) [19].

Masticatory activity is the result of the action of three jaw muscles: the masseter, the temporalis and the medial pterygoid, which contribute 43%, 36% and 21% of the force produced respectively.

BTXa blocks the release of acetylcholine at the cholinergic synapses, leading to their relaxation at therapeutic doses, and has therefore been considered as a potentially effective therapy for controlling symptoms secondary to muscle activity in bruxism patients. Moreover, the analgesic properties of botulinum toxin may contribute to the improvement of pain associated with bruxism [12].

The administration of BTXa determines a reduction in the intensity of contraction, as it reduces the intensity of rhythmic masticatory muscle activity (RMMA) during sleep, but does not interact with its genesis, because it is a consequence of micro-awakenings, i.e.: a physiological activity of the muscles during sleep determined by the reticular-ascending excitation system of the brainstem, which contributes to the increase in activity in motor and autonomic-cardiac neuronal networks.

The action of BTXa therefore only interacts with the last phase of an episode of sleep bruxism, reducing the intensity of contraction of the neuromuscular plate, peripherally, while it has no effect on its genesis, located in the central nervous system.

It is believed that this reduction in the intensity of muscle contraction during sleep may be responsible for the improvement in subjective symptoms such as morning muscle stiffness and pain, but the mechanism responsible

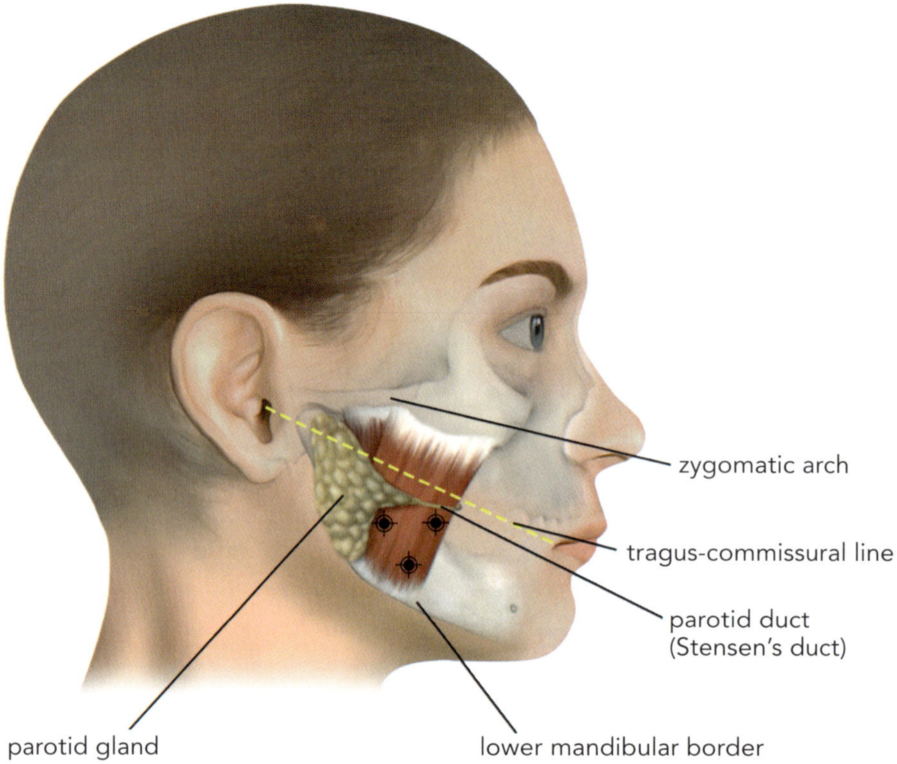

Figure 8 Masseter muscle injection sites

VIDEO 10.1

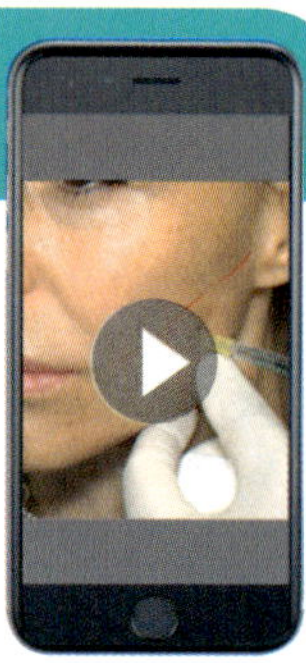

Treatment of bruxism

for the effectiveness of botulinum toxin injection has yet to be fully understood [20].

The use of BTXa in bruxism is an off-label therapy. There is not yet enough evidence in literature to define a standardised approach, so no clinical protocols or recommended dosages are available.

Consequently, the incomplete understanding of the pharmacological activity of botulinum toxin results in a lack of clinical protocols and standardisation of doses and dilutions of toxins available in the pharmacopoeia and on the market. This has led to extensive variability in the protocols repor-

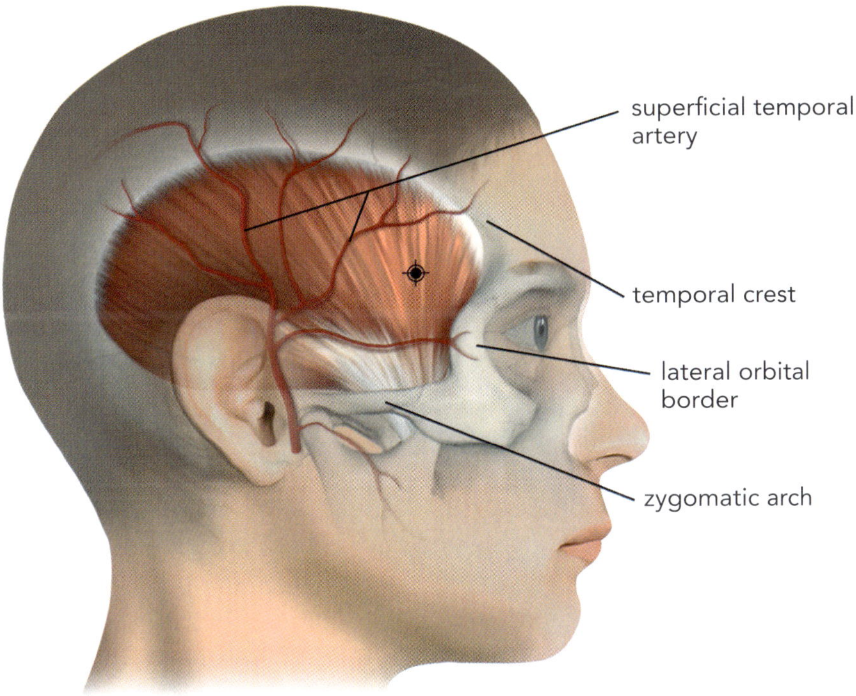

Figure 9 Temporalis muscle injection sites (anterior portion)

ted by the different studies found in literature, with dosages ranging from 8 to 100 Botox Units (BUCs) used to treat the masseter muscle and up to 25 BUCs injected into the temporalis muscle, while injection into the medial pterygoid muscle is rarely reported (figs. 8-9) [21].

The difference in dosage between the two muscles is due to their size, as the masseter muscles, being larger, require more units of BoNT-A to achieve the therapeutic effect.

The effect of BTX-A is transient and limited to the area around the injection, as are the most common adverse effects of treatment that remain local, such as sensitivity and mild skin reaction at the injection site. More rarely, reversible adverse effects such as headache, dysphonia, dysphagia and xerostomia have been reported [22].

Bibliography

1. Jost W, Valerius K (2012). Pictorial atlas of botulinum toxin injection: dosage, localization, application. Surrey (UK), Quintessence Publishing.
2. Albanese A, Bhatia K, Bressman SB, Delong MR, Fahn S, Fung VS, Hallett M, Jankovic J, Jinnah HA, Klein C, Lang AE, Mink JW, Teller JK. Phenomenology and classification of dystonia: a consensus update. Mov Disord. 2013 Jun 15;28(7):863-73.
3. Karp BI, Alter K. Botulinum Toxin Treatment of Blepharospasm, Orofacial/Oromandibular Dystonia, and Hemifacial Spasm. Semin Neurol. 2016 Feb;36(1):84-91.
4. Hassell TJW, Charles D. Treatment of Blepharospasm and Oromandibular Dystonia with Botulinum Toxins. Toxins (Basel). 2020 Apr 22;12(4):269.
5. Anandan C, Jankovic J. Botulinum Toxin in Movement Disorders: An Update. Toxins (Basel). 2021 Jan 8;13(1):42.
6. Simpson DM, Hallett M, Ashman EJ, Comella CL, Green MW, Gronseth GS, Armstrong MJ, Gloss D, Potrebic S, Jankovic J, Karp BP, Naumann M, So YT, Yablon SA. Practice guideline update summary: Botulinum neurotoxin for the treatment of blepharospasm, cervical dystonia, adult spasticity, and headache: Report of the Guideline Development Subcommittee of the American Academy of Neurology. Neurology. 2016 May 10;86(19):1818-26.
7. Green KE, Rastall D, Eggenberger E. Treatment of Blepharospasm/Hemifacial Spasm. Curr Treat Options Neurol. 2017 Sep 30;19(11):41.
8. Kenney C, Jankovic J. Botulinum toxin in the treatment of blepharospasm and hemifacial spasm. J Neural Transm (Vienna). 2008;115(4):585-91.
9. Dressler D, Altavista MC, Altenmueller E, Bhidayasiri R, Bohlega S, Chana P, Chung TM, Colosimo C, Fheodoroff K, Garcia-Ruiz PJ, Jeon B, Jin L, Kanovsky P, Milanov I, Micheli F, Orlova O, Pandey S, Pirtosek Z, Relja M, Rosales R, Sagástegui-Rodríguez JA, Shahidi GA, Timerbaeva S, Wan X, Walter U, Saberi FA. Consensus guidelines for botulinum toxin therapy: general algorithms and dosing tables for dystonia and spasticity. J Neural Transm (Vienna). 2021 Feb 26. Epub ahead of print.
10. Rodrigues FB, Duarte GS, Marques RE, Castelão M, Ferreira J, Sampaio C, Moore AP, Costa J. Botulinum toxin type A therapy for cervical dystonia. Cochrane Database Syst Rev. 2020 Nov 12;11:CD003633.
11. Comella CL. Systematic review of botulinum toxin treatment for oromandibular dystonia. Toxicon. 2018 Jun 1;147:96-99.
12. Serrera-Figallo MA, Ruiz-de-León-Hernández G, Torres-Lagares D, Castro-Araya A, Torres-Ferrerosa O, Hernández-Pacheco E, Gutierrez-Perez JL. Use of Botulinum Toxin in Orofacial Clinical Practice. Toxins (Basel). 2020 Feb 11;12(2):112.
13. Singh H, Nene Y, Mehta TR, Govindarajan R. Efficacy of Botulinum Toxin for Treating Sialorrhea in Neuromuscular Conditions. Front Neurol. 2020 Jun 10;11:513.
14. Jost WH, Bäumer T, Laskawi R, Slawek J, Spittau B, Steffen A, Winterholler

M, Bavikatte G. Therapy of Sialorrhea with Botulinum Neurotoxin. Neurol Ther. 2019 Dec;8(2):273-288.
15. Bendtsen L, Sacco S, Ashina M, Mitsikostas D, Ahmed F, Pozo-Rosich P, Martelletti P. Guideline on the use of onabotulinumtoxinA in chronic migraine: a consensus statement from the European Headache Federation. J Headache Pain. 2018 Sep 26;19(1):91.
16. Do TP, Hvedstrup J, Schytz HW. Botulinum toxin: A review of the mode of action in migraine. Acta Neurol Scand. 2018 May;137(5):442-451.
17. Blumenfeld AM, Silberstein SD, Dodick DW, Aurora SK, Brin MF, Binder WJ. Insights into the Functional Anatomy Behind the PREEMPT Injection Paradigm: Guidance on Achieving Optimal Outcomes. Headache. 2017 May;57(5):766-777.
18. Shim YJ, Lee HJ, Park KJ, Kim HT, Hong IH, Kim ST. Botulinum Toxin Therapy for Managing Sleep Bruxism: A Randomized and Placebo-Controlled Trial. Toxins (Basel). 2020 Mar 9;12(3):168.
19. Kumar A, Spivakovsky S. Bruxism- is botulinum toxin an effective treatment? Evid Based Dent. 2018 Jun;19(2):59.
20. De la Torre Canales G, Câmara-Souza MB, do Amaral CF, Garcia RC, Manfredini D. Is there enough evidence to use botulinum toxin injections for bruxism management? A systematic literature review. Clin Oral Investig. 2017 Apr;21(3):727-734.
21. Ågren M, Sahin C, Pettersson M. The effect of botulinum toxin injections on bruxism: A systematic review. J Oral Rehabil. 2020 Mar;47(3):395-402.
22. Fernández-Núñez T, et al. Efficacy of botulinum toxin in the treatment of bruxism: Systematic review. Med Oral Patol Oral Cir Bucal. 2019 Jul 1;24(4):e416-e424.

11

PARTICULAR USES OF BOTULINUM TOXIN

Claudia Ledda, Giovanni Brunelli

ANAL FISSURES

Claudia Ledda

Anal fissures are linear tears along the long axis of the distal anoderm of the anal canal, located along the posterior midline or, more rarely, along the anterior midline, extending below the serrated line. The most common symptoms are rectal bleeding, pain during and after defecation and nocturnal pain [1-2].

A distinction is made between acute and chronic fissures when they last more than six weeks. Acute fissures are treated with conservative methods, such as changes in diet, and tend to heal within 1-2 weeks [1].

The aetiology of fissures is unknown but hypertonia and/or spasm of the internal anal sphincter seems to be involved [1,3]. Precipitating factors may be trauma caused by altered bowel movements, constipation or diarrhoea, hypertonia of the internal anal sphincter, sexual abuse or natural delivery during birth. An anal fissure can lead to complications such as hypertrophy of the anal papilla, a sentinel skin tag or a mucosal defect exposing the internal sphincter [2].

The prevalence is of one in 100,000 people per year [3], there does not appear to be a gender-based prevalence and it is more common in young and middle-aged adults [2].

Treatment aims to reduce the pressure on the internal anal sphincter during rest. For many years, the gold standard has been surgery, using techniques such as anal dilatation, posterior midline sphincterotomy and lateral midline sphincterotomy. The gold standard is represented by internal lateral sphincterotomy with a success rate of more than 95% [3]. However, these surgical techniques are accompanied by a high rate of post-operative faecal incontinence. Consequently, the decision has been made to try alternative, less invasive therapies, such as locally applied nitrates and calcium channel blockers and botulinum toxin injection [1].

According to the recommendations of the American Society of Colon and Rectal Surgeons, the American College of Gastroenterology and the Association of Coloproctology of Great Britain and Ireland, initial treatment should be non-invasive, with topical treatments of nitrates or calcium channel blockers. For cases refractory to non-invasive treatment, injection of botulinum toxin into the internal anal sphincter is recommended. The recommended dosage according to the Association of Coloproctology of Great Britain and Ireland is 20-25 U in two separate doses injected into the internal anal sphincter on either side of the anal fissure. According to the study by Sekmen et al., it is preferable to inject 50 U of botulinum into the internal anal sphincter at the 6 and 12 o'clock position (anterior and posterior), rather than lateral injections. The authors found less post-procedure pain and better results, and recommend the use of ultrasound guidance [2].

Botulinum toxin is not more effective

than internal lateral sphincterotomy, but it is a minimally invasive alternative therapy with a lower rate of side effects than the surgical option [1,3]. Botulinum toxin is able to achieve a temporary chemical sphincterotomy and reduce the firmness of the internal anal sphincter. It also seems to increase microcirculation, resulting in improved pain and healing of the fissure.
Despite its widespread use for the treatment of this condition, there are no standardised treatment protocols and there is a great deal of heterogeneity in the literature published on the results of treatment. In a meta-analysis aimed at assessing the cure rate achieved with the toxin and the patient characteristics that can influence it, a higher cure rate was found in female patients, with only one anal fissure and a shorter duration of symptoms. The authors suggested the use of the toxin in the earliest stages of the disease, before chronic fissure fibrosis sets in. Furthermore, the results of the studies considered in the meta-analysis showed a low rate of side effects, characterised by transient gas and faecal incontinence. More serious side effects such as bruising, perianal abscesses or perianal thrombosis may occur in a small number of patients.
The doses of botulinum toxin used in the various randomised clinical trials vary from 5 to 150 U [3].

DEPRESSION

Claudia Ledda

According to the World Health Organization, depression is one of the major causes of disability in the world, with an estimated 300 million sufferers. Despite the high prevalence and considerable disability attributed to this condition, a significant proportion of patients do not respond adequately to the treatments currently available [4].
For the first time, in 2006, it was observed that the injection of botulinum toxin into the glabellar area to treat glabellar wrinkles, also known as thinker's lines, had a positive effect on the symptoms of depression.
The contraction of the corrugator muscle, which appears to be overactive in depressed patients, of the depressor supercilii and of the procerus muscle causes the formation of glabellar wrinkles and is important for the expression of negative emotions (sadness, anger, fear). One of the most common uses of botulinum toxin in aesthetic medicine is precisely the treatment of these wrinkles, and it seems to influence emotions and their perception, as well as changing the appearance of the face, making it look more youthful. The paralysis of the corrugator muscle increases the feeling of well-being and reduces irritability, mo-

odiness and anxiety; it can also delay the understanding of sentences and concepts with negative emotional connotations [4,5].

Prior to this evidence, it had already been observed that botulinum injections in the face are able to influence the perception of emotional stimuli; this hypothesis is also supported by functional magnetic resonance imaging studies, which have shown a reduction in the activation of the amygdala (part of the limbic circuits) during imitation or exposure to negative emotional stimuli, i.e.: the amygdala becomes less responsive to negative stimuli [6-8].

Since 2012, five randomised clinical trials have been conducted, demonstrating efficacy and superiority of botulinum toxin over placebo on the persistent symptoms of depression (Magid et al. found a benefit for up to six months following treatment), with some patients even showing a remission of symptoms. The evidence of effectiveness of botulinum toxin is promising for use as additional therapy in unipolar depression. There are also some studies in male patients with depression showing similar efficacy to women, and some studies suggesting a positive effect in patients with bipolar disorder, social anxiety disorder and borderline personality disorder [4]. In 2019, efficacy was also demonstrated in an animal model (rodent): a single facial injection of botulinum toxin induced a persistent improvement in the symptoms of depression and increased serotonin levels [6].

The studies completed to date present some weaknesses: the difficulty in conducting a double-blind study (the effect of the toxin is evident to the patient), the lower representation of the male sex in the samples of patients enrolled and the small number of total patients (4,5,9). Nevertheless, the results are promising.

The mechanism of action by which botulinum toxin inoculated into the glabellar area improves depressive symptoms is still unclear, and there are several hypotheses, which we will discuss in detail. The first hypothesis is the aesthetic effect of treatment with the toxin, which induces greater self-esteem and a positive perception of the body, leading to an improvement in mood. Nevertheless, the improvement was demonstrated beyond the duration of the aesthetic effect in patients who had no wrinkles at baseline and even in cases where patients were not satisfied with the aesthetic effect obtained; this hypothesis would therefore not appear to be the main mechanism of action [4,6]. Moreover, improved scores on the Beck Depression Inventory Scale (BDI) do not correlate with improved scores on the Rosenberg scale of self-esteem [4].

Another hypothesis is that a more positive facial expression, due to paralysis of the corrugator muscle (also known as the "mourning muscle"), is responsible for positive social feedback, i.e.: that a more pleasant facial expression improves social interactions, thereby increasing self-esteem and improving mood [4,7].

However, the most popular hypothesis continues to be the "facial feedback hypothesis" (FFH), i.e.: the ability to reduce the symptoms of depression by interrupting the circuits of feedback from the face to the central nervous system that reinforce and maintain negative emotions [4]. FFH is based on the hypothesis that emotional experiences and expressions are able to influence each other through feedback circuits: communication between facial muscles and the emotional centres of the brain is therefore bidirectional [6,8]. According to Finzi and Rosenthal's thesis, mimic muscles are essential in the transmission and encoding of information sent to the emotional brain circuitry (emotional proprioception) [7].

In addition, locally injected botulinum toxin in animals seems to be able to reach the central nervous system via axonal and trans-synaptic transport and may, therefore, have a central effect; it cannot be ruled out that a similar mechanism exists in humans [4,6]. Botulinum toxin inhibits the release of acetylcholine, a neurotransmitter that is increased in patients suffering from depression [4].

Interestingly, an improvement in the symptoms of depression was also observed in patients treated with botulinum toxin for non-aesthetic purposes, such as migraine, limb spasticity, cervical dystonia, blepharospasm and hyperhidrosis; this finding suggests the existence of an additional mechanism of action, differing from FFH and the emotional proprioception hypothesis. Possible causes include action due to the reduction of muscle tension, efficacy due to improvement of the underlying pathology for which treatment with botulinum toxin was indicated, axonal/trans-synaptic transport of the toxin and its possible central effects [9].

The first studies used 29 units of onabotulinumtoxinA (onaBoNTA) in women in five injection sites: 7 U in the procerus muscle, 6 U in the medial corrugator supercilii muscle, bilaterally, and 5 U in the lateral supercilii corrugator, bilaterally; 2 U were added in men, but it is acceptable to increase the number of units due to the more hyperplasic muscle structure, for each injection site. The frontalis muscle may be involved in the expression of negative emotions, such as sadness or fear, but it is also involved in the expression of surprise, sometimes associated with positive emotions, so its treatment may have a positive or negative outcome. Other potentially treatable muscles involved in the expression of negative emotions are the depressor anguli oris muscle and the mentalis muscle, which makes the surface of the chin uneven when over contracted, giving the skin an orange peel appearance, also known as "popply chin" [4].

On the contrary, paralysis of the orbicularis muscle for the treatment of periocular wrinkles, also known as "crow's feet", or blepharospasm, would seem to have negative effects on mood, given the involvement of this muscle in the spontaneous smile also known as the Duchenne smile, a smile which consists of lifting the cheeks, squinting the eyes and lifting the corners of the lips, an involuntary reaction which shows the real emotion of joy; its paralysis could therefore block the feedback circuits involved in the emotions of happiness [4,9].

The only side effects reported after glabellar botulinum toxin injection were local irritation immediately after injection and brief episodes of headache in the weeks following the injection [10].

There are numerous advantages of using botulinum toxin in the treatment of depression: the effects of a single treatment session last about three to four months, reducing healthcare costs compared to the daily use of antidepressants and increasing patient compliance; locally injected botulinum toxin is safe and has very high tolerability, with few side effects, and there are very few interactions with other drugs [4,10]. Although its use seems to be highly beneficial, botulinum toxin injections into the glabellar site for the treatment of depression is still an off-label use, unlike its use for aesthetic purposes.

VAGINISMUS

Giovanni Brunelli

Among the many off-label indications for botulinum toxin, that for the treatment of female sexual function disorders plays an important, though not yet widespread, role.

This is certainly not the place to discuss sexual dysfunction in detail, but it seems only appropriate to mention two of the psycho-emotional aspects of this group of pathologies caused by numerous contingent factors, namely:

- dyspareunia, defined as pain felt in the vagina or pelvis during sexual intercourse;
- vaginismus, i.e.: involuntary muscle spasm often caused by preventive and anticipatory fear of the aforementioned pain.

While dyspareunia often has pathological aspects related to inflammatory, infectious, muscular, hormonal or iatrogenic situations, the causes of vaginismus are more often psychological and can have their roots in early childhood. Traumatic memories of attempted penetration or sexual abuse may be at the root of the disorder, but often there is no correlation with negative sexual experiences. In other cases, a vicious circle develops, in which fear of penetration causes a spastic contracture of the perineum muscles, which almost always makes penetration impossible.

Vaginismus is estimated to affect about 2% of post-pubertal women, but some clinical studies estimate that this percentage can be as high as 15% in women who have frequent gynaecological examinations and report the problem. The true incidence of this condition remains difficult to calculate, however, partly because of the feeling of shame that prevents patients from

TABLE 1 - CLASSIFICATION OF VAGINISMUS

Grade 1	The patient is able to relax for pelvic examination
Grade 2	The patient is unable to relax for pelvic examination
Grade 3	The patient retracts early and contracts the buttocks, lifting them off the couch
Grade 4	The patient has a general defensive reaction: she raises her buttocks, squeezes her thighs together and moves away from the examiner, making the examination impossible
Grade 5 (Pacik)	General reaction, as in grade 4, with associated visceral reactions such as palpitations, hyperventilation, sweating, general trembling, uncontrollable cloning, screaming, desire to get off the couch, feeling faint, nausea, vomiting or, in extreme cases, desire to attack the examiner

talking to their doctor about it.

Vaginismus is defined as a persistent and recurrent difficulty in introducing a penis, a finger, or any object into the vagina, despite the woman having a strong desire to do so. It consists of an involuntary and reflex contraction of the muscles of the perineum, vulva and vaginal orifice (i.e.: the outer third of the vagina), associated with a phobia of coitus, which makes penetration and, in severe cases, even a simple digital exploration or insertion of a tampon during a gynaecological examination very painful, if not impossible.

In primary vaginismus, the patient has never experienced penetration, while in secondary vaginismus, the patient has had non-painful intercourse before the onset of the disease; in this case the causes may be inflammatory, infectious, traumatic, post-surgical, genital and/or pelvic pathologies or the onset of menopause.

It is one of the possible causes of the termination of the marriage, as it prevents sexual intercourse from taking place normally.

The most commonly accepted classification is Lamont's four-grade classification, modified by Pacik with the addition of a fifth grade, as shown in the table 1.

From a therapeutic point of view, vaginismus can be approached in various ways; individual and/or couples psychological therapy is extremely valuable, using autogenic training and muscle relaxation techniques. Kegel exercises and the use of progressive vaginal dilators can also be useful. Surgery is almost never indicated, except in the case of a particularly rigid or unperforated hymen. From a

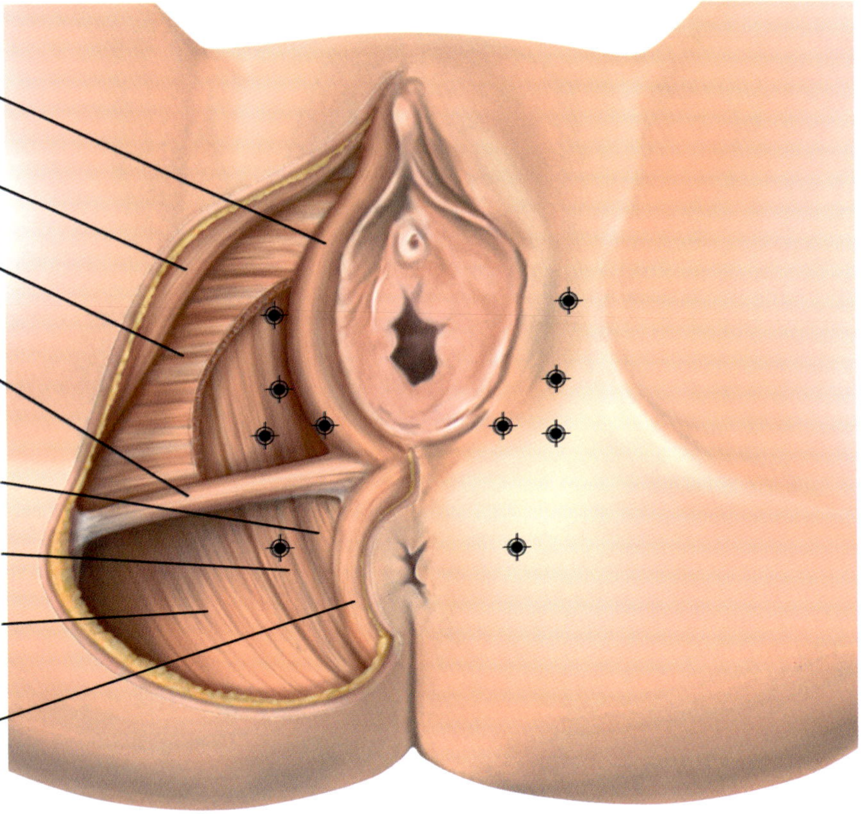

Figure 1 Injection points for the treatment of vaginismus with botulinum toxin

pharmaceutical point of view, antidepressants, tranquilisers and muscle relaxants can be used.

In cases of severe vaginismus, botulinum toxin may represent an alternative capable, in certain cases, of curing this disease. The first case described in literature by Brin and Vapnek dates back to 1997, but not many articles have been published on this subject.

Treatment with botulinum can be carried out, in a good percentage of cases, without anaesthetic, except for the application of commonly available anaesthetic creams half an hour before treatment; in the most difficult cases, when the patient will not allow the examiner her to approach her at all, it is necessary to proceed with injection with the aid of sedation.

The pelvic floor muscles must be injected, in particular:

- the bulbospongiosus (or bulbocavernosus) muscles which, in the female, surround the vagina and the terminal portion of the urethra and which, during contraction, cause the vaginal orifice to narrow;
- the levator ani muscle, which in turn is subdivided into the pubococcygeal, puborectalis and iliococcygeal bundles (fig. 1).

The treatment can be carried out with all types of botulinum on the market (Ona-, Abo- and Incobotulinum), naturally using the classic unit conversion factors depending on the product chosen, using a normal insulin syringe with a 25 G needle or even smaller.
In literature, doses vary from as low as 50 units (150) up to 150 units and more. The reader is referred to specialist articles on this subject.
The results are usually highly satisfactory; the vast majority of women are able to engage in sexual intercourse about a week after injection with botulinum toxin.
Treatment with botulinum successfully breaks the vicious circle (fear of penetration-anxiety-rejection by the partner) and the couple can, again with the help of psychological therapy, dilators, etc., begin to have a healthy and normal sex life.
In more difficult cases, subsequent sessions may be necessary.

Bibliography

1. Yiannakopoulou E. Botulinum toxin and anal fissure: efficacy and safety systematic review. Int J Colorectal Dis. 2012 Jan;27(1):1-9.
2. Sekmen U, Paksoy M. The Efficacy of Botulinum Toxin Injection Site in Chronic Anal Fissure Healing. Niger J Clin Pract. 2020 Dec;23(12):1639-1642.
3. Soltany S, Hemmati HR, Toussy JA, Salehi D, Toosi PA. Therapeutic properties of botulinum toxin on chronic anal fissure treatment and the patient factors role. J Family Med Prim Care. 2020 Mar 26;9(3):1562-1566.
4. Wollmer MA, Magid M, Kruger THC., Finzi E. (2020) The Use of Botulinum Toxin for Treatment of Depression. In: Whitcup SM, Hallett M (eds). Botulinum Toxin Therapy. Handbook of Experimental Pharmacology, vol 263. Springer.
5. Kruger TH, Wollmer MA. Depression. An emerging indication for botulinum toxin treatment. Toxicon. 2015 Dec 1;107(Pt A):154-7.
6. Schulze J, Neumann I, Magid M, Finzi E, Sinke C, Wollmer MA, Krüger THC. Botulinum toxin for the management of depression: An updated review of the evidence and meta-analysis. J Psychiatr Res. 2021 Mar; 135:332-340.
7. França K, Lotti T. Botulinum toxin for the treatment of depression. Dermatol Ther. 2017 Mar;30(2).
8. Finzi E. Update: Botulinum Toxin for Depression: More Than Skin Deep. Dermatol Surg. 2018 Oct;44(10):1363-1365.
9. Makunts T, Wollmer MA, Abagyan R. Postmarketing safety surveillance data reveals antidepressant effects of botulinum toxin across various indications and injection sites. Sci Rep. 2020 Jul 30;10(1):12851.
10. Parsaik AK, Mascarenhas SS, Hashmi A, Prokop LJ, John V, Okusaga O, Singh B. Role of Botulinum Toxin in Depression. J Psychiatr Pract. 2016 Mar;22(2):99-110.
11. Shafik A, El-Sibai O. Vaginismus: results of treatment with botulin toxin. J Obstet Gynaecol. 2000;20(3):300-302.
12. Brin MF, Vapnek JM. Treatment of vaginismus with botulinum toxin injections. Lancet. 1997;349(9047):252-253.

13. Pacik PT. Vaginismus: review of current concepts and treatment using botox injections, bupivacaine injections, and progressive dilation with the patient under anesthesia. Aesthetic Plast Surg. 2011;35(6):1160-1164.

14. Dick B, Natale C, Reddy A, Akula KP, Yousif A, Hellstrom WJG. Application of Botulinum Neurotoxin in Female Sexual and Genitourinary Dysfunction: A Review of Current Practices. Sex Med Rev. 2021;9(1):57-63.

12

THE FUTURE OF BOTULINUM TOXIN

Giuseppe Sito

There is no doubt that botulinum toxin (BoNT) is one of the most successful and stable products ever to be developed in the world of pharmaceuticals. Since Alan Scott's first publication in the 1970s [1], the use of BoNT products in the world of therapeutic and aesthetic treatments has grown year by year. The use of the products first authorised in the late 1980s, almost 30 years ago, has continued to grow, without ever stopping. There is no denying their ability to bring real benefit to patients in a multitude of ways and to improve the quality of life for countless people. While they are not life-saving drugs, BoNT products are now essential in many branches of neurology, urology and pain therapy. New uses that demonstrate clinically significant value in treating patients are regularly identified.

The actual size of the market for BoNT products is notoriously hard to determine. While data on their use in therapeutics is collected regularly, no comparable data exists for the aesthetic medicine market. Estimates in the order of $2 billion are currently available and look set to grow to $20 billion over the next decade.

In reality, however, the potential profits could be described as unlimited, given the countless new uses that have been highlighted.

Initially there were just two products, Oculinum and Dysport. Oculinum, launched by Alan Scott through his company Oculinum Inc., was created in the USA, on the West Coast, at the Smith-Kettlewell Institute. Dysport, pioneered by doctors and the Centre for Applied Microbiology and Research, had been created in the UK after several UK doctors had trained with Alan Scott and realised the product's huge potential for treating difficult diseases, such as strabismus, which had only been previously treatable with surgery [2]. Oculinum was purchased by Allergan soon after its approval in the US and became Botox. The background to Oculinum has recently been described [3]. Botox became established in the US and shortly afterwards in Europe and the rest of the world. Dysport only reached the US in 2009, for many reasons that have still to be described, but this allowed Allergan to have a virtual monopoly for several years and the brand to establish itself globally. Both of these first-generation serotype A products contain the active neurotoxin, which is found in aggregate form with a number of other natural proteins, often referred to as neurotoxin-associated proteins (NAPs). Despite arguments put forward by practitioners over the years, these neurotoxin-associated proteins remain separate from active BoNT upon rehydration in vials prior to injection [4] and show no known effect with respect to the pharmaceutical action of the products. Moreover, no harmful effects related to their presence have been identified so far. This obviously goes against the role that neurotoxin-associated proteins play when the toxin is ingested as poison in food [5].

After the first years of use of the two type A products, it was many years before another BoNT-based product

became available on the market. What people often fail to realise or what they rarely talk about is the fact that another serotype, type F, was the subject of clinical trials in several countries long before the advent of the Neurobloc type B product [6]. There are several publications on the use of the F-type, but due to its relatively short duration of action, the product was never marketed. Nor was Neurobloc a generally successful product, mainly due to the high doses required and the appearance of immunoresistance following prolonged use in many patients. The reason BoNT type B is required in such high doses has only recently been explained and is linked to inefficiencies in one of the human-specific receptors. The product has been bought and sold several times by the companies that own it.
In the early 2000s, a new serotype A product was created in Germany by the Merz company. Their product, Xeomin, was developed outside Merz in the initial phase, but then authorised for the first time in Germany in 2005. Xeomin gradually became available in many other countries.
The product is characterised by the fact that it is free of complex proteins and, due to the high concentration of the human serum albumin stabiliser, can be stored at room temperature (<25 °C). This means that Xeomin could be considered a second-generation BoNT-based drug after the initial complex A-type products.
The three main products, Botox, Dysport and Xeomin, dominate the international market.

Botulinum toxin products worldwide

However, other products have gradually established themselves in some countries and have gained market shares, with notable exceptions in Europe and the United States, where they are unavailable. Four of these products come from Asia, three from South Korea (tabs. 1-2).
The oldest of these BoNT products of Asian origin is CBTXA from the Lanzhou Institute in China (since 1997). This product is unique in the world because it uses dextran and gelatine as stabilisers, instead of the traditional HSA found in all but one other product. The presence of these stabilisers poses a degree of risk to the product that is not the case with all other BoNT products, namely the possibility of anaphylactic shock as a reaction to gelatine [7]. Significant side effects have been reported for this Chinese product [8].
The three Korean BoNT products were developed, as claimed by these companies, as "copies" of Botox. Their formulas are the same as or similar to those of Botox, but the manufacturing processes are different and they use different strains of production organisms [9]. Clinical studies conducted on these products were published rather late and frequently show that the units of potency of the products are different. Comparative clinical studies in the field of aesthetics with the same dosage of Botox have often revealed significant differences in results. This only emphasises what is stated in prescriptive information and product documentation around the world, basically that the units of potency of each

TABLE 1 - BOTULINUM TOXIN PRODUCTS OF ASIAN ORIGIN

Product™	Company	Country	Bacterial production strain	Process	U/vial specific per product	Excipients (in vial)
BTXA/Prosigne	Lanzhou Institute	China	Hall	Crystallization, dialysis	50/100 U	5 mg gelatine
Redux/Lantox/ Lanzox	Biological Products/ Hugh Source Internatio-nal					25 mg dextran 25 mg saccharose
Meditoxin	MedyTox Inc.	South Korea	Hall	Acid precipit.	50/100/ 200 U	0,5 mg HSA
Neuronox/Siax/ Botulift/Cunox				Dialysis		0,9 mg NaCl
Innotox	MedyTox Inc.	South Korea	Hall	Unknown	25/50 U	No human serum albumin or animal products
Botulax/Zentox	Hugel Pharma	South Korea	CBFC26	Protamine sulphate	50/100/ 200 U	0,5 mg HSA
Regenox				DEAE Sepharose		0,9 mg NaCl
Nabota/Evosyal	Daewoong	South Korea	Hall	High-Pure Technology®	100 U	0,5 mg HSA
(DWP 450)	Pharma-ceutical Co. Ltd			(patented)		0,9 mg NaCl

Source: Toxin Science Limited, 2015. Updated to end of 2015

TABLE 2 - NEW LOCAL BOTULINUM TOXIN PRODUCTS

Product™	Company	Country	U/vial specific per product	Excipients (in vial)
Masport	Masoondarou	Iran	500 U	0,5 mg HSA 2,5 mg lactose
Relatox/Relatoks	Microgen	Russia	50/100 U	Gelatine
BOTOgenie	Bio-Med Pvt. Ltd	India	50/100 U	5 mg lactose
BTXA	Intas Pharmaceuticals Ltd	India	100 U	Unknown

Source: Toxin Science Limited, 2015. Updated to end of 2015

product are specific to that product and are not interchangeable. This is clearly proven by studies that use apparently "identical" units of two different products, but describe results in clinical trials that are superior or inferior to each other.

In addition to the Asian toxins now available, there are other regional products that have limited use in various countries. Typical examples are shown in table 3. As yet, there is no clinical data on these products in literature and very limited information is available on the company websites. In some cases, there is a video on the specific use of the product on YouTube. There is no information available on exactly why these regional products have been developed, but it is believed that the main reason is to provide a much cheaper alternative to major branded products through local production. One area of work that specifically addresses the aesthetic treatment sector is the development of so-called "topical" toxin products. Several companies have been active in this field for many years (tab. 3), the best known of which is the Californian company Revance, which has been operational since 2002. Data published on their RT001 product has proven its limited effectiveness in treating targeted areas of the face. [10]. In addition, the mechanism used to transport BoNT through the dermal layers is highly inefficient, given the very high doses of active BoNT that are required to be effective. The company has been the subject of much speculation and fluctuation in financial stocks following the publication of their data over the years, but there is still no certainty that topical BoNT used for aesthetic purposes will reach the market and, more importantly, prove useful and effective in the long term. Other companies that advertise their work on topical toxins have not yet provided any substantial data on any clinical trials. Lastly, the

TABLE 3 - DEVELOPMENT OF TOPICAL BOTULINUM TOXIN PRODUCTS WORLDWIDE

Company	Country	Product name	Technology	Clinical data published
Revance	United States	RT001-RTT150	TransMTS®	Yes
Transdermal Corp.	Canada	CosmeTox	InParT (mixed micellar/ nanoparticle ionic)	Yes
Anterios	United States	ANT-1207 lotion	Unknown	No
Malvern Cosmeceutics Ltd	United Kingdom	MCL005-2 gel	Unknown	No

Source: Toxin Science Limited, 2015. Updated to end of 2015

field of modified BoNT molecules with new or improved properties has been in the limelight for several years. The company Syntaxin, which originated from the Centre for Applied Microbiology and Research and is now owned by Ipsen, has made considerable progress in the field, with publications dating back 20 years.

The main molecules under investigation are termed secretion suppressors (STIs) and use modified BoNT molecules to transfer their activity to different cell types where BoNT is not normally active [11]. Syntaxin molecules are currently in the early stages of clinical trials, but the doses of these modified molecules necessary to take effect are considerably higher than those of native BoNT. Consequently, issues such as the development of immunogenic responses will be more significant than with biological molecules.

Initially with just a very few products, the global BoNT market has grown significantly and now includes a wide range of both international and local products, along with a substantial amount of research and development into new products for specific and targeted uses. The future of BoNT is therefore as bright today as it was right when it first came into use more than 30 years ago.

Bibliography

1. Scott AB, Rosenbaum A, Collins CC. Pharmacologic weakening of extraocular muscles. Invest Ophthalmol. 1973;12(12):924-927.
2. Elston JS, Russell RW. Effect of treatment with botulinum toxin on neurogenic blepharospasm. Br Med J (Clin Res Ed). 1985;290 (6485):1857-1859.

3. Pickett A. Historical aspects of botulinum toxin used clinically: part I: is that the right serotype? Botulinum J. 2013;2(3/4):176.
4. Eisele KH, Fink K, Vey M, Taylor HV. Studies on the dissociation of botulinum neurotoxin type A complexes. Toxicon. 2011;57(4):555-565.
5. Fujinaga Y, Sugawara Y, Matsumura T. Uptake of botulinum neurotoxin in the intestine. Curr Top Microbiol Immunol. 2013;364:45-59.
6. Pickett A. Historical aspects of botulinum toxin used clinically: Part II: overcoming resistance. Botulinum J. 2015;3(1):34-40.
7. Kamin W, Staubach P, et al. Anaphylaxis after vaccination due to hypersensitivity to gelatin. Klin Padiatr. 2006;218(2):92-94.
8. Careta MF, Delgado L, Patriota R. Report of Allergic Reaction After Application of Botulinum Toxin. Aesthet Surg J. 2015;35(5):NP102-NP105.
9. Kim BJ, Kwon HH, Park SY, et al. Double-blind, randomized non-inferiority trial of a novel botulinum toxin A processed from the strain CBFC26, compared with onabotulinumtoxin A in the treatment of glabellar lines. J Eur Acad Dermatol Venereol. 2014;28(12):1761-1767.
10. Glogau R, Blitzer A, Brandt F, Kane M, Monheit GD, Waugh JM. Results of a randomized, double-blind, placebo-controlled study to evaluate the efficacy and safety of a botulinum toxin type A topical gel for the treatment of moderate-to-severe lateral canthal lines. J Drugs Dermatol. 2012;11(1):38-45.
11. Masuyer G, Chaddock JA, Foster KA, Acharya KR. Engineered botulinum neurotoxins as new therapeutics. Annu Rev Pharmacol Toxicol. 2014;54:27-51.

APPENDIX

TIPS FOR A PERFECT BOTULINUM SESSION

Maria Vittoria Giatti et al.

1) Planning the treatment with a global approach:
- patient requests
- psychological assessment
- objectification of real needs
- anatomical-physiological study
- analysis of the clinical case
- formulation of an appropriate and personalised medical treatment plan

2) Patient selection:
- medical history,
- absolute or temporary contraindications

3) Patient assessment, dynamic and static

4) Acquisition of informed consent

5) Mapping

6) Acquisition of videos/photographs

7) Choice of the type of toxin, dilution, technique and dose

8) Post-treatment prescriptions

9) Scheduling a check-up (possible touch-ups, symmetrisation, progress checks) and/or a new session

10) Coretta handling of any complications

INFORMED CONSENT

Giovanni Brunelli

Informed consent is a fundamental and indispensable part of the medical procedure, without which we are not allowed to perform any kind of treatment on our patients.

The only exception is in the case of a patient who, for one or more reasons, is at risk of dying but is not in full possession of their faculties.

Informed consent must be given in writing or on video or, in the case of people with disabilities, using devices that enable them to communicate.

It must be included in the medical records or in the electronic health records and can be revoked at any time.

Informed consent requirements

Informed consent must meet several requirements, as follows:

- it must be given by an individual who is in full possession of their faculties;
- it must include a set of information that is true, complete and appropriate to the degree of understanding of the patient concerned.

It must also be:

- personal, meaning that it cannot be delegated to relatives or third parties, except in the exercise of guardianship of incapacitated patients or of parental authority in the case of patients who are minors;
- explicit (can never be inferred);
- specific, meaning that it must relate solely to the service that is envisaged. Conduct other than that for which consent has been given is not legitimate, except in cases where a state of necessity can be established;
- informed, meaning that it must follow adequate, complete and understood information and, at the time it is given, the patient must be in full possession of their faculties;
- free and will not be considered valid if it is coerced or acquired by deception or error. It must be aimed at preserving or recovering physical or psychological well-being; the patient's decision-making capacity must be verified on a case-by-case basis, ascertaining whether the patient is able to communicate with the caregiver(s) and whether they show signs of understanding the information, understand the alternatives and persist in the conclusions drawn;
- current, it must be persistent at the time of the medical procedure.

The information must be:

- truthful, meaning that it cannot be gi-

ven in misleading phrases or half-truths;
- complete, meaning that the patient must be given all the comparative elements to make their decision, those elements that may be considered reasonably necessary and useful, leaving aside what does not affect the risk factors and is not related to the success of the treatment;
- understood by the patient, being given in everyday terms and not with mere technical data. The information must be comprehensible, so that the patient is able to understand the possible alternatives and make free and prudent choices.

Informed consent is the last step in the interaction between doctor and patient before moving on to the practicalities of the procedure. It is signed at the end of the preliminary interview and must therefore contain the methods of performance, the probable benefits, the possible side effects, the possible early and late complications and the treatment alternatives, including abstention from treatment, and consent to the acquisition and storage of photographic and/or video material.

Informed consent for on-label and off-label use of botulinum toxin

In this case, it is important for the informed consent to clearly state what botulinum toxin is and what the treatment options and their probable duration are.

At the time of writing this chapter, only three types of toxin are marketed in Italy for outpatient aesthetic use (excluding hospital use).

The three molecules are called Onabotulinum, Abobotulinum, and Incobotulinum; they differ in terms of the presence of certain accompanying proteins and the method of storage.

The use of Onabotulinum and Incobotulinum are currently authorised for use in the treatment of forehead and glabellar lines and periocular wrinkles (crow's feet), while Abobotulinum is authorised only for glabellar lines and periocular wrinkles, but not for forehead lines. The use of Abobotulinum is authorised in all cases under 65 years of age and in patients with an aesthetic defect that has a psychological impact. On-label use concerns these areas only.

As we know, however, the indications for the use of the toxin are now numerous and range from the treatment of the middle and lower thirds of the face to the neck, hyperhidrosis, pathological scars and a series of dermatological conditions. In all these cases, which are supported by extensive, international, indexed literature, botulinum is used off-label, i.e. not indicated in the package leaflet and under the direct responsibility of the doctor; of course the patient must be informed of this and must accept it.

Informed consent must indicate:
- contraindications; hypersensitivity to botulinum toxin type A or to one of

the excipients, certain diseases such as myasthenia gravis, Eaton-Lambert syndrome or ALS, possible interactions with other drugs, pregnancy and breastfeeding;
- possible side effects, even if only related to the injection, such as erythema, swelling or bruising;
- complications, such as drooping of the eyebrow or eyelid, headache and other minor and very uncommon symptoms; all possible complications are transient and leave no permanent evidence;
- the existence of rare "non-responders", i.e.: patients who are not sensitive to treatment with botulinum, which cannot be predicted in advance.

There are various informed consent forms available on the web from the various scientific societies. It is possible to use one of these consent forms or to write your own, as long as the basic points are respected.

CONSENT TO TREATMENT WITH BOTULINUM TOXIN

Giuseppe Sito

I am aware that the injection of botulinum toxin for the elimination of wrinkles is a relatively novel treatment, although it has been used for years in neurology, against muscle spasms.

The practitioner has explained to me that most of what has been written and said about this method in newspapers and magazines, on television, etc. is intended to create headlines. I am aware of the nature, purpose and limitations of the method, as well as the possibility to ask for clarification about the procedure, its limitations and possible complications.

I acknowledge and accept the following:

1. like any other aesthetic treatment, botulinum toxin injections allow a certain improvement, not perfection;
2. the end result may not be evident until two weeks after treatment;
3. several applications are sometimes necessary to achieve the best possible result. Each application has its own specific cost;
4. observance of the post-op recommendations (frequent contraction of the muscles concerned for one hour, then standing for 4-6 hours, no alcohol, use of sun lamps or sunbathing for 48 hours, no massage of the treated areas for 48

hours) is essential to obtain the best possible result and to limit the occurrence of side effects;

5. temporary drooping of one eyelid and one eyebrow may occur. These episodes are quite rare (1-5%), perceptible only to the patient, and disappear spontaneously. An upright position will help avoid these problems.

The effect of botulinum toxin injections is temporary (approximately 3-8 months). However, in some patients, results can be cumulative.

Although complications are rare, I am aware that the following problems may occur:

1. slight infiltration of subcutaneous blood, resulting in the appearance of bruises lasting several days;

2. a feeling of heaviness in the area treated;

3. slight stinging of the eyes with a dry sensation.

In extremely rare and resistant cases, botulinum toxin does not result in any real improvement. There is no way of predicting this absence of reaction. Additional injections are usually all that is needed. The practitioner injects a medium amount of product, but in some patients, particularly men and women with intense muscular activity, a greater amount of product is required.

Additional applications have an extra cost. I agree that Dr [name of aesthetic practitioner] or designated personnel may take photographs during the procedure and use this material for educational purposes or in medical publications, as long as my identity is not revealed.

By signing this document, I declare that I understand the purpose, limitations and possible complications of botulinum toxin injections and that I wish to proceed with the treatment.

Patient ______________________________

Practitioner ______________________________

Witness ______________________________

Date ____________________